INFERTILITY

PRACTICAL PATHWAYS IN OBSTETRICS & GYNECOLOGY

Marcelle I. Cedars, MD

Professor and Director
Division of Reproductive Endocrinology
University of California, San Francisco
San Francisco, California

McGRAW-HILL
Medical Publishing Division
New York   Chicago   San Francisco   Lisbon   London   Madrid   Mexico City   Milan
New Delhi   San Juan   Seoul   Singapore   Sydney   Toronto

The **McGraw·Hill** Companies

Infertility

2 3 4 5 6 7 8 9 0   DOC/DOC   0 9 8 7 6 5

ISBN 0-07-139931-3

This book was set in Melior by International Typesetting and Composition.
The editors were Andrea Seils and Michelle Watt.
The production supervisor was Richard Ruzycka.
Project management was provided by International Typesetting and Composition.
The cover designer was Mary McKeon.
RR Donnelley was printer and binder.

This book is printed on acid-free paper.

Library of Congress Cataloging-in-Publication Data

Infertility / [edited by] Marcelle Cedars.
     p. ; cm.
  Includes bibliographical references and index.
  ISBN 0-07-139931-3 (alk. paper)
  1. Infertility. I. Cedars, Marcelle.
  [DNLM: 1. Infertility—diagnosis. 2. Infertility—therapy. 3. Reproductive Techniques, Assisted. WP 570 I4301 2005]
  RC889.I542 2005
  618.1'78—dc22

                                                      2004056462

This book is dedicated to my family, especially Daniel and Ariana, and to all those investigators and clinicians who work tirelessly to improve the care and caring of infertile couples

Contents

Contributors

Ruben Alvero, MD
Associate Professor
University of Colorado Health
  Sciences Center
Aurora, Colorado

Linda D. Applegarth, EdD
Clinical Assistant Professor of Psychology
Departments of Obstetrics and Gynecology
  and Psychology
Director of Psychological Services
Institute for Reproductive Medicine
Weill Medical College of Cornell University
New York, New York

Nancy L. Bossert, PhD, HCLD (ABB)
Assistant Laboratory Director
Reproductive Medicine Center
University of Minnesota
Minneapolis, Minnesota

Marcelle I. Cedars, MD
Professor and Director
Division of Reproductive Endocrinology
University of California, San Francisco
San Francisco, California

Susan L. Crockin, JD
Private Practice
Newton, Massachusetts

Alan H. DeCherney, MD
Professor
Department of Obstetrics and Gynecology

David Geffen School of Medicine
University of California, Los Angeles
Los Angeles, California

Christopher J. DeJonge, PhD, HCLD (ABB)
Professor
Department of Obstetrics, Gynecology and
  Women's Health
Director of Laboratories, Reproductive
  Medicine Center
University of Minnesota
Minneapolis, Minnesota

Karen E. Dumser, JD
Associate
Law Office of Susan L. Crockin
Newton, Massachusetts

Marc A. Fritz, MD
Professor and Chief
Reproductive Endocrinology and Infertility
Department of Obstetrics and Gynecology
University of North Carolina School
  of Medicine
Chapel Hill, North Carolina

Elena Gates, MD
Clinical Professor & Interim Chair
Department of Obstetrics, Gynecology and
  Reproductive Science
University of California, San Francisco
San Francisco, California

ix

David Guzick, MD, PhD
Office of the Dean
University of Rochester Medical Center
Rochester, New York

Heather Hoddleston, MD
Fellow
Division of Reproductive Endocrinology
Department of Obstetrics and Gynecology
Brigham and Women's Hospital
Harvard Medical School
Boston, Massachusetts

Mark D. Hornstein, MD
Director
Division of Reproductive Endocrinology
Department of Obstetrics and Gynecology
Brigham and Women's Hospital
Harvard Medical School
Boston, Massachusetts

David Keefe, MD
Director
Division of Reproductive Medicine
Brown University School of Medicine
Women and Infants' Hospital
Providence, Rhode Island
Tufts–New England Medical Center
Boston, Massachusetts

Ashim V. Kumar, MD
Fellow
Reproductive Endocrinology and Infertility
Department of Obstetrics and Gynecology
David Geffen School of Medicine
University of California, Los Angeles
Los Angeles, California

William H. Kutteh, MD, PhD, HCLD
Professor, Obstetrics and Gynecology
Director, Reproductive Endocrinology,
  Infertility, and Genetics

Director, Reproductive Immunology
University of Tennessee
Fertility Associates of Memphis
Memphis, Tennessee

Danielle Lane, MD
Clinical Fellow
Division of Reproductive Endocrinology
  and Infertility
Department of Obstetrics, Gynecology and
  Reproductive Sciences
University of California, San Francisco
San Francisco, California

Bill L. Lasley, PhD
Population, Health, and Reproduction
School of Veterinary Medicine
Center for Health and the Environment
Department of Obstetrics and Gynecology
University of California, Davis
Davis, California

Kenneth K. Moghadam, MD
Clinical Instructor/Fellow
Department of Obstetrics and Gynecology
Division of Reproductive Endocrinology
  and Infertility
University of Cincinnati School of
  Medicine
Cincinnati, Ohio

Renee A. Reijo Pera, PhD
Associate Professor
Associate Director, Center for
  Reproductive Sciences
Co-Director, Program in Human Stem
  Cell Biology
Department of Obstetrics, Gynecology, and
  Reproductive Sciences
University of California, San Francisco
San Francisco, California

Mitchell P. Rosen, MD
Fellow
Division of Reproductive Endocrinology and
    Reproductive Sciences
Department of Obstetrics, Gynecology, and
    Reproductive Sciences
University of California, San Francisco
San Francisco, California

Jane I. Ruman, MD
Fellow
Reproductive Endocrinology
Columbia University of Physicians &
    Surgeons
New York

Mark V. Sauer, MD
Professor & Vice Chairman
Department of Obstetrics and Gynecology
Columbia University College of
    Physicians & Surgeons
Chief, Division of Reproductive
    Endocrinology & Infertility
Columbia Presbyterian Medical Center
New York, New York

William D. Schlaff, MD
Professor and Vice Chairman
Director, Division of Reproductive
    Endocrinology
University of Colorado Health
    Sciences Center
Aurora, Colorado

Shehua Shen, MD, ELD (ABB)
Director, Embryology Laboratory
Center for Reproductive Health
Assistant Adjunct Professor

Department of Obstetrics, Gynecology, and
    Reproductive Sciences
University of California, San Francisco
San Francisco, California

Susan E. Shideler, PhD
Center for Health and the Environment
University of California, Davis
Davis, California

Sae H. Sohn, MD
Assistant Clinical Professor
Center for Reproductive Health
University of California, San Francisco
San Francisco, California

Paul J. Turek, MD
Associate Professor in-residence
Departments of Urology and Obstetrics,
    Gynecology, and Reproductive Sciences
Center of Reproductive Health
University of California, San Francisco
San Francisco, California

Tracey L. Telles, MD
Assistant Clinical Professor
Fertility Group
University of California, San Francisco
San Francisco, California

Michael Thomas, MD
Associate Professor
Director, Division of Reproductive
    Endocrinology and Infertility
Department of Obstetrics and Gynecology
University of Cincinnati School of
    Medicine
Cincinnati, Ohio

Preface

Advances in the field of reproductive medicine and infertilility are made at an increasingly rapid rate. For those of us who care for infertile couples, our job becomes both easier and harder. Our job is made easier by the development of new, effective treatment strategies that may offer hope to our patients. However, the complexity of treatments and the significant impact these treatments may have on personal and social norms makes treatment more difficult for both our patients and ourselves. The rapid explosion in reproductive genetics is only now beginning to have its impact felt in our field. The application of this new knowledge to our field offers great promise for the future, but must be introduced after careful study and consideration.

In the chapters that follow, I have attempted to present both the history—the tried and true knowledge that guides our decision-making—and the future. As we approach patients, our approach will be increasingly multi-disciplinary. The involvement of those with expertise in genetics and psychology will be critical. And, for those in this field, our patients and society, we will increasingly involve those with expertise in ethics and the law. It is with this broad brush that I have painted a picture of current infertility care.

Introduction

Nearly five million American women aged 15 to 44 years report difficulty or delay in achieving a live birth. The percentage of affected women has not increased despite increased public awareness of this problem. What has changed is the number of women (couples) seeking medical attention. Each year, approximately 1.3 million of these women seek medical advice or treatment. This number has increased because of significant demographic changes in our society. These include the aging of the "baby boom" generation leading to an increased size of the reproductive age population. More importantly is the change in society with more women seeking careers and delaying fertility. In fact, the number that has changed is the number of *nulligravid* women with infertility, in other words, the women who have never had a child and are now infertile. There is a false sense by many that modern reproduction can overcome *all* factors, including those associated with age.

The chief female categories of infertility are ovulatory disorders (25%) and tubal disease (20 to 25%), including endometriosis (10%). Male infertility is the primary category in approximately 25% of cases and contributes to a further 15 to 25% of the remaining cases. Infertility remains "unexplained" in up to 20% of cases. These cases are unexplained only in that our current methods do not identify a critical factor. Although recent developments have improved the effectiveness of conventional specific therapies, the overall prognosis for childbirth is not better than 50%. This can be explained by the presence of unexplained factors that persist after conventional therapy. A further reason is the limited access in many jurisdictions to artificial reproductive technologies.

Most couples are not infertile, but rather *subfertile*. This distinction is critical as there is a small chance that conception and birth may occur without treatment. The effectiveness of treatment can therefore only be determined by randomized clinical trials preferably comparing the pertinent treatment to no-treatment or placebo. A second choice for the control group would be use of a standard active treatment for the "control." Ideally, this treatment should have been confirmed previously by randomized controlled trials. Less convincing data are generated by cohort and case series. Unfortunately, these later study designs comprise a major share of available literature in this field. This lack of convincing data regarding treatment approaches makes care of these couples even more difficult. Each treatment option has many costs: emotional, physical, and financial, oftentimes without clear documentation of success. It is thus important to evaluate and treat couples with a comprehensive approach taking into consideration expected benefits, unwanted side-effects, and costs in dollars and time.

Time is a critically important factor for couples seeking fertility, as the age of the female partner is the number one prognosticator for success. After age, the duration of infertility plays a large role in considering treatment options. Thus, a prompt, efficient evaluation is likely to be most beneficial to the infertile couple. Diagnostic assessment is indicated for couples attempting pregnancy and who fail to conceive following 12 or more months of regular, unprotected intercourse. This timeframe is selected since 85 to 90% of normally fertile couples conceive in this interval of time. This "delay" will thus save many couples unnecessary testing and evaluation. Earlier assessment *is* indicated in women over 35 years of age, women with irregular menstrual cycles, or those with a high risk for tubal disease and/or endometriosis. The current focus of diagnostic testing is on a limited panel of specific investigations rather than a broad screen of tests.

It is important to remember that there is, in most couples, the chance for spontaneous conception. Recent studies estimate the average prognosis for live birth without treatment at 25 to 40% during the three years after the first infertility consultation. This translates into a cycle fecundity rate of 0.7 to 1% per month. The presence of endometriosis, abnormal sperm, or tubal disease independently reduced the chance of spontaneous pregnancy and live birth by approximately 0.5 for each variable. Infertility for greater than 3 years, female age greater than 30 years, and primary infertility were important negative prognostic factors.

Evaluation should focus on known causes of infertility/subfertility. Hence, the first section of this text will describe normal female and male physiology and the relevant investigation of the infertile couple. Attention will be paid to recent reviews of the literature and the development of a time and cost-sensitive evaluation.

Treatment should be diagnosis specific, if possible. The second section of this text therefore delves more deeply into specific etiologies of infertility and appropriate diagnostic and therapeutic interventions.

Assisted reproductive technologies (ART), the art of taking fertilization outside the human body, deserves special consideration and will be considered in depth in the third section of the text. Although only a small percentage of all infertile couples will actually need ART, the dramatic advances in the last quarter century (yes, Louise Brown—the first "IVF baby"—celebrated her 25th birthday in the summer of 2003) and the strong media interest have made ART a central focus for the infertile practice and for patients. ART remains the only option for some patients and the "final" option for couples who fail simpler modalities.

SOCIAL ISSUES

The field of infertility is complicated by the personal and ***emotional*** nature of the desire for parenthood. Treating couples *as* couples, rather than focusing "blame" (which couples do themselves all too often) is one way in which the physician can help. It is also crucial to give accurate and fair assessments for success so that couples can make informed decisions. Psychologic support should be available to all couples and couples considering any reproduction with third parties (donors or surrogates) should be required to meet with a psychologist. There may be many times within the fertility evaluation and treatment when couples should have a discussion regarding long-term goals: to have a child to raise as their own, to have a pregnancy to share, to share genetic traits. Each of these may or may not be achieved via adoption, donor gametes, or only with further treatment. The option of child-free living should also be included in any discussion. At times couples must be advised to stop treatment if the likelihood for success is quite low. Frequently this is a very difficult time for both the patient and the physician, but fruitless treatment should be avoided.

The potential benefit relative to potential ***cost*** (financial, physical, and emotional) must all be considered. A review of 45 reports on unexplained infertility estimated the marginal costs of treatment at $7143, $15,823, and $46,391 respectively for CC/IUI, FSH/IUI, and IVF treatment compared with untreated pregnancy rates equivalent to 1.3% per month.[1] The treatment effects are generally small. Treatment may only hasten conception in those couples who would eventually conceive in any case. Given this, the high rate of multiple gestation and its incumbent medical and social risks must be considered and every attempt should be made to limit this complication. In most cases, simple treatments should be considered before complex treatment.

This field is also complicated by the many ***ethical*** boundaries that are approached. There are issues of defining "the family" and parentage, issues about "abandoned" embryos, and about how far couples and society should go to procreate. Most recently, the issue has become public as the government has faced the critically important decision of use of "disposed" embryos from IVF for creation of stem cells. The potential

Introduction

for this technology is not proven but appears to be great; however, as with the restriction on funding for IVF research, politics has all too often entered into this field. The results are not always positive for patients or society at large.

Thus, in the final section of the text, we will hear from experts in psychology, law, and ethics. This is truly a field where caring for patients requires all the skills of a clinician: healing, caring, teaching, and discovering.

REFERENCE

1 Guzick DS, Sullivan MW, Adamson GD, Cedars MI, Falk RJ, Peterson EP, Steinkampf MP. Efficacy of treatment for unexplained infertility. *Fertil Steril* 70(2):207–213, 1998.

INFERTILITY

1 Evaluation of the Female: Ovulation

Marc A. Fritz

Introduction

Infertility may result from a wide variety of causes. One of the most important and common causes is the failure to ovulate or *anovulation*. Tests of ovulation are therefore an integral part of the evaluation of every infertile couple. Because most such tests are noninvasive and involve relatively little cost, a test of ovulation also is usually one of the first steps in the evaluation of infertility. After first documenting anovulation, the same techniques may then be used to determine the effectiveness of any ovulation induction treatment strategy.

Any of a number of different methods may be used to determine if and when ovulation occurs. All are based on one or another of the hormonal events that characterize the normal ovulatory menstrual cycle, or on the effects that those hormones have at various sites within the reproductive system. This chapter will briefly outline the characteristics and key features of the normal menstrual cycle, describe each of the tests of ovulation commonly used in clinical practice, and discuss their interpretation and potential pitfalls.

Guiding Questions

DOES THE PATIENT OVULATE?

- At what interval do you have periods? How many days from the first day of one period to the first day of the next?
- How many days do you bleed?
- If you didn't have a calendar, could you predict a period was coming?

1

CAN YOU DOCUMENT
OVULATION?

• What techniques are available for documentation of ovulation?
  BBT charting
  Serum progesterone
  Urinary LH monitoring
  Endometrial biopsy
  Trasvaginal ultrasound

The Menstrual Cycle

To understand the various tests of ovulation and how and when to use and interpret them, one must first have a firm, if only very basic, understanding of the major events in the normal menstrual cycle.

NORMAL CYCLE
CHARACTERISTICS

The follicular phase of the ovarian cycle spans the interval from onset of menses to ovulation. In general, variations in overall cycle length reflect differences in the length of the follicular phase. In normal ovulatory cycles, the follicular phase generally varies between 12 and 20 days in duration. The luteal phase of the ovarian cycle spans the interval from ovulation to onset of the next menses. In contrast to the follicular phase, the length of the luteal phase is remarkably consistent and from 13 to 15 days in duration. Cycles in which the follicular or luteal phase duration falls outside of these ranges generally are best considered abnormal.

KEY POINT

Fertile cycles should fall between 25 and 35 days in length.

To achieve optimum reproductive efficiency, menstrual cycles generally should last no less than 25 days and no more than 35 days in duration. Cycles that are shorter than 25 days in length typically exhibit either an abnormally short follicular or luteal phase and are less likely to be fertile than those of normal length. Cycles longer than 35 days in duration also decrease fertility, if only by reducing the number of opportunities to conceive within a given interval of time. The average and also most common cycle length is 28 days, but a great many normally fertile women have cycles that are slightly shorter or longer than 28 days in duration.

THE OVARIAN CYCLE

The stimulus for the initiation of follicular growth is unknown, but the earliest stages are independent of pituitary gonadotropin stimulation and are ongoing, even in prepubertal girls, pregnant women, and in those using oral contraceptives. Initial follicular growth occurs in a continuous series of waves that to some extent overlap, and each wave contains a group or cohort of follicles. The cohort recruited to participate in each new menstrual cycle is that which happens, by chance, to reach the stage of development at which it first becomes sensitive to cyclic changes in the circulating concentration of follicle-stimulating hormone (FSH). As one cycle draws to a close and another begins, FSH levels rise sufficiently to support further follicular growth and development[1,2] (Fig. 1-1).

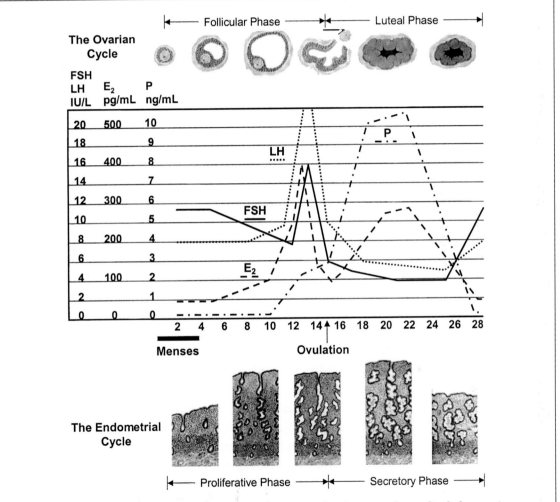

Figure 1-1: The normal menstrual cycle. Temporal relationship between the cyclical changes in serum concentrations of follicle-stimulating hormone (FSH), luteinizing hormone (LH), estradiol (E_2), and progesterone (P) and the stages of ovarian follicular and endometrial development across the normal ovulatory menstrual cycle.

As each cycle begins, FSH stimulates granulosa cells in the newly recruited follicles to proliferate and produce increasing quantities of estrogen and inhibin B. Serum levels of the two hormones rise progressively, the combined negative feedback effects of both on pituitary FSH secretion increase, and serum FSH levels steadily declines. Decreasing FSH concentrations, in concert with other complex intraovarian regulatory mechanisms involving other peptide hormones and growth factors, effectively withdraws support from all but a single "selected" follicle. The larger complement of granulosa cells in the dominant follicle and advanced development of its local microvasculature help allow it to remain sensitive to declining levels of FSH and therefore to further grow and mature while all other less mature follicles in the cohort lapse into atresia.[1–3]

After its selection, the dominant follicle quickly becomes the primary source of circulating estrogen. Estrogen levels rise steadily, slowly at first, then more rapidly, and peak approximately 24–36 h before ovulation (Fig. 1-1). Once estradiol levels reach a critical threshold concentration (approximately 200 pg/mL) and remain elevated for the requisite interval (approximately 50 h), they exert a "positive feedback" effect on the pituitary and trigger the midcycle "surge" in luteinizing hormone (LH) that induces ovulation and thus ends the "follicular phase" of the ovarian cycle. A midcycle spike in FSH levels accompanies the LH surge because the two pituitary hormones share the same hypothalamic releasing factor, gonadotropin-releasing hormone (GnRH).[1,2]

At midcycle, the preovulatory follicle "luteinizes" and becomes the corpus luteum, thus marking the transition to the "luteal phase" of the ovarian cycle. Now, in addition to estrogen, the corpus luteum also produces large amounts of progesterone. Levels of both steroid hormones rise steadily to reach their highest luteal phase concentrations 7–8 days after ovulation (Fig. 1-1). As estrogen and progesterone levels rise, their negative feedback effects cause FSH and LH concentrations to fall again to basal levels. Unless pregnancy occurs, the corpus luteum is destined to regress in a form of programmed cell death. As it does, serum concentrations of estrogen and progesterone steadily decline, ultimately reaching the baseline concentrations observed at the beginning of a new cycle. Decreasing levels of negative feedback allow FSH concentrations to rise again and recruit a new cohort of follicles (Fig. 1-1).[1,2]

KEY POINT

Follicle recruitment is an ongoing process. Development of the dominant follicle requires a complex interplay among the hypothalamus, the pituitary, and the ovary.

In conception cycles, the embryo arrives and implants sometime between 6 and 10 days after ovulation, just as the corpus luteum reaches full maturity and peak functional capacity.[4,5] Human chorionic gonadotropin (hCG) produced by the invading trophoblast "rescues" the corpus luteum, preventing its otherwise inevitable demise. Rapidly rising hCG concentrations stimulate the corpus luteum to maintain high levels of estrogen and progesterone production in early pregnancy. Gradually, the growing placenta develops sufficient functional capacity to assume that responsibility and pregnancy becomes independent of the corpus luteum. Normally, this "luteal-placental shift" in steroid hormone production is functionally completed by the end of the seventh week of pregnancy (menstrual dates).

THE ENDOMETRIAL CYCLE

During the preovulatory or follicular phase of the ovarian cycle, estrogen secreted first by the newly emerging cohort of follicles and later by the one selected and dominant follicle serves to stimulate renewed growth and proliferation of the functional layer of the endometrium that was shed in the immediately preceding menstrual period. The follicular phase of the ovarian cycle thus coincides with the "proliferative phase" of the endometrial cycle (Fig. 1-1). The endometrium gradually increases in thickness and reaches full development as estrogen levels peak just before ovulation.

After ovulation, in response to the rising levels of progesterone, the endometrium organizes, matures, and releases secretions into the uterine cavity, in preparation for the anticipated arrival of an embryo. The luteal phase of the ovarian cycle thus coincides with the "secretory phase" of the endometrial cycle (Fig. 1-1). The endometrium becomes "receptive" to implantation at midluteal phase, just as corpus luteum progesterone and estrogen production reaches its highest level.[4,5] Thereafter, unless pregnancy occurs, the corpus luteum regresses and steroid hormone concentration steadily decline. Support for the endometrium is thus withdrawn and menses ensues.

In conception cycles, hCG-stimulated sustained high levels of corpus luteum steroid hormone production ensure that the endometrium remains stable during early pregnancy. Ultimately, under continuous stimulation by progesterone and estrogen, first derived from the corpus luteum and later from the placenta, the secretory endometrium is again transformed to become the decidua.

INTERVAL OF HIGHEST FERTILITY

Normal sperm can survive in the female reproductive tract and retain the ability to fertilize an egg for at least 3 and up to 5 days, but an oocyte can be successfully fertilized for only approximately 12–24 h after it is released.[6] Consequently, in virtually all conception cycles, intercourse occurs sometime within the 6-day interval ending on the day of ovulation.[7,8] The probability of conception increases progressively during that time and abruptly declines to near zero thereafter.[7,8] Careful studies suggest that the probability of conception is highest when coitus occurs on the day before ovulation occurs (approximately 0.30).[8] However, given the inherent variability in the length of menstrual cycles and the time of ovulation, even in regularly menstruating women, the time of ovulation cannot be predicted accurately based on cycle characteristics alone.[9]

Timed coitus commonly is recommended as a means to improve the likelihood of pregnancy for infertile couples, even though there are little data to demonstrate its effectiveness. Although some tests of ovulation can help to define the time of ovulation, they should not necessarily be used for this purpose without specific reason. Scheduled intercourse clearly can add to the already significant stress of infertility. Moreover, much of the interval of peak fertility during the menstrual cycle may be inadvertently excluded while awaiting the appropriate "signal." The approximate temporal relationship among the midcycle LH surge, the time of ovulation, and the intervals during which various tests may predict or detect ovulation is shown in Fig. 1-2. However, for most couples, the simple recommendation for intercourse approximately twice per week can avoid an unnecessary source of stress while also helping to ensure that coitus occurs during the interval of highest fertility.[10] For couples who have infrequent intercourse, by preference or circumstance, timed coitus may be an appropriate recommendation.

KEY POINT

The most fertile time during the menstrual cycle actually begins BEFORE ovulation. Recommendation for intercourse every other day, beginning approximately 6 days before expected ovulation, may be the simplest advice for many couples.

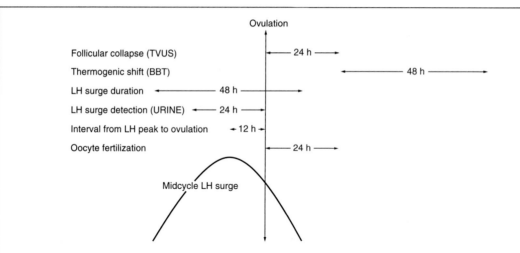

Figure 1-2: Temporal relationships with time of ovulation. Approximate temporal relationship between the midcycle LH surge, the time of ovulation, and the intervals during which various tests may predict or detect ovulation. TVUS, transvaginal ultrasound examinations; BBT, basal body temperature.

Tests of Ovulation

In the evaluation of the infertile couple, a wide variety of methods or tests may be chosen to determine if, when, and how well a woman ovulates. The tests of ovulation commonly used in clinical practice, their criteria, and relative advantages and disadvantages are summarized in Table 1-1. Each will be considered in detail, in order of increasing complexity and cost. Although any of these methods may provide evidence of ovulation, none proves that ovulation or egg release has actually occurred. The only positive proof of ovulation is pregnancy.

MENSTRUAL HISTORY   Menstrual history alone often provides a substantial amount of useful information. Ovulatory menstrual cycles typically are regular, predictable, and last approximately 1 month. In ovulatory women, menses generally are consistent in the amount, character, and duration of flow, and often are preceded by a recognizable pattern of premenstrual symptoms or molimina. The converse also is most often true. Menses in anovulatory women generally are somewhat irregular, unpredictable, less frequent,

Table 1-1. **TESTS OF OVULATION**

Test	Criteria	Advantages	Disadvantages
Menstrual history	Regular, predictable cycles at 25–35-day interval Consistent flow characteristics and premenstrual molimina	No cost Noninvasive	Subjective Unreliable in infertile women
Natural family planning methods	Cyclic changes in cervical mucus characteristics	No cost Noninvasive	Subjective Unreliable Unacceptable to many women
Basal body temperature	Biphasic pattern	Low cost Noninvasive Defines approximate time of ovulation Defines approximate follicular and luteal phase duration	May become tedious over time Interpretation frequently uncertain Defines approximate time of ovulation only after interval of highest fertility has passed
Serum progesterone concentration	Luteal phase concentration >3 ng/mL	Modest cost Minimally invasive Simple and objective Highly accurate if properly timed	Correct interpretation requires proper timing Cannot define time of ovulation
Monitoring urine LH excretion	Detection of LH surge	Modest cost Relatively simple, objective, and reliable Accurately defines the interval of highest fertility, in advance of ovulation Accurately defines follicular and luteal phase duration	May become costly and tedious over time Self-testing must be performed according to specific instructions May yield false negative or equivocal results
Endometrial biopsy	"Secretory" histology	Objective Highly accurate if properly timed Specifically confirms or excludes diagnoses of endometrial hyperplasia or chronic endometritis	Moderately high cost Invasive May be associated with significant discomfort Cannot define time of ovulation Associated risks greater than with other methods

(continued)

Table 1-1. TESTS OF OVULATION *(CONTINUED)*

TEST	CRITERIA	ADVANTAGES	DISADVANTAGES
Serial transvaginal ultrasound examinations	Observation of progressive preovulatory follicular growth and subsequent follicle collapse, increased internal echo density, and increased volume of cul-de-sac fluid	Defines the size and number of antral follicles Accurately defines time of ovulation during interval of highest fertility Accurately defines follicular and luteal phase duration Best evidence that ovulation actually occurs	High cost Moderately invasive Requires frequent office visits Requires a highly trained and experienced examiner

typically vary in the amount and duration of flow, and generally are not associated with any consistent pattern of premenstrual symptoms.

The regularity, predictability, and consistency of menses in normally cycling women result from ovulation, or more specifically, from the organized sequence of hormonal events that characterizes the ovulatory cycle. Women who have grossly infrequent, irregular, or unpredictable menstrual periods almost certainly do not ovulate frequently or regularly enough to maximize their chances to achieve pregnancy and do not require more formal or sophisticated testing to prove what is already quite obvious.

NATURAL FAMILY PLANNING METHODS

Many women are familiar with "natural family planning" methods of determining if and when ovulation occurs. The technique centers on the detection of ovulation via self-monitoring of the amount and consistency of cervical mucus across the cycle.[11] Estrogen stimulates cervical mucus production and as estrogen levels rise, mucus becomes more abundant, clear, and watery, and more easily penetrated by sperm.[12] In contrast, progesterone inhibits cervical mucus production and renders it thick, cloudy, and more jelly-like in consistency.

A regular and predictable pattern of mucus production suggests normal ovulation, but many women find self-monitoring of their mucus production and characteristics cumbersome, unpleasant, or difficult to interpret.[11] Moreover, not all ovulatory women experience cyclical changes in the amount and character of cervical mucus sufficient to allow confident interpretation. Whereas the information provided by menstrual history and cervical mucus changes can be helpful, careful evaluation of the infertile couple requires more objective and definitive evidence of ovulation.

BASAL BODY TEMPERATURE

Basal body temperature (BBT) is body temperature under "basal" conditions, meaning when completely at rest, such as during sleep. Although 98.6°F generally is considered as normal body temperature, basal temperature is actually somewhat lower, typically below 98.0°F. As a test of ovulation, BBT recordings are based on the fact that progesterone is a "thermogenic" hormone. As progesterone levels rise after ovulation, BBT also increases. The effects are to some extent concentration dependent, but more qualitative than quantitative; any progesterone level above approximately 3 ng/mL will raise BBT. The thermogenic shift in BBT that follows ovulation is subtle but nonetheless distinct and generally easy to detect when BBT is carefully monitored and recorded on a daily basis.[13] Synthetic progestational agents (medroxyprogesterone acetate, norethindrone acetate) that are commonly used to induce menses in amenorrheic women have similar thermogenic properties and also raise BBT.

METHODOLOGY For practical purposes, BBT monitoring involves recording oral temperature each morning, immediately on awakening and before arising. Women who work nights or have rotating shifts should be advised to take their temperature after the longest uninterrupted interval of sleep each day. Traditionally, BBT is measured using a specially designed glass/mercury BBT thermometer that looks, acts, and works just like any standard fever thermometer, but has an expanded scale that typically ranges from 96.0 to 100.0°F, marked in tenths of one degree. The expanded scale provides the means for highly accurate temperature recordings and to detect the subtle shift in BBT that occurs after ovulation. More modern electronic thermometers may be suitable alternatives, but only if they have the necessary accuracy and precision.

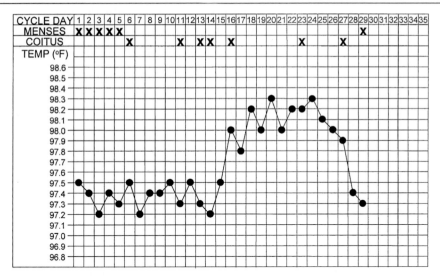

Figure 1-3: Basal body temperature recording. A typical basal body temperature graph demonstrating the classical biphasic pattern observed in an ovulatory menstrual cycle, also indicating the times of coitus and days of menses.

BBT recordings are easiest to interpret when temperatures are plotted on graph paper. In ovulatory women, a "biphasic" pattern usually is readily evident (Fig. 1-3).[13] During the follicular phase of the cycle, BBT generally fluctuates 0.1–0.5 degrees around an average in the range between 97.0 and 97.5°F. Once progesterone concentrations rise above the thermogenic threshold, BBT increases by 0.4–0.6 of a degree or more over the previous average, usually somewhat abruptly. During the luteal phase of the cycle, BBT remains elevated, with fluctuations as before, until again falling to baseline levels just before or after the onset of menses. The ideal BBT recording is clearly biphasic and reveals a cycle between 25 and 35 days in length, with menses beginning 12 days or more after the rise in temperature. When pregnancy occurs in a monitored cycle, onset of menses is delayed and BBT remains elevated, reflecting the sustained production of progesterone by the corpus luteum stimulated by hCG.

INTERVAL OF HIGHEST FERTILITY IN MONITORED CYCLES In addition to providing objective evidence of ovulation, BBT recordings also can help to determine approximately when ovulation occurs. Unfortunately, the temporal relationship between the thermogenic shift in BBT and ovulation is frequently misunderstood. BBT generally falls to its lowest level just before ovulation, but the nadir in BBT cannot be reliably identified until after temperature rises.[14] The normal range of daily fluctuations in BBT makes the temperature on any given morning difficult to interpret with confidence. What on one morning may look like the preovulatory nadir in BBT or the beginning of the thermogenic shift that follows ovulation often will be recognized as only another temperature fluctuation on the next day. The progesterone-mediated thermogenic shift in BBT generally occurs 1–3 days *after* the midcycle LH surge and 1–2 days *after* ovulation occurs.[15] The rise in BBT is fairly easy to identify when it is sharply defined. However, a more gradual "stair-step" increase in temperature is not uncommon and more difficult to interpret. A shift in BBT almost always becomes apparent in ovulatory cycles, but frequently can be recognized only days later and long after ovulation has occurred.

Given the temporal relationship among the midcycle LH surge, ovulation, and the thermogenic shift in BBT, the interval of highest fertility in BBT-monitored cycles spans the 7-day interval immediately *before* the midcycle rise in temperature (Table 1-2).

Table 1-2. **INTERVAL OF HIGHEST FERTILITY IN MONITORED CYCLES, ACCORDING TO METHOD**

METHOD	OPTIMUM TIME FOR COITUS OR INSEMINATION
Basal body temperature	Within the 7-day interval immediately preceding the postovulatory thermogenic shift
Monitoring urine LH excretion	Within the 3-day interval beginning with the day on which a midcycle LH surge is detected. The day following detection of the LH surge is likely to be the single one most fertile day
Serial transvaginal ultrasound examinations	Within the interval beginning on the day the lead preovulatory follicle reaches a size consistent with full maturity (variable, depending on whether follicular development is spontaneous or induced by treatment with clomiphene citrate or exogenous gonadotropins) and ending approximately 24 h after observation of follicular collapse Approximately 36 h after injection, when exogenous hCG is used to induce ovulation

Once a biphasic pattern becomes clearly evident, the most fertile interval is already passed. One way to avoid the inevitable uncertainties in predicting the time of ovulation in BBT-monitored cycles is to review a series of recordings, noting the earliest and latest days of the cycle on which the temperature shift has occurred. When there is reason for such recommendations, coital timing can be optimized by suggesting alternate day intercourse during the interval beginning 7 days before the earliest observed rise and ending on the day of the latest observed shift in BBT.

ADVANTAGES AND DISADVANTAGES   As a test of ovulation in the infertile couple, the principle advantage that BBT charting has over other methods is its relatively low cost. A BBT thermometer can be purchased in any full-service pharmacy, typically costs between 10 and 15 dollars, and can be used to monitor cycles indefinitely without additional expense. BBT recordings also can help to identify an abnormally long follicular phase or short luteal phase that might otherwise be undetected, and for which treatment may help to improve fertility.

BBT monitoring is easy and noninvasive, but can become rather tiresome over time. For some it can also increase stress as a daily reminder of unsuccessful efforts to conceive, each day beginning with thoughts of a family not yet realized. Moreover, some women menstruate regularly and predictably, but do not exhibit a clearly biphasic BBT pattern. Under such circumstances, an alternative method should be used to objectively document ovulation before assuming that treatment is required. In recent years, BBT charting has become less popular as most physicians have come to prefer more reliable or efficient tests of ovulation as described below. Nevertheless, BBT recording remains useful and may still be the best method for couples that are reluctant or unable to begin a more formal and costly evaluation.

SERUM PROGESTERONE CONCENTRATION

Another common method for evaluating ovulation in infertile women is to measure the serum progesterone concentration. Progesterone is not produced in any significant quantity before the midcycle LH surge. Serum progesterone levels generally remain below 1 ng/mL during the follicular phase of the cycle, rise slightly on the day of the LH surge, and increase dramatically only after ovulation has occurred (Fig. 1-1). During the luteal phase of the cycle, the serum progesterone concentration increases steadily, peaks 7–8 days after ovulation, and then declines over the days preceding menses (Fig. 1-1). Drawing a blood sample to determine the serum progesterone concentration is a simple, effective, and very common test of ovulation. In general, any serum progesterone concentration greater than 3 ng/mL provides reliable evidence that ovulation has occurred.[16]

METHODOLOGY   When best to measure the serum progesterone concentration to document ovulation deserves specific discussion. One popular recommendation is to perform the test on cycle day 21, with cycle day 1 defined as the first day of menses. In the ideal and classical 28-day menstrual cycle in which ovulation occurs on or about cycle day 14, day 21 falls during the midluteal phase, approximately 1 week after ovulation and 1 week before the onset of the next menstrual period, just when serum progesterone levels should be at their highest. However, any regular menstrual cycle length between 25 and 35 days is completely normal; ovulation may thus occur as early as cycle day 10 or as late as cycle day 22 in a normal cycle. If ovulation occurs on cycle day 10, day 21 will fall 11 days after ovulation, at a time when progesterone concentrations have already begun to decline. If ovulation occurs on cycle day 22, day 21 will fall just before ovulation, when the serum progesterone level has not yet begun to rise. Consequently, when the serum progesterone concentration is chosen as the method to document ovulation, the best time to test is not always cycle day 21 and depends on the overall length of the menstrual cycle. Confident interpretation of the serum progesterone level may not be possible until menses has again occurred and the time of sampling can be more clearly defined. Sampling only after observing a sustained elevation in BBT helps to ensure appropriate timing, but if BBT is clearly biphasic, a serum progesterone measurement also may be redundant and unnecessary.

Serum progesterone levels have been used not only to document that ovulation has occurred but also to assess the "quality" of luteal function and of the cycle overall. The amount and duration of progesterone production certainly do reflect the functional capacity of the corpus luteum, but an accurate assessment requires daily serum progesterone determinations that are both costly and clearly impractical.[17,18] Some have suggested the sum of a series of progesterone determinations as an alternative, but recommendations have varied.[19,20] A single "low" midluteal phase serum progesterone level is one popular criterion for the diagnosis of "luteal phase deficiency" or a "luteal phase defect" (LPD), a disorder that is perhaps best viewed as a subtle form of ovulatory dysfunction.[16,20,21] However, a judgment based on a single test, no matter how well timed, has numerous pitfalls and cannot reliably define the quality of the cycle.

There is no consensus regarding the minimum serum progesterone concentration that confirms normal luteal function. A level greater than 10 ng/mL is one widely used standard,[20] but the concentrations observed in normal and abnormal cycles and in conception and nonconception cycles in both fertile and infertile women vary widely and overlap to a large extent.[21] One obvious explanation for such observations is that corpus luteum progesterone secretion is pulsatile in nature.[22] Careful studies in women have clearly demonstrated that progesterone levels fluctuate widely during the luteal phase, closely correlating with distinct pulses in pituitary LH release.[22] Progesterone levels as low as 5 and as high as 40 ng/mL may be observed within an interval of only hours. Some have suggested that sampling during the morning hours when concentrations generally are highest and less erratic may minimize the influence of pulsatile progesterone secretion,[23] but these observations effectively invalidate the use of serum progesterone concentrations for anything more than documenting that ovulation has occurred.

ADVANTAGES AND DISADVANTAGES A properly timed measurement of the serum progesterone concentration is one of the simplest, most reliable, and popular methods to evaluate ovulation. The test is minimally invasive, widely available, highly accurate if not overinterpreted, requires little time, and is reasonably cost-effective, typically costing between 20 and 40 dollars. Unlike BBT recordings, serum progesterone cannot be used to determine when ovulation occurs; it can only indicate that it did. When more detailed information is required, as in couples whose treatment requires a carefully timed artificial insemination with partner or donor sperm, an alternative method must be employed.

**MONITORING URINE
LH EXCRETION**

A wide variety of different commercial products now available allow women to determine if they ovulate, and more precisely when, in advance of the actual event. Generally known as "ovulation predictor kits" or "LH kits," these products are all designed to detect the midcycle LH surge in urine, thereby identifying the hormonal trigger for ovulation and informing the user that release of an egg is imminent. Ovulation predictor kits take advantage of recent advances in hormone measurement technology, reducing what was once a very labor-intensive process in the hospital laboratory to one or two simple steps that typically require less than 5 min time in the home. They have become extremely popular in recent years and are now widely used by both patients and physicians alike.

METHODOLOGY   The midcycle LH surge that ovulation predictor kits are designed to detect is a relatively brief event, lasting between 48 and 50 h from start to finish. Once LH is released from the pituitary gland into the blood, it has a very short half-life and is rapidly cleared from the body, primarily via the urine. Ovulation predictor kits yield a positive result when the urinary LH concentration exceeds a threshold level normally seen only during the LH surge. In most cycles, the test will be positive on only a single day, occasionally on two consecutive days. Therefore, to reliably detect the LH surge, testing must be done on a daily basis. The usual recommendation is to begin testing 2 or 3 days before the surge is expected, based on the overall length of the cycle and observations in previous cycles; all commercial products include detailed instructions that explain how and when to perform the test. The first positive test provides all of the information of importance; there is no benefit from continuing to test on subsequent days. Any left over tests in the kit are better saved for use in a subsequent cycle.

The results of tests to determine the urine LH concentration are sensitive to both the volume of fluid intake and time of day. There is no need to restrict fluid intake, but patients should be advised to avoid drinking large volumes of fluid a short time before they plan to test. Logically, the first morning void would be an ideal specimen to test because it typically is the most concentrated. However, careful studies have shown that when testing is performed once daily, the most efficient time to test is in the late afternoon or early evening (3:00–8:00 p.m.).[24] LH surges often begin in the early morning hours and cannot be detected in urine for several hours thereafter. Consequently, urinary LH concentrations may not yet be sufficient to yield a positive test in the first morning void, and because the LH surge lasts only a relatively brief time, may again fall to levels below the threshold of the test by the following morning. Testing more than once a day decreases the frequency of false negative results (failure to detect the LH surge in an ovulatory cycle), but more frequent testing also increases cost. If performed once a day in the late afternoon or early evening, tests can be expected to detect the LH surge in approximately 90% of ovulatory cycles. Although true false positive tests (detection of an LH surge in an anovulatory cycle) are generally rare, equivocal or "borderline" results are not altogether uncommon and can be both confusing and frustrating.

The accuracy and cost of the many different ovulation predictor kits on the market vary. All are useful and reasonably reliable, but some are better and easier to use than others.[25,26] The best products available are those that have been rigorously and scientifically validated; with these, the first positive result predicts that ovulation will occur within the following 24–48 h, with greater than 90% probability.[24,25] The choice of product may vary with the goals of testing. If one is simply trying to determine if and approximately when ovulation is occurring so that intercourse might be focused during the interval when conception is most likely, any of the products available in most pharmacies will suffice. However, when more precise information is needed, as in couples whose treatment requires a carefully timed artificial insemination with the sperm of the partner or an anonymous donor, the attendant logistic demands and costs involved justify using the best and most accurate products available.

INTERVAL OF HIGHEST FERTILITY IN MONITORED CYCLES Ovulation generally follows within 18–24 h after detection of the urine LH surge and almost always within 48 h.[24] Consequently, the interval of highest fertility includes the day of LH surge detection and the following 2 days. The day *after* the first positive test generally should be the one best day for timed intercourse or to perform an artificial insemination, when it is indicated (Table 1-2).[24,27]

Advantages and Disadvantages   Monitoring urine LH excretion is a noninvasive test of ovulation that is widely and readily available, requires relatively little time and effort, and invites the patient to become actively and directly involved in her care. The many different products available contain between five and nine individual tests and range in cost between 20 and 50 dollars. Monitoring urinary LH excretion is thus comparable to a serum progesterone concentration in cost and similar to BBT recordings in the demands made on the patient. Accurate identification of the midcycle LH surge also provides the means to define exactly the length of the follicular and the luteal phase and thus to identify otherwise unrecognized abnormalities of the cycle that may benefit from treatment.

Over time, like BBT recordings, the method can become costly, tedious, and frustrating, particularly when testing fails to clearly identify the LH surge, or does so falsely. The greatest advantage that an ovulation predictor kit has over most other tests of ovulation is the ability to accurately determine when ovulation occurs, in advance of the actual event. Monitoring urine LH excretion may thus be reserved for women who ovulate (based on menstrual history, BBT recordings, or an appropriately timed serum progesterone concentration), when knowing the precise time of ovulation clearly will improve the likelihood of success, as in those who have infrequent intercourse or when treatment includes artificial insemination.

ENDOMETRIAL BIOPSY

Endometrial biopsy is one of the classic tests of ovulation and is based on the characteristic histologic changes that progesterone induces in its principal target tissue. An endometrial tissue specimen obtained during the preovulatory or follicular phase of the menstrual cycle exhibits a "proliferative" pattern, reflecting the growth inducing effects of increasing levels of estrogen produced first by the cohort of developing follicles and later by the single dominant follicle. An endometrial tissue specimen obtained during the postovulatory or luteal phase of the cycle exhibits a "secretory" pattern, reflecting the maturational influence of progesterone secreted from the corpus luteum. Ovulatory women have a proliferative endometrium before ovulation and develop a secretory endometrium after ovulation occurs. In contrast, anovulatory women are always in the follicular phase. Consequently, their endometrium is always proliferative, and may even display hyperplastic changes if an unopposed estrogenic stimulus is allowed to persist for an extended interval of time. A tissue specimen revealing a secretory endometrium therefore implies the presence of progesterone and provides indirect but reliable and objective evidence of recent ovulation. Treatment with exogenous progesterone or a synthetic progestin will also convert a proliferative endometrium to a secretory histologic pattern.

METHODOLOGY To be an effective test of ovulation, endometrial biopsy must be properly timed to ensure it is performed during what should be the secretory phase of the endometrial cycle. The overall length of the menstrual cycle and the latest acceptable time of ovulation must be considered in the same way and for the same reasons discussed earlier with regard to the timing of serum progesterone measurements.

Endometrial biopsy is a relatively simple office procedure; most commonly performed using any one of the many disposable plastic aspiration cannulas now widely available. The narrow caliber of such instruments generally permits passage through even a nulliparous cervix without need for a tenaculum or preliminary sounding or dilation. Endometrial biopsy generally does not require sedation or anesthetic, but either or both may be used for procedures that are technically difficult or for patients who are extremely anxious. Endometrial biopsy typically requires less than a minute to perform and generally is very well tolerated, most often causing only modest cramping during and for a short time afterward. A "vaso-vagal reaction," characterized by bradycardia, nausea, and orthostatic hypotension is an occasional complication. The reaction generally is self-limited and usually does not require specific treatment. Pretreatment with a nonsteroidal anti-inflammatory drug helps to reduce any pain or cramping associated with endometrial biopsy. A paracervical block also is effective, but may cause as much or more discomfort as the biopsy procedure itself.

The histologic features of the secretory endometrium change with the duration of progesterone exposure, in a classical sequence that is generally well defined. The temporally dependent pattern of postovulatory endometrial maturation is sufficiently predictable to allow experienced pathologists to "date" the endometrium, offering a retrospective estimate of how many days have passed since ovulation occurred.[28] The observed "date" (based on the most advanced changes observed) may then be compared to the actual day of sampling. Traditionally, the day of biopsy has been estimated by counting backward from onset of the next menstrual period, assuming that menses began on the 14th postovulatory day. However, the day of sampling is more accurately defined by the number of days elapsed since detection of the LH surge.[29] Agreement between the histologic date and the sampling date, within a 2-day interval, generally is considered normal. A histologic endometrial date more than 2 days "out of phase" with the defined day of sampling has been the traditional criterion for the diagnosis of LPD.[24]

In the past, LPD has been identified more often in women with unexplained infertility or advanced reproductive age (age over 35 years) than in those with tubal factor infertility or in normally fertile women.[30,31] The abnormality also has been observed more commonly in women with primary infertility than in those who have conceived before, and more frequently in women with history of recurrent early pregnancy loss than in those with a normal obstetrical history.[32,33] However, endometrial dating, and even the very concept of LPD, has become highly controversial in recent years. The methods used to establish the traditional dating criteria have been challenged, primarily because tissue specimens were obtained from an infertile population, not from normally fertile women. Moreover, the day of sampling was defined by onset of the next menses, and biopsy itself may affect when menses next begins, or when it is perceived to start. More recent studies have further and seriously undermined the validity of endometrial dating. Several have demonstrated that even normally fertile women occasionally exhibit evidence of LPD.[34,35] Others have shown that the histologic date of any given tissue specimen can vary widely among different pathologists, or even when reexamined by the same pathologist.[36,37] Recent careful, systematic studies also have revealed that the classical histologic features used for dating the endometrium are much less temporally discrete than was originally described. Consequently, few any longer regard endometrial dating as a reliable indicator of the quality of luteal function.

In recent years, a great many studies have sought to define the cascade of molecular events involved in the implantation process.

A number of endometrial proteins that are expressed specifically during the putative implantation window have been identified and investigated, but none has yet been validated as a reliable marker of "endometrial receptivity."[38,39] If and when that occurs, endometrial biopsy might once again be regarded as offering unique and valuable information beyond that provided by other tests of ovulation.

ADVANTAGES AND DISADVANTAGES A well-timed endometrial biopsy is an effective test of ovulation, but has rather limited and specific indications. For women with chronic anovulation of long duration in whom the possibility of endometrial hyperplasia must be suspected, biopsy can identify or exclude endometrial hyperplasia that requires specific treatment. In those with history of recurrent early pregnancy loss, biopsy can reveal a chronic endometritis not otherwise detected. In the past but no longer, biopsy was considered the "gold standard" of methods for the diagnosis of LPD. Consequently, as a test of ovulation, endometrial biopsy is difficult to justify. The procedure is invasive and may cause significant discomfort. Although small, the risks of biopsy still are clearly greater than those associated with any other method. Endometrial biopsy also is very expensive, with costs relating to the procedure and histologic interpretation commonly approaching or exceeding the sum of 500 dollars. Most importantly, endometrial biopsy provides no more useful information than can be obtained from BBT recordings, monitoring urine LH excretion, or measuring the serum progesterone concentration. Consequently, biopsy generally should be reserved for women in whom endometrial hyperplasia or chronic endometritis is strongly suspected and must be excluded.

TRANSVAGINAL ULTRASOUND EXAMINATIONS The last and most complicated test of ovulation involves a series of transvaginal ultrasound (TVUS) examinations, ideally performed in the physician's office. The method is based on direct observation of a characteristic sequence of changes in the ovulatory follicle, just prior to and immediately after egg release. Serial TVUS examinations performed over the week or so before expected ovulation provide the means to observe the latter stages of follicular development and the early stages of corpus luteum development. Although still not providing positive proof that an egg was in fact released, serial TVUS examinations offer detailed information concerning the size and number of preovulatory follicles and provide the most accurate estimate of when ovulation occurs.

METHODOLOGY   With modern ultrasound technology, the ovaries generally can be easily and clearly imaged to include the size and number of antral follicles that each contains. A carefully timed series of TVUS examinations, performed on a daily or alternate day schedule beginning 3–5 days before the expected time of ovulation, provides the means to follow the growth and subsequent collapse of the preovulatory follicle directly. Over the days immediately preceding ovulation, the preovulatory follicle typically grows at a predictable pace, approximately 2 mm per day (range 1–3 mm/day). Soon after ovulation, a characteristic pattern of changes may be observed. The follicle abruptly decreases in size, its margins become less distinct, the density of internal echoes increases, and the volume of cul-de-sac fluid increases.[40] When urinary LH excretion also is monitored, evidence of ovulation generally will be observed within approximately 48 h after detection of the midcycle LH surge.[24]

Abnormal patterns of follicle development also may become apparent. The dominant follicle may not grow at a normal pace, it may collapse before it reaches a size consistent with full maturity, or it may continue to grow but fail to rupture, persisting as a cyst long after the LH surge has occurred.[41,42] Such observations suggest subtle forms of ovulatory dysfunction that cannot be detected with any other method, but these abnormalities also are relatively rare, except perhaps in women with otherwise unexplained infertility. Serial TVUS examinations to monitor the size and number of developing follicles are essential to ensure the safety and effectiveness of treatment when exogenous gonadotropins are used to induce ovulation. However, there is otherwise seldom a reason to study cycle characteristics in such exacting detail. Treatments to correct subtle disorders of follicular development are the same as those generally recommended for couples with unexplained infertility. Consequently, diagnosis has little or no significant impact on subsequent treatment.

INTERVAL OF HIGHEST FERTILITY IN MONITORED CYCLES   Given that the oocyte can be fertilized for only approximately 12–24 h after ovulation and considering the typical longevity of sperm in the female reproductive tract, the interval coinciding with highest fertility in cycles monitored with serial TVUS examinations generally begins when the preovulatory follicle first reaches a size consistent with full maturity and ends approximately 24 h after observing follicular collapse (Table 1-2). Unfortunately, the size of a mature preovulatory follicle may vary considerably and even depends to some extent on whether follicular development is spontaneous (range 17–26 mm) or induced by treatment with clomiphene citrate (range 19–30 mm) or exogenous gonadotropins (range 15–22 mm). When hCG is used as a surrogate LH surge to induce ovulation, ovulation generally follows 24–48 h later. Consequently, the optimum time for intercourse includes the 3-day interval beginning with hCG administration, and when indicated, artificial insemination is best performed approximately 36 h after hCG injection (Table 1-2).[43]

KEY POINT

There are many tests for ovulation. The selection of any one test can best be determined by the information sought with testing, e.g., confirmation of ovulation, timing of intercourse or insemination, and adequacy of ovulation.

ADVANTAGES AND DISADVANTAGES   For those with the necessary training and experience, TVUS examinations are easy to perform, typically are associated with little or no significant discomfort, and generally take only a few minutes to accomplish. Serial TVUS examinations provide detailed information about the pace and quality of follicular development, accurately define the time of ovulation, and offer the most definitive evidence that ovulation has in fact occurred. As a test of ovulation, serial TVUS examinations also have distinct disadvantages. Chief among these is the need for frequent office visits within an interval of a few to several days and the substantial expense associated with such visits and examinations, each typically costing between 100 and 200 dollars or more. Consequently, serial TVUS examinations generally should be reserved for those in whom the safety or effectiveness of treatment hinges on the detailed information the method offers.

Summary

Evaluation of ovulation is an important part of any infertility investigation. All of the different tests of ovulation are useful and no one test is necessarily best. Some are very simple, noninvasive, and inexpensive. Others are relatively more complicated, invasive, and costly. A few provide the means to determine not only if ovulation occurs, but also when, with varying accuracy.

The best choice among the tests of ovulation varies with the information required (Fig. 1-4). No testing may be necessary in women whose menstrual history clearly indicates that ovulation seldom if ever occurs. However, when there is reason for strong suspicion of endometrial hyperplasia, cancer, or chronic endometritis, endometrial biopsy may be prudent. When cycles are regular and predictable and the only objective is to document ovulation, BBT or a timed serum progesterone concentration generally will suffice. When circumstances also require accurate prediction of the time of ovulation, as in couples who have infrequent intercourse or when treatment includes artificial insemination, monitoring urine LH excretion with an ovulation predictor kit is the most cost-effective and appropriate choice. In those who require insemination but cannot reliably detect a midcycle uLH surge, serial TVUS examinations can be used to obtain the necessary information. Ultimately, the test of ovulation must be tailored to meet the needs of the individual patient.

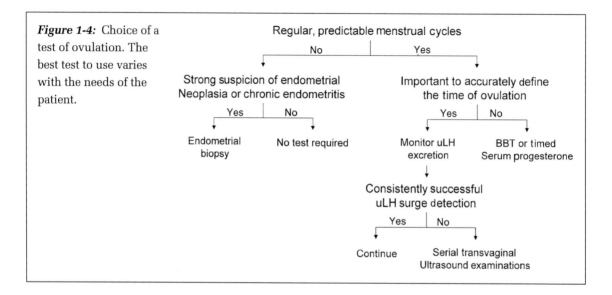

Figure 1-4: Choice of a test of ovulation. The best test to use varies with the needs of the patient.

Discussion of Cases

CASE 1

You are evaluating a 29-year-old patient for preconception counseling. She is a long-standing patient of yours and has an unremarkable medical and surgical history. She has never tried to conceive. Prior to sending the patient for routine blood screening (e.g., type and Rh, antibody screen), you begin your evaluation.

How would you evaluate the patient's ovulatory status and counsel her regarding attempts at conception?

History The patient reports menarche at age 12. Since that time she has had regular, cyclic, predictable periods at a 29–30-day interval lasting for 5 days.

Do you believe this patient is ovulatory?

Yes

Does this patient need any testing at this time to document ovulatory status?

No

How would you advise her to time her intercourse?

The patient likely ovulates around the 15th day of her cycle. She should start having intercourse around cycle day 12 and continue on a daily, or every other day, pattern until day 17. Given the time that sperm will survive in the reproductive tract, sperm will be available for fertilization without expensive monitoring.

CASE 2

You are evaluating a healthy 26-year-old nulligravid woman and her husband who have been trying unsuccessfully to conceive since discontinuation of oral contraception 2 years ago.

History Treatment with oral contraceptives began at age 14 for control of menstrual irregularity and was discontinued to attempt pregnancy. Her menstrual periods during treatment with oral contraceptives were regular, predictable, light, and relatively brief. Since discontinuing the pill, like before treatment began, her menses have been irregular, occurring once every 6–8 weeks, vary in the duration and character of flow, and are sometimes but not always preceded by premenstrual symptoms of breast tenderness, irritability, and transient weight gain. Her dysmenorrhea is generally mild, greater when menstrual flow is heaviest, and has not changed in severity over time. She denies any known past episodes of pelvic infection or exposure to sexually transmitted infections, and has had no previous pelvic or abdominal surgery. She is taking no medications and denies any allergies. She further denies any symptoms of pelvic pain, hirsutism, acne, galactorrhea, or dyspareunia. She is employed as a nurse in your hospital where she works rotating shifts in a surgical ward. She exercises for 30 min two to three times per week and has intercourse approximately three to four times each month.

Her husband is a healthy 28-year-old male, has not fathered any children, and has no history of medical illnesses or surgery, current treatment with medications, or allergies. He is employed as a long-haul truck driver and is frequently away from home for intervals of 7–10 days. A recent urologic examination revealed no abnormalities and a semen analysis was normal in all parameters.

Physical Examination   Physical examination reveals a normal-appearing adult female measuring 65 in. in height and weighing 120 lb. Examination of the thyroid, breasts, abdomen, and external genitalia reveals no abnormalities. Speculum examination reveals a normal-appearing vagina and cervix. On bimanual examination, her uterus is of normal size and shape, freely mobile, and nontender; palpation of the adnexa demonstrates no mass or tenderness.

What is the most likely cause of the couple's infertility and what testing, if any, is required to confirm your impression?

- **Ovulatory dysfunction**
- **No tests of ovulation are needed at this time.**

The patient's long history of oligomenorrhea, variable flow characteristics, and the inconsistent observations of premenstrual molimina clearly indicate that although she likely does ovulate occasionally, she does not do so with any regularity or predictability. Moreover, the couple's opportunities to conceive, even when ovulation may occur, are quite limited by their conflicting schedules and frequent intervals apart.

The patient's past medical history and physical examination suggest that abnormalities of her reproductive anatomy are relatively unlikely and her husband's normal semen analysis largely excludes any serious male factor.

There is no need for any specific tests of ovulation at this time because the menstrual history alone is sufficient to establish a diagnosis of ovulatory dysfunction. An endometrial biopsy is unnecessary because there is no reason for strong suspicion of endometrial neoplasia or chronic endometritis. The patient is young, used oral contraception for an extended interval of years until recently, and has no complaints of abnormally prolonged or heavy bleeding. Furthermore, her menstrual history suggests that she likely does ovulate, albeit infrequently, and she has never had a pelvic infection.

What is your recommendation for initial management?

- **Measurement of serum thyroid-stimulation hormone (TSH) and prolactin.**
- **Both results are in normal ranges.**

Given that thyroid abnormalities and hyperprolactinemia have been excluded (either of which would require specific treatment), you recommend that treatment to induce ovulation begin with clomiphene citrate, 50 mg/day, cycle days 5 through 9.

What testing, if any, would you now recommend as ovulation induction begins?

- **Timed serum progesterone measurement, on cycle day 24 or 25.**

The probability is high that the patient will respond to clomiphene citrate treatment, at a dose of 50, 100, or 150 mg/day, but the dose required to achieve ovulation cannot be confidently predicted. You want the treatment trial to proceed in an orderly and efficient fashion that will establish normal, regular, ovulatory cycles as quickly as possible, using the minimum dose required to minimize costs and any associated risks. If she does not respond to your initial treatment regimen, you want to be able to increase to the next dosage level without wasting time, and therefore want to apply a test of ovulation that will clearly indicate whether your treatment regimen successfully induced ovulation.

At this point in time, you need only to know whether treatment did or did not induce ovulation as intended. The obvious choices are BBT recordings or a timed serum progesterone measurement. Given that the patient works rotating shifts and sleeps at different times of day, often within a single menstrual cycle, and does not have a well-established daily regimen, reliable BBT recordings may be difficult to obtain. BBT recordings could be used, but your legitimate concerns lead you to conclude that a timed serum progesterone measurement is perhaps the best initial test to apply.

You do not yet know if ovulation will occur, much less when. However, you know that when clomiphene citrate treatment is successful, ovulation rarely occurs before the 5th day or later than the 12th day, and most commonly occurs between the 7th and 9th days, after the last dose of medication (cycle days 14–21, when medication is administered on cycles days 5 through 9). You want to avoid the very early and late luteal phases when equivocal or "borderline" results are more likely and more difficult to interpret confidently (because serum progesterone concentrations are normally relatively low). If treatment is successful, the targeted days for the test will fall somewhere between 3 and 11 days after ovulation and yield clear evidence of a response. If treatment is not successful, that too will be clear, allowing you to advance to the next higher dose of clomiphene citrate without undue delay.

The patient follows your advice, follows the prescribed treatment regimen, and returns on cycle day 25 for the timed serum progesterone measurement you recommended. Treatment was tolerated without difficulty.

- Spontaneous menses began on cycle day 32.
- The serum progesterone concentration was 12.0 ng/mL.

What is your interpretation and what counseling and recommendations would you now offer?

- **The test result (>3.0 ng/mL) clearly indicates that treatment was successful and that ovulation very likely occurred.**
- **Continue current treatment.**
- **Monitor urinary LH excretion in the next treatment cycle and record the test results.**

To ensure that the treatment regimen is truly successful and that the clomiphene-induced cycle has normal characteristics, you would like to know whether the luteal phase is of normal duration. In addition, because the couple has conflicting schedules and long intervals apart, accurate identification of the time of ovulation may also allow the couple the opportunity to adjust their schedules to avoid conflicts during those times when conception is most likely. Both goals can be achieved by monitoring urinary LH excretion with a commercial "ovulation predictor" kit or by serial transvaginal ultrasound examinations. The first of these two options is far less costly and logistically demanding.

The test should be performed once daily, in the afternoon or evening hours, beginning on approximately cycle day 12 and continuing until cycle day 20 or until the test first becomes positive. The interval of highest fertility will begin on the day of the first positive test and end 2 days later.

The patient again follows your advice, and later reports the following observations:

- The test was negative on cycle days 12–15, but clearly positive on cycle day 16.
- Menses began 15 days later, on cycle day 31.

What is your interpretation and what counseling and recommendations would you now offer?

- **The current treatment regimen is effective.**
- **Continue treatment.**
- **Expect ovulation to occur between cycle days 15 and 19 (within 2 days of that observed in the monitored cycle), with the interval of highest fertility likely to fall in the interval between cycle days 13 and 20.**
- **Consider continued monitoring of urinary LH excretion.**
- **Expand evaluation (to include assessment of her reproductive anatomy) if conception does not occur within a minimum of three and a maximum of six treatment cycles, assuming that the couple's schedules offer the opportunity to conceive.**

The LH surge was detected within the interval expected and the luteal phase duration (14 days) was normal. There is no need to change the treatment regimen. Once an effective clomiphene treatment regimen has been established, one generally can anticipate a similar response in subsequent similar treatment cycles, with minor variations.

In light of the couple's conflicting schedules and long intervals apart, it may be helpful, if it is not also intrusive, to continue monitoring of urinary LH excretion so as to even more accurately define her interval of highest fertility in each treatment cycle (the 3 days beginning on the day of LH surge detection with the day after the surge being the day on which the probability of conception will be highest).

The largest majority of pregnancies that result from clomiphene treatment alone occur within the first three to four treatment cycles, and virtually all will occur within six cycles of treatment. Other fertility factors should be excluded when semen quality is normal (as previously documented) and conception does not occur within the expected interval despite successful ovulation induction.

If menses had begun before cycle day 30, how would you interpret the observation and what recommendations would you offer?

- **Although ovulation likely did occur, treatment has not yet established a truly normal ovulatory cycle.**
- **Increase the dose of clomiphene citrate to 100 mg daily, cycle days 5–9, for the next cycle of treatment.**
- **Monitor urinary LH excretion in the same way as previously instructed.**

The observation would have represented objective evidence of a short luteal phase (<13 days duration), a subtle manifestation of ovulatory dysfunction that may result in decreased cycle fecundability (probability of achieving pregnancy per cycle), or increased risk of spontaneous abortion. Despite the subtle abnormality in cycle characteristics, response at the next higher dose of clomiphene is very likely and continued monitoring to determine the time of ovulation and confirm that treatment was truly successful is therefore reasonable and justified.

If the patient failed to detect a midcycle LH surge by cycle day 20, but nonetheless observed onset of a spontaneous menses between cycle days 26 and 36, how would you interpret the observations and what recommendations would you offer?

- **The patient did ovulate, but simply failed to detect the midcycle LH surge.**
- **Continue the current treatment regimen.**

The alternative explanation, that she failed to ovulate despite receiving the same treatment that was proven successful in the preceding cycle and yet menstruated within the expected interval, is much less likely. Another cycle of observation should allow a confident conclusion.

If the patient failed to detect a midcycle LH surge by cycle day 20 and remained amenorrheic beyond cycle day 35, how would you interpret the observations and what recommendations would you offer?

- **There would be three distinct possibilities to consider in your interpretation.**
  - **The patient may have ovulated in a timely fashion but failed to detect the midcycle LH surge and conceived.**
  - **She may have ovulated, but sometime after testing ended on cycle day 20, and if so, may have conceived.**
  - **She may have failed to ovulate altogether (least likely, in light of her response to the same treatment in the preceding cycle).**
- **Pregnancy test and serum progesterone measurement to differentiate among the three possible explanations. Recommendations will vary in accordance with the test results.**

If the pregnancy test is positive, the intended goal was achieved, regardless whether ovulation occurred before or after cycle day 20.

If the pregnancy test is negative and the serum progesterone concentration indicates that ovulation clearly did occur (>3.0 ng/mL), onset of menses may be expected within 2 weeks.

If menses does not begin within the following 2 weeks, the pregnancy test should be repeated to confirm reasonable expectations that the patient has conceived, because that is the most obvious explanation for a prolonged delay of menses after documented ovulation.

If menses does begin, as expected, within the following 2 weeks but after cycle day 36, ovulation did occur but treatment clearly has not yet effectively established regular, predictable, timely ovulation (because the cycle exceeded 35 days in total duration). A recommendation to advance to the next higher dose of clomiphene in the following cycle is therefore justified. Because earlier ovulation in response to a higher dose of treatment can be reasonably expected, you may choose to recommend that the patient again monitor her urinary LH excretion, for the same reasons and in the same way as previously instructed.

If the pregnancy test is negative and the serum progesterone concentration indicates that ovulation did not occur (<3.0 ng/mL), treatment even more clearly has failed to achieve its goal. A recommendation to advance to the next higher dose of clomiphene in the following cycle is again justified.

You may choose to repeat a timed serum progesterone measurement, again on cycle day 24 or 25, to evaluate the patient's response to the new, higher-dose treatment regimen, as before.

Alternatively, in the interests of efficiency, you might choose to recommend continued monitoring of urinary LH excretion to evaluate the response to treatment and at the same time, define the time of ovulation and the length of the luteal phase. In general, however, to avoid frustration and unnecessary cost, monitoring urinary LH excretion is best postponed until there is evidence that treatment has successfully induced ovulation.

REFERENCES

1 Macklon NS, Fauser BC. Follicle development during the normal menstrual cycle. *Maturitas* 30:181, 1998.

2 Chabbert Buffet N, Djakoure C, Maitre SC, et al. Regulation of the human menstrual cycle. *Front Neuroendocrinol* 19:151–186, 1998.

3 Zeleznik AJ. Follicle selection in primates: "many are called but few are chosen". *Bio Reprod* 65:655, 2001.

4 Wilcox AJ, Baird DD, Weinberg CR. Time of implantation of the conceptus and loss of pregnancy. *N Engl J Med* 340:1796, 1999.

5 Nikas G. Endometrial receptivity: changes in cell-surface morphology. *Semin Reprod Med* 18:229, 2000.

6 Wilcox AJ, Weinberg CR, Baird DD. Post-ovulatory ageing of the human oocyte and embryo failure. *Hum Reprod* 13:394, 1998.

7 Wilcox AJ, Weinberg CR, Baird DD. Timing of sexual intercourse in relation to ovulation. Effects on the probability of conception, survival of the pregnancy, and sex of the baby. *N Engl J Med* 333:1517, 1995.

8 Dunson DB, Baird DD, Wilcox AJ, et al. Day-specific probabilities of clinical pregnancy based on two studies with imperfect measures of ovulation. *Hum Reprod* 14:1835, 1999.

9 Wilcox AJ, Dunson D, Baird DD. The timing of the "fertile window" in the menstrual cycle: day specific estimates from a prospective study. *Br Med J* 321:1259, 2000.

10 Agarwal SK, Haney AF. Does recommending timed intercourse really help the infertile couple? *Obstet Gynecol* 84:307, 1994.

11 Tommaselli GA, Guida M, Palomba S, et al. The importance of user compliance on the effectiveness of natural family planning programs. *Gynecol Endocrinol* 14:81, 2000.

12 Katz DF, Slade DA, Nakajima ST. Analysis of pre-ovulatory changes in cervical mucus hydration and sperm penetrability. *Adv Contracept* 13:143, 1997.

13 Bates GW, Garza DE, Garza MM. Clinical manifestations of hormonal changes in the menstrual cycle. *Obstet Gynecol Clin North Am* 17:299, 1990.

14 Quagliarello J, Arny M. Inaccuracy of basal body temperature charts in predicting urinary luteinizing hormone surges. *Fertil Steril* 45:334, 1986.

15 Luciano AA, Peluso J, Koch E, et al. Temporal relationship and reliability of the clinical, hormonal, and ultrasonographic indices of ovulation in infertile women. *Obstet Gynecol* 75:412, 1990.

16 Wathen NC, Perry L, Lilford RJ, et al. Interpretation of single progesterone measurement in diagnosis of anovulation and defective luteal phase: observations on analysis of the normal range. *Br Med J* 288:7, 1984.

17 Soules MR, McLachlan RI, Ek M, et al. Luteal phase deficiency: characterization of reproductive hormones over the menstrual cycle. *J Clin Endocrinol Metab* 69:804, 1989.

18 Li TC, Lenton EA, Dockery P, et al. A comparison of some clinical and endocrinological features between cycles with normal and defective luteal phases in women with unexplained infertility. *Hum Reprod* 5:805, 1990.

19 Abraham GE, Margoulis GB, Marshall JR. Evaluation of ovulation and corpus luteum function using measurements of plasma progesterone. *Obstet Gynecol* 44:522, 1974.

20 Jordan J, Craig K, Clifton DK, et al. Luteal phase defect: the sensitivity and specificity of diagnostic methods in common clinical use. *Fertil Steril* 62:54, 1994.

21 Hull MGR, Savage PE, Bromham DR, et al. The value of a single serum progesterone measurement in the midluteal phase as a criterion of a potentially fertile cycle ("ovulation") derived from treated and untreated conception cycles. *Fertil Steril* 37:355, 1982.

22 Filicori M, Butler JP, Crowley WR Jr. Neuroendocrine regulation of the corpus luteum in the human: evidence for pulsatile progesterone secretion. *J Clin Endocrinol Metab* 73:1638, 1984.

23 Syrop CH, Hammond MG. Diurnal variations in midluteal serum progesterone measurements. *Fertil Steril* 47:67, 1987.

24 Miller PB, Soules MR. The usefulness of a urinary LH kit for ovulation prediction during menstrual cycles of normal women. *Obstet Gynecol* 87:13, 1996.

25 Nielsen MS, Barton SD, Hatasaka HH, et al. Comparison of several one-step home urinary luteinizing hormone detection test kits to OvuQuick. *Fertil Steril* 76:384, 2001.

26 Martinez AR, Bernardus RE, Vermeiden JP, et al. Reliability of home urinary LH tests for timing of insemination: a consumer's study. *Hum Reprod* 7:751, 1992.

27 Martinez AR, Bernardus RE, Vermeiden JP, et al. Time schedules of intrauterine insemination after urinary luteinizing hormone surge detection and pregnancy results. *Gynecol Endocrinol* 8:1, 1994.

28 Noyes RW, Hertig AI, Rock J. Dating the endometrial biopsy. *Fertil Steril* 1:3, 1950.

29 Shoupe D, Mishell DR Jr, Lacarra M, et al. Correlation of endometrial maturation with four methods of estimating day of ovulation. *Obstet Gynecol* 73:88, 1989.

30 Graf MJ, Reyniak JV, Battle Mutter P, et al. Histologic evaluation of the luteal phase in women following follicle aspiration for oocyte retrieval. *Fertil Steril* 49:616, 1988.

31 Lessey BA, Castelbaum AJ, Sawin SJ, et al. Integrins as markers of uterine receptivity in women with primary unexplained infertility. *Fertil Steril* 63:535, 1995.

32 Jones GS. Luteal phase insufficiency. *Clin Obstet Gynecol* 44:255, 1974.

33 Fritz MA. Inadequate luteal function and recurrent abortion: diagnosis and treatment of luteal phase deficiency. *Semin Reprod Endocrinol* 6:129, 1988.

34 Li TC, Dockery P, Cooke ID. Endometrial development in the luteal phase of women with various types of infertility: comparison with women of normal fertility. *Hum Reprod* 6:325, 1991.

35 Davis OK, Berkeley AS, Naus GJ, et al. The incidence of luteal phase defect in normal, fertile women, determined by serial endometrial biopsies. *Fertil Steril* 51:582, 1989.

36 Scott RT, Snyder RR, Bagnall JW, et al. Evaluation of the impact of intraobserver variability on endometrial dating and the diagnosis of luteal phase defects. *Fertil Steril* 60:652, 1993.

37 Duggan MA, Brashert P, Ostor A, et al. The accuracy and interobserver reproducibility of endometrial dating. *Pathology* 33:292, 2001.

38 Lessey BA. Endometrial integrins and the establishment of uterine receptivity. *Hum Reprod* 13(Suppl 3):247, 1998.

39 Lindhard A, Bentin-Ley U, Ravn V, et al. Biochemical evaluation of endometrial function at the time of implantation. *Fertil Steril* 78:221, 2002.

40 Ecochard R, Marret H, Rabilloud M, et al. Sensitivity and specificity of ultrasound indices of ovulation in spontaneous cycles. *Eur J Obstet Gynecol Reprod Biol* 91:59, 2000.

41 Petsos P, Chandler C, Oak M, et al. The assessment of ovulation by a combination of ultrasound and detailed serial hormone profiles in 35 women with long-standing unexplained infertility. *Clin Endocrinol* 22:739, 1985.

42 Daly DC, Soto-Albors C, Walters C, et al. Ultrasonographic assessment of luteinized unruptured follicle syndrome in unexplained infertility. *Fertil Steril* 43:62, 1985.

43 Irons DW, Singh M. Evaluation of transvaginal sonography combined with a urinary luteinizing hormone monitor in timing donor insemination. *Hum Reprod* 9:1859, 1994.

Evaluation of the Female: Tubal Function

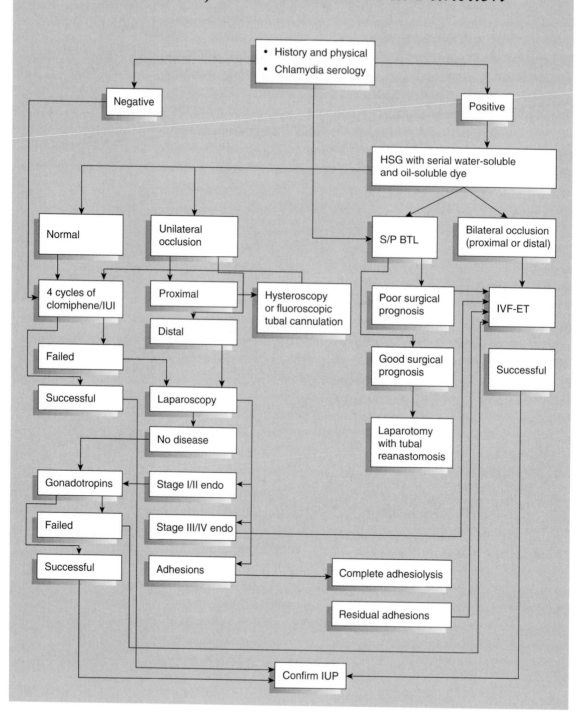

2 Evaluation of the Female: Tubal Function

Ashim V. Kumar
Alan H. DeCherney

Introduction

The prevalence of tubal disease in infertile couples varies from 20 to 30% depending on the population. Therefore, most gynecologists will encounter this diagnosis frequently. However, there is considerable controversy regarding the diagnostic evaluation and treatment for infertility secondary to tubal disease. With a focus on the evaluation of tubal function, we will present the treatment options, our recommendations, and the available data (Chaps. 10 and 13 elaborate on surgical management and assisted reproductive technologies, respectively). The workup and the management plan should be customized to each patient. With advances in assisted reproductive technologies, the algorithm has evolved and the overall prognosis for tubal factor infertility has improved.

The fallopian tubes develop from the separated cranial ends of the paramesonephric (Müllerian) ducts in the absence of Müllerian-inhibiting substance. The fallopian tubes not only facilitate the proovarian transport of sperm and the prouterine transport of the embryo, but also function in oocyte capture, fertilization, and embryo growth. For conception to occur, the mucosa must serve as an incubator while the cilia and the muscularis provide conveyance. Any form of intraluminal lesion resulting from congenital anomalies, proinflammatory states, direct cytotoxicity, or immunopathology can lead to tubal dysfunction.

Etiology

INFECTION

The majority of tubal disease is secondary to infection, specifically pelvic inflammatory disease (PID). Other possible causes of infection include ruptured appendix, septic abortion, or postoperative complications. Inflammatory conditions such as endometriosis and surgery can also lead to tubal occlusion due to adhesions. Infrequently, an embryologic defect is the source of the infertility. Lastly, the etiology may be iatrogenic, a tubal ligation.

The incidence of acute PID is approximately 10–13 per 1000 women aged 15–19 and increases to 20 per 1000 in women aged 20–24.[1] The rising prevalence of sexually transmitted infections (STIs) has led to an increasing incidence of PID. The incidence is higher in women with intrauterine devices (IUDs) and after instrumentation (e.g., D&C). The rate of infertility due to PID is 12%, 23%, and 54% after one, two, and three episodes of PID, respectively.[1]

Unfortunately, patients with acute PID can present with a multitude of complaints and less than 50% present with the classic symptoms of pain, fever, and lower genital tract infection. Therefore, one must use the minimum criteria set forth by the Centers for Disease Control (CDC); the triad consists of cervical motion tenderness, adnexal tenderness, and lower abdominal tenderness. The diagnosis should be made with a minimum of suspicion. Treatment should follow the CDC guidelines be it outpatient or inpatient.[2]

Although pelvic inflammatory disease may be due to a multitude of organisms, *Chlamydia trachomatis* is the predominant cause of infertility.[3] The insidious onset of disease allows for tubal damage before initiation of antibiotic treatment; occasionally the infection may be subclinical and remain in the fallopian tubes for months prior to diagnosis and treatment. This is in contrast to the rapid onset of PID due to *Neisseria gonorrhea*. It is suspected that Chlamydial infection damages tubal mucosa through immunopathologic mechanism as opposed to the cytotoxicity associated with *N. gonorrhea*. Other potential pathogens include *Mycoplasma hominis* and endogenous aerobic or anaerobic bacteria. In developing nations, pelvic tuberculosis is the cause of approximately 40% of tubal factor infertility.[4]

The risk of infertility due to tubal disease is not increased with unruptured appendix. Nevertheless, women with a ruptured appendix had a relative risk of tubal infertility of 4.8 in the nulliparous and 3.2 in those with previous pregnancies.[5] Early detection and treatment can prevent the reproductive sequelae.

Postoperative infection, from peritonitis to abscesses, can lead to adhesion formation severely affecting the pelvic architecture. The infection rate varies from 1 to 15% in gynecologic surgery.[6] To keep the rate at a minimum, the gynecologic surgeons should monitor their postoperative infection rate.[5] Use of prophylactic antibiotics can also decrease the rate.

Septic abortions are a major risk factor for tubal factor infertility. A preoperative examination should include evaluation for bacterial vaginosis and cervicitis. Cultures or serology should be done at this time and results reviewed prior to procedures. We routinely use prophylactic antibiotics after a dilation and evacuation.

INFLAMMATION/ ADHESIONS

Although there is controversy over the potential for minimal or mild endometriosis (stage I or II) to cause infertility, the resulting proinflammatory state can lead to adhesive disease causing subfertility. The dramatic distortion caused by stage III or IV endometriosis does not lead to any skepticism regarding its role in infertility.

Surgically induced tissue trauma can also lead to a proinflammatory state and thus adhesions. The rate of postoperative adhesions is approximately 75%.[7] Laparoscopic approach does not preclude the sequelae of adhesions. The use of adhesion barriers (e.g., Interceed) reduce the adhesions by 50%, on average.[8] Resection of adhesions does increase infertility rates, but if severe disease is present, *in vitro* fertilization-embryo transfer (IVF-ET) may be the only option.

CONGENITAL ANOMALIES

In utero deithylstilbestrol (DES) exposure has been associated with abnormalities such as short, tortuous tubes and shriveled fimbria with small os.[9] Salpingits isthmica nodosa denotes a diverticula of the isthmic tubal mucosa into the muscularis or underneath the serosa. Although there is conflicting evidence as to the congenital versus infectious nature of the diverticulum, it is clearly associated with infertility and ectopic gestation.[10] Other anomalies such as accessory tubal ostia and elongated fimbria-ovarica syndrome have been associated with infertility.

Guiding Questions

APPROACHING THE PATIENT

- What is the overall likelihood that the patient has tubal disease?
  (a) Age of patient
  (b) Primary versus secondary infertility
  (c) Duration of the infertility
  (d) History of IUD use
  (e) Pelvic pain
- Is the patient at risk for or has a history of sexually transmitted infections or pelvic inflammatory disease been documented?
  (a) Age at first coitus
  (b) Number of sexual partners
- What is the surgical history?
  (a) Prior tubal surgery for ectopic gestation or adhesions
  (b) Any pelvic procedures
  (c) Prior D&C (screen for septic abortions)
  (d) History of appendectomy
- Were there any infectious complications after surgery?
- Is there dysmenorrhea or dyspareunia suggestive of endometriosis?
- Is there a history of DES exposure *in utero*?

The history and physical examination can expose important risk factors to guide the workup. The objective is to concentrate on the potential etiologies listed above. The same is true for the physical examination. The guiding questions outline the pertinent aspects of the patient's history.

The physician should examine the patient for signs of infection. The cervix should be inspected for cervicitis. Look for signs of PID including cervical motion tenderness and adnexal tenderness. A wet prep should not be overlooked. A cervical culture is a good practice. A rectovaginal examination should be done to illicit for signs of endometriosis such as uterosacral tenderness and nodularity. Chlamydia antibody testing (CAT) should be used to determine if the patient has ever been exposed. Numerous studies support the association of CAT with tubal disease with one retrospective analysis reporting sensitivity and specificity of 92 and 70%, respectively.[11]

If the patient has cervicitis or acute PID, she should be treated as per the CDC guidelines (available at www.cdc.gov). For patients without risk factors for tubal disease or in whom another etiology (e.g., anovulation or male factor) for infertility has been identified, it is acceptable to attempt three to four cycles of clomiphene citrate (CC) with intrauterine insemination (IUI) prior to tubal evaluation. The other option is to evaluate the fallopian tubes with a hysterosalpingogram (HSG) as a part of the initial evaluation in all patients. Individuals at low risk for tubal disease are older, have a short duration of infertility, no prior history of sexually transmitted infections (STIs) or PID, no dysmenorrhea or dyspareunia, no prior surgeries, a history of previous pregnancy, and a negative CAT. If the patient is at low risk for disease or no other source for infertility has been isolated, we recommend proceeding with HSG. If patient is at high risk or there is the possibility of existing disease, a laparoscopic evaluation is preferable. Salpingoscopy or hysteroscopy with falloposcopy can be done during the laparoscopy and can add to the prognostic value of the procedure.

What's the Evidence?

There are no well-designed studies evaluating the workup for tubal infertility. A number of studies have been done to determine the validity or prognostic value of the individual tests. It is perilous to compare the studies with each other to determine the relative effectiveness of the procedures because the patient inclusion and exclusion criteria as well as the endpoints can vary a great deal.

Mol et al. conducted a cost-effective analysis of various combinations of empiric treatment and Chlamydia antibody testing, hysterosalpingography, and laparoscopy based on data from more than 2000 patients from the Canadian Infertility Treatment Evaluation Study.[12] Of the 13 algorithms studied, the two most cost-effective strategies involved initial CAT or HSG followed by immediate or delayed laparoscopy depending on probability of tubal pathology, and ultimately *in vitro* fertilization if low likelihood of live birth.

If clomiphene/IUI was attempted prior to HSG, tubal condition should be evaluated with HSG if the patient fails to conceive. If tubal patency was confirmed by HSG, one should proceed to laparoscopy on failure with four cycles of clomiphene/IUI.

Traditionally, the diagnosis of tubal factor infertility is based on two tests. Hysterosalpingogram offers substantial information with little risk and is relatively simple. Nonetheless, definitive evaluation of the fallopian tube is through laparoscopy and chromopertubation. Recent advances in microendoscopy facilitate direct visualization of the tubal lumen; falloposcopy and salpingoscopy (not in routine usage) can play an important role in the diagnostic workup. Procedures which evaluate tubal function such as radionucleotide hysterosalpingography are not in routine clinical use. Tubal insufflation is of historical interest but is rarely used today due to difficulty in interpretation of the results. Ultrasonography and sonohysterogram are poor tests for tubal patency.[13]

For the initial evaluation of the fallopian tubes, an HSG is a quick and inexpensive test with low risk for the patient. The hysterosalpingogram can detect tubal occlusion, mobility, mucosal lesions from previous infections or tubal endometriosis, hydrosalpinx, salpingitis isthmica nodosa, adhesions, and tubal anomalies such as accessory ostia and diverticula. However, a metaanalysis reported that the sensitivity of the HSG for tubal occlusion and adhesions was 65%.[14] A frequently cited confounder is tubal spasms. As an added benefit, HSG with oil-soluble medium can increase the fertility rate.[15] Pain, infection, and intravasation of dye into the vascular system are rare complications.

An HSG is usually performed after the cessation of menses and before ovulation to prevent interruption of unrecognized pregnancy. Although there are little data to support the practice, some physicians use prophylactic antibiotics (e.g., doxycycline 100 mg bid × 3 days starting 1 day prior to HSG). It is prudent to check for bacterial vaginosis and cervicitis prior to the procedure. Use of nonsteroidal anti-inflammatory drug (NSAID) (e.g., ibuprofen), to inhibit prostaglandin synthesis, prior to procedure, can improve patient comfort. Although water-soluble medium is better tolerated by the patient and offers improved resolution, oil-soluble medium improves fecundity. In order to obtain advantages of both media, some use a serial approach with the water-soluble medium first followed by the oil-soluble medium. Contraindications to HSG include suspected STI (cervicitis or PID), possible pregnancy, or allergy to the contrast medium. There is a 1–3% risk of acute pelvic infection requiring hospitalization after the procedure.

There are two procedures which allow for direct visualization of the lumen of the fallopian tube, salpingoscopy (transfimbrial) and falloposcopy (transcervical). Salpingoscopy is the direct assessment of the ampullary tubal epithelium using a hysteroscope during laparoscopy or laparotomy. It is used to detect intraluminal adhesions or epithelial damage and has good prognostic value. The procedure is relatively easy to perform and does not require additional equipment. The lack of ability to evaluate the entire tube is its major shortfall. In a patient undergoing laparoscopy, the surgeon should consider this adjunctive procedure.

Falloposcopy is a transvaginal microendoscopic technique which can evaluate the entire length of the fallopian tube. Tubal recanalization can be performed during this procedure. Therefore, it has the potential to be therapeutic for patients with proximal tubal obstruction. Unfortunately, falloposcopy requires significant technical skill and additional equipment.[16] A large multicenter study revealed that less than 57% of patients received a full fallopscopic assessment.[17] Tubal recanalization or fallopian tube catheterization was successful in 53% of tubes compared to success rates of 71–92% reported for fluoroscopic guided procedure.[18,19] Ironically, pregnancy rates were higher for hysteroscopic cannulation—compared to radiographic cannulation—and approach 50%.[20] Falloposcopy has selected indications for the infertility workup and can be a useful therapeutic procedure in the armament of a reproductive surgeon.

For those with a normal HSG, the initial management includes four cycles of clomiphene/IUI. If unilateral proximal obstruction is found without other disease, a radiologist can attempt fluoroscopic tubal canalization. Clomiphene/IUI is an acceptable alternative in those wishing to avoid procedures. In the event that intrapelvic disease is found concurrent to unilateral obstruction or the patient has failed several cycles of clomiphene/IUI and a laparoscopy is planned, it would be practical to perform a hysteroscopy with tubal recanalization at the same time.

KEY POINT

Do not forego laparoscopic evaluation if patient fails to conceive with ovulation induction and intrauterine insemination.

However, if a unilateral distal obstruction is found, a laparoscopic fimbrioplasty or neosalpingostomy is the procedure of choice depending on the specific pathology present. Again, if the patient desires to avoid surgery, she may attempt to conceive with several cycles of clomiphene/IUI. For those with bilateral occlusion, IVF-ET is the best option. Exceptions would include a patient status post bilateral tubal ligation (S/P BTL) and a surgeon experienced with microsurgical tubal reanastomosis.

However, maternal age and/or presence of a sperm factor may make laparoscopic evaluation less cost-effective if chances for pregnancy with continued insemination without assisted reproduction are diminished.

Although there is controversy regarding the need for laparoscopy, a laparoscopic evaluation of the pelvis is an important tool in elucidating the cause of infertility due to the suboptimal sensitivity and specificity of an HSG. Laparoscopy with chromopertubation is the gold standard for evaluating tubal disease. Additional benefits include evaluation and treatment of other intrapelvic pathology such as endometriosis or adhesions. The optimal timing of laparoscopy is after failure to conceive with four to six cycles of clomiphene/IUI.[21] However, if the patient has significant risk factors for intrapelvic pathology such as history of PID, prior pelvic surgery, or symptoms and signs consistent with endometriosis or adhesions, it would be prudent to perform the procedure during the initial workup and forego the HSG.

The laparoscopy should be performed during the follicular phase to avoid interruption of pregnancy and to facilitate evaluation of endometrial cavity if hysteroscopy is done concomitantly. Potential findings need to be discussed with the patient prior to the procedure and informed consent should be obtained for possible lysis of adhesions, resection/ablation of endometriosis, fimbrioplasty, neosalpingostomy, or salpingectomy (for hydrosalpinx in preparation for IVF). The presence of a hydrosalpinx can adversely affect pregnancy rates in IVF; salpingectomy can restore the pregnancy rate (PR). The same is not true for simple drainage of hydrosalpinx because of the high likelihood of recurrence. For agglutinated fimbriae, the treatment of choice is fimbrioplasty (deagglutination with grasping forceps) over neosalpingostomy (creating new os with scissors/electrocoagulator).[22]

KEY POINT

It is thus always important to include the evaluation of all aspects of the fertility evaluation when making treatment decisions.

If the laparoscopy fails to reveal any pathology, the patient should attempt several cycles of clomiphene/IUI or gonadotropins/IUI depending on prior treatment, current laboratory findings, and her wishes for aggressive or conservative management. Minimal or mild endometriosis should be ablated and/or resected followed by ovulation induction/IUI as outlined above. If severe (stage III or IV) endometriosis is found, the patient should be directed toward IVF-ET. In cases of successful salpingoovariolysis, the patient may attempt OI/IUI; if unsuccessful, the patient should be counseled that the highest pregnancy rate will be obtained via IVF-ET.

Treatment

Assisted reproductive technology (ART) and surgery are the two main treatment options. The stepwise approach to ART discussed here starts with clomiphene/IUI, progresses to gonadotropins/IUI, and then IVF-ET. The surgical options consist of hysteroscopic tubal recanalization, laparoscopic adhesiolysis, fimbrioplasty or neosalpingostomy, and tubal reanastomosis.

Ovulation induction and intrauterine insemination can increase the per cycle fecundity after surgery or in those who choose to forego surgery. In patients with poor surgical prognosis (e.g., bilateral tubal occlusion) or after failure of other therapies, IVF-ET remains the decisive option.

The management of a patient who desires fertility after bilateral tubal ligation is very controversial. Historically, laparotomy with microsurgical tubal reanastomosis offered the best results with subsequent pregnancy rates over 1 year reported from 50 to 80%. The success is highly dependent on the experience of the surgeon. Recently, some have proposed a laparoscopic approach, but the data are scarce. The workup preceding surgery is dependent on the surgeon. Some prefer an HSG to evaluate proximal tubal length, while others prefer laparoscopy to also determine if other disease is present.

With the dramatic improvement in the per cycle pregnancy rate in IVF-ET, many physicians prefer assisted reproductive technologies rather than surgery. Pregnancy rates for tubal factor approach 50% per cycle.

Ultimately, the evaluation of a patient's tubal function must be tailored to the individual. A good knowledge of the fundamentals allows the physician to successfully navigate the management algorithm to minimize the emotional and financial strain on the patient while yielding the highest likelihood of success, a pregnancy.

Discussion of Cases

CASE 1

The patient is a 27-year-old female who complains of infertility. She and her partner have been attempting conception for the past 16 months. The patient states that she has not used any form of contraception since her relationship started 3 years ago. She further reports that she has regular menses and mild dysmenorrhea that responds to NSAIDs. Physical examination was normal with no cervical motion or adnexal tenderness. The wet prep and culture were negative for signs of infection.

In addition to day 3 follicle-stimulating hormone (FSH), estradiol, and semen analysis, what other test will impact the management plan?

Chlamydia antibody testing. FSH, estradiol, and semen analysis were normal. CAT was positive.

Should you attempt three to four cycles of clomiphene/IUI or evaluate tubal patency with HSG?

HSG should be obtained due to the long history of infertility (3 years without contraceptive use), young age, the absence of other pathology, and positive CAT. An HSG is obtained and shows right-sided proximal tubal obstruction and a patent left tube.

Is this a spasm or a true obstruction? Do you recommend a selective salpingoscopy, a falloposcopy, or several cycles of clomiphene/IUI to the patient?

Any one of the options stated above is appropriate. A selective salpingoscopy is done revealing a true proximal tubal occlusion. Tubal recanalization, however, is successful during the procedure. The patient undergoes six cycles of clomiphene/IUI and fails to conceive.

Should you proceed with gonadotropins/IUI or evaluate the pelvis with a laparoscopy?

Laparoscopy should be performed after failure to achieve pregnancy after four to six cycles of clomiphene/IUI. A laparoscopy reveals extensive adhesions and severe endometriosis.

Should the patient undergo laparotomy with lysis of adhesions and resection/ablation of endometriosis or IVF-ET?

IVF-ET. With severe endometriosis and extensive adhesions, IVF-ET would offer the best pregnancy rates and avoid the risks of surgery.

CASE 2

A 37-year-old female G2P2 is referred to your clinic for evaluation of a 14-month history of secondary infertility. The patient states she has been taking oral contraceptive pills (OCP) since her last pregnancy 5 years ago. She stopped OCP use 14 months ago in order to conceive. She presented to her primary care physician (PCP) 5 months ago complaining of infertility. The PCP ordered day 3 FSH, estradiol, and a semen analysis because the patient desired to be aggressive in the workup. She subsequently underwent two cycles of clomiphene citrate with timed intercourse without success. The patient asks for your recommendation.

Do you encourage that she continue with several more cycles of clomiphene citrate with intrauterine insemination, go to gonadotropins/IUI, HSG, or have a laparoscopic evaluation of the pelvis?

Continue with several more cycle of CC/IUI. The patient attempts three more cycles with CC/IUI and fails to become pregnant.

Should she have an HSG, a laparoscopy, or gonadotropins/IUI?

The patient's tubal patency should be evaluated with an HSG. The HSG reveals bilaterally patent tubes with no intrauterine filling defects. The patient undergoes gonadotropin/ IUI and becomes pregnant on the second cycle.

REFERENCES

1 Westrom L. Incidence, prevalence, and trends of acute pelvic inflammatory disease and its consequences in industrialized countries. *Am J Obstet Gynecol* 138(7 Pt 2):880, 1980.

2 Workowski KA, Berman SM. CDC sexually transmitted diseases treatment guidelines. *Clin Infect Dis* 35(Suppl 2):S135, 2002.

3 Westrom LV. Chlamydia and its effect on reproduction. *JBr Fertil Soc* 1(1):23, 1996.

4 Parikh FR, Nadkarni SG, Kamat SA, et al. Genital tuberculosis—a major factor causing infertility in Indian women. *Fertil Steril* 67(3):497, 1997.

5 Mueller BA, Daling JR, Moore DE, et al. Appendectomy and the risk of tubal infertility. *N Engl J Med* 315(24):1506, 1986.

6 Evaldson GR, Frederici H, Jullig C, et al. Hospital-associated infections in obstetrics and gynecology. Effects of surveillance. *Acta Obstet Gynecol Scand* 71(1):54, 1992.

7 DeCherney AH, Mezer HC. The nature of posttuboplasty pelvic adhesions as determined by early and late laparoscopy. *Fertil Steril* 41:643, 1984.

8 Nordic Adhesion Prevention Group. The efficacy of Interceed for prevention of reformation of postoperative adhesions on ovaries, fallopian tubes, and fimbriae in microsurgical operation for fertility: a multicenter study. *Fertil Steril* 63:709, 1995.

9 Decherney AH, Cholst I, Naftolin F. Structure and function of the fallopian tubes following exposure to deithylstilbestrol (DES) during gestation. *Fertil Steril* 36(6):741, 1981.

10 Saracoglu FO, Mungan T, Tanzer F. Salpingitis isthmica nodosa in infertility and ectopic pregnancy. *Gynecol Obstet Invest* 34(4):202, 1992.

11 Johnson NP, Taylor K, Nadgir AA, Chinn DJ, et al. Can diagnostic laparoscopy be avoided in routine investigation for infertility. *Br J Obstet Gynecol* 107(2):174, 2000.

12 Mol BW, Collins JA, van der Veen F, Bossuyt PM. Cost-effectiveness of hysterosalpingography, laparoscopy, and Chlamydia antibody testing in subfertile couples. *Fertil Steril* 75(3):571, 2001.

13 Holz K, Becker R, Schurmann R. Ultrasound in the investigation of tubal patency. A meta-analysis of three comparative studies of Echovist-200 including 1007 women. *Zentralbl Gynakol* 119(8):366, 1997.

14 Swart P, Mol BW, van der Veen F, van Beurden M, et al. The accuracy of hysterosalpingography in the diagnosis of tubal pathology: a meta-analysis. *Fertil Steril* 64(3):486, 1995.

15 Vandekerckhove P, Watson A, Lilford R, et al. Oil-soluble versus water-soluble media for assessing tubal patency with hystersalpingography or laparoscopy in subfertile women. *Cochrane Database Syst Rev* 2:CD000092, 2000.

16 Surrey ES. Microendoscopy of the human fallopian tube. *J Am Assoc Gynecol Laparosc* 6(4):383, 1999.

17 Rimbach S, Bastert G, Wallwiener D. Technical results of falloposcopy for infertility diagnosis in a large multicentre study. *Hum Reprod* 16(5):925, 2001.

18 Schill T, Bauer O, Felberbaum R, et al. Transcervical falloscopic dilatation of proximal tubal occlusion. Is there an indication? *Hum Reprod* 14(Suppl 1):137, 1999.

19 Thurmond AS, Machan LS, Maubon AJ. A review of selective salpingography and fallopian tube catheterization. *Radiographics* 20(6):1759, 2000.

20 Honore GM, Holden AE, Schenken RS. Pathophysiology and management of proximal tubal blockage. *Fertil Steril* 71(5):785, 1999.

21 Hammond MG. Monitoring techniques for improved pregnancy rates during clomiphene ovulation induction. *Fertil Steril* 42(4):499, 1984.

22 Oh ST. Tubal patency and conception rates with three methods of laparoscopic terminal neosalpingostomy. *J Am Assoc Gynecol Laparosc* 3(4):519, 1996.

Uterine Function/Defects

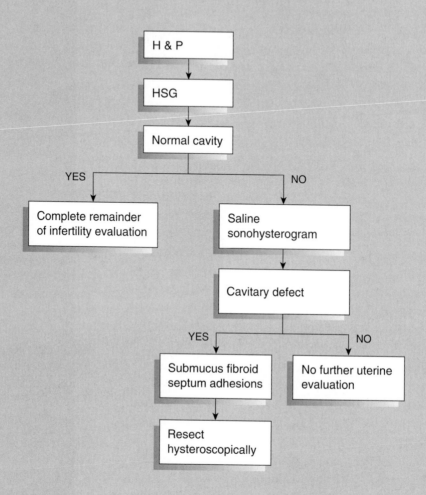

3 Uterine Function/Defects

Ruben Alvero
William D. Schlaff

Introduction

While uterine anomalies are clearly overrepresented in the infertile population, there is a great deal of controversy with regard to the degree to which they cause reproductive dysfunction. Very few controlled studies have actually been performed to evaluate the association, and even where the design has been appropriate, adequate numbers of subjects are unusual in these studies. There is more substantial evidence that anatomically abnormal uteri are associated with pregnancy wastage than with infertility *per se*. The absence of controlled studies is especially striking in those studies where an operative intervention takes place since it is not clear what the reproductive outcome would have been if there had not been a surgical procedure. Nevertheless, where no other clear infertility diagnosis can be assigned, it is possible that correcting the anatomical anomaly may improve reproductive competence. Since endometrial receptivity remains a largely uncertain process, the biological plausibility for an anatomic disturbance to implantation is also unclear. Ongoing research in this area will, in the future, help to expose areas for successful and specific intervention. In the short run, a combination of surgical and hormonal manipulations may in part ameliorate poor reproductive performance.

As with all other aspects of medicine, a good history and physical is the first step in appropriate diagnosis and treatment of uterine malformations. In the field of infertility the patient will usually present with one of two symptoms: inability to achieve pregnancy or inability to maintain a pregnancy. It has already been noted that

49

the influence of uterine abnormalities on infertility *per se* is controversial, but all other diagnoses having been excluded, evaluation of the uterine cavity is an important aspect in the evaluation of infertility. Those patients presenting with recurrent spontaneous abortion will also require some assessment of the uterus and the endometrial cavity. The history of progressively abnormal uterine bleeding may be associated with cavitary defects such as endometrial polyps or submucus fibroids. In addition, the possibility of chronic endometritis should be entertained in cases of abnormal bleeding and an endometrial biopsy should be performed.

Guiding Questions

EVALUATING UTERINE ABNORMALITIES

ASSESSING INFERTILE PATIENTS

- When did the patient begin to menstruate? If the patient has primary amenorrhea, has her secondary sexual development been appropriate?
- What has the patient's menstrual pattern been like? Is it unusually heavy or light? Especially if heavy, is the pelvic examination consistent with uterine fibroids?
- Has the patient had any surgical procedures such as a dilation and curettage (D&C) performed?
- Is the patient in an age group where her mother might have been exposed to diethylstilbestrol (DES)?
- Has the patient lived in an area where tuberculosis is endemic?

ASSESSING PATIENTS WITH RECURENT SPONTANEOUS ABORTION

- How many pregnancies has the patient lost? In which trimesters did the pregnancy losses occur?
- Did the patient have a D&C in association with the pregnancy loss?
- If the patient has had a live birth, at what gestational age did it occur?
- Does the patient have anatomic findings on pelvic examination such as cervical duplication that would suggest Müllerian abnormality?

Uterine Receptivity

Uterine receptivity is a complex concept that to date has been very poorly evaluated in the human. While the current clinical evaluation involves macroscopic approaches such as the history and physical, imaging studies, and microscopic evaluations such as the endometrial biopsy, the actual implantation process involves a complex series of molecular interactions leading to apposition, attachment, and ultimately invasion of the endometrial tissues. Much of the translational research necessary to determine the impact of congenital or acquired uterine abnormalities on the process of implantation is, at best, incomplete. It is clear that apposition and attachment of the blastocyst to the endometrial lining involves the sequential appearance of pinopodes and cell adhesion molecules that are involved in the cross talk and recognition so that attachment may begin to take place. A number of growth factors and cytokines such as epidermal growth factor, leukemia inhibiting factor, colony stimulation factor I, and interleukins are involved in the communication necessary for implantation to occur.[1] During the invasive phase of implantation, transforming growth factor beta (TGF beta), insulin-like growth factor binding protein 1 (IGFBP1), fibronectin, laminin, and tissue inhibitor of metalloproteases (TIMP) are thought to be associated with implantation largely because of their sequential appearance in the late luteal phase of the menstrual cycle. Disruption of the appropriate sequential appearance of these molecular factors in the process of implantation by acquired or congenital abnormalities of the uterus is very poorly defined at this point and constitutes a significant opportunity for research in this area of infertility. Since uterine anomalies are also associated with pregnancy wastage, research into the process of placental invasion and early development in pregnancy is also needed.

The Uterus and Aging

An emerging concept in endometrial receptivity and uterine function is that women of advanced reproductive age appear to have minimal compromise with regard to their ability to achieve a pregnancy. While earlier studies[2] suggested that pregnancy rates were reduced in women over the age of 40 receiving donor oocytes and that this compromise was corrected by increasing progesterone supplementation, it is now well established that women over the age of 50 can easily achieve pregnancy via donated oocytes and that these pregnancy outcomes are similar to younger donor recipients.[3] While older women appear to experience gestational diabetes, preeclampsia, and cesarean delivery, the proportion of women with singleton gestations and term delivery is similar to younger *in vitro* fertilization (IVF) patients using their own or donated oocytes. In what is perhaps the largest cohort of women over the age of 50 undergoing donor oocyteIVF, Richard Paulsen and colleagues describe a clinical pregnancy rate of 45.5% with a live birth rate of 37.2%. The gestational age of delivery for singletons in this cohort was 38.4 weeks gestation with mean delivery at 35.8 weeks for twins and 32.2 weeks for triplets. Therefore, it appears that those factors responsible for normal pregnancy development at the *uterine* level are not disrupted by the process of aging to any great extent.

Congenital Uterine Anomalies

LATERAL FUSION DEFECTS

Disruption in either growth of the Müllerian ducts or fusion of the developed ducts is responsible for the majority of the congenital anomalies of the uterus.[4] Embryologically, the abnormalities are thought to occur at the eighth week of intrauterine development. The overwhelming majority of patients with congenital uterine anomalies have a normal karyotype of 46,XX and, because of their distribution in the population, it is believed that they are of polygenic origin. The American Fertility Society (AFS), as the American Society for Reproductive Medicine (ASRM) was called at the time, in an attempt to standardize the classification of uterine anomalies, published criteria for their diagnosis in 1988 (Fig. 3-1).[5] Prior to the use of this reporting system, there were significant inconsistencies in defining Müllerian anomalies, which confused the reproductive implications of individual abnormalities.

In a review of the world's literature on the prevalence and distribution of uterine anomalies, Nahum in 1998[6] was able to evaluate the prevalence of these disorders in over 570,000 fertile women as well as 6512 infertility patients. He discovered that the prevalence of uterine malformations was 1 in 594 fertile women as compared to 1 in 28 infertility patients. This finding,

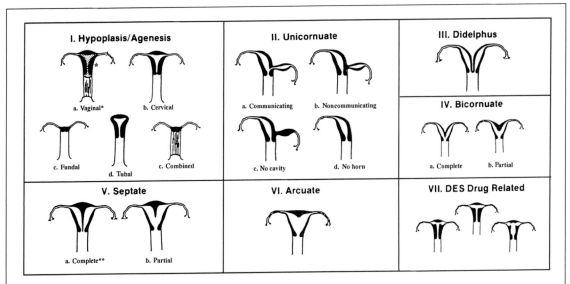

Figure 3-1: The American Fertility Society classification of Müllerian anomalies.

which suggested that congenital uterine anomalies were 21 times more prevalent among infertile women, was highly statistically significant. In reviewing the distribution of anomalies in both fertile and infertile women he found that 7% of the uterine anomalies were arcuate, 34% septate, 39% bicornuate, 11% didelphic, and 5% unicornuate. Additionally, he found that approximately 4% of the patients in the general population had a range of hypoplastic uteri consistent with varying degrees of Müllerian agenesis. When comparing the fertile and infertile populations, Nahum discovered that bicornuate and didelphic uteri were proportionately less common in the infertility population as compared to unicornuate uteri which were overrepresented by a factor of almost three. Arcuate and septate uteri were present proportionally in both fertile and infertile populations, suggesting that these abnormalities do not contribute to infertility. As will be seen subsequently, however, septate uteri may be associated with increased rates of pregnancy wastage. While this review may have been susceptible to the type of classification error that the ASRM was attempting to avoid, Nahum attempted to include only those studies that had been explicit with regard to type of Müllerian anomaly.

Despite the limitations of the studies heretofore performed with regard to uterine malformations, the current conventional wisdom is that for vertical Müllerian anomalies, the less severe the abnormality, the more significant the miscarriage rate. Therefore, the partial uterine septum has the highest rate of pregnancy wastage, followed by the bicornuate uterus, then by the complete septum, and finally the uterus didelphus.[4] The arcuate uterus is a benign anomaly with no reproductive implications.[5] The unicornuate uterus is unique in that infertility has been associated with the disorder in addition to late obstetric complications.[6,7] Workers in this area who have noted decreased fertility rate in the unicornuate uterus attribute this to abnormal uterine musculature as well as possible compromised uterine vasculature, although few data actually exist.

Because of the close embryologic development of the Müllerian system and the urinary tract, coexisting renal abnormalities are very common. Relatively recent studies looking at the distribution of the abnormalities and their association with specific types of congenital anomalies are lacking. In general, however, it appears that renal abnormalities are more commonly associated with class I and II anomalies (hypoplasia/agenesis and unicornuate uterus) than with other types.[8] There appears to be no increased incidence in patients with anomalies associated with *in utero* DES exposure.

The data are very poor with regard to the appropriate intervention for Müllerian anomalies as regards infertility. Studies in this field are often uncontrolled and, despite the availability of a standardized classification system, variable criteria are used for diagnosis. The consensus, however, of most practitioners, is that congenital anomalies of the Müllerian tract do not have an impact on fertility, but do increase pregnancy wastage. The abnormality associated with the greatest impact on miscarriage rates is the partial uterine septum. The bicornuate uterus is also thought to be associated with increased wastage. Unfortunately, controversy surrounds surgical correction of this defect using the so-called Strassman procedure and no reasonable recommendation can be made either way as regards its use. Although circumstantial evidence points to enhanced infertility in unicornuate uterus, the only recommended surgical intervention consists of removing the noncommunicating uterine horns with functional endometrium if they exist. Similarly, no advocacy exists for surgical correction of the didelphic uterus.

THE SEPTATE UTERUS The septate uterus (Fig. 3-2) deserves special recognition because of its association with the highest incidence of pregnancy complications. As previously noted, the uterine septum is not likely to be associated with infertility, but is associated with recurrent spontaneous abortion, malpresentation, and growth abnormalities in the fetus. Histologically, the septum consists of fibromuscular tissue with varying amounts of connective tissue and muscle fibers.[4] Additionally, the endometrium overlying the septum has been shown to have defective sensitivity to cyclical hormonal stimulation. The majority of the pregnancy wastage that takes place in patients with a septate uterus appears to be between the mid first trimester and early second trimester of pregnancy.

Treatment of the septate uterus in these patients has been shown to improve reproductive outcome in multiple series. In their review of 16 papers available in the world's literature, Homer and colleagues compared pregnancy wastage both before and after

Figure 3-2:
Hysteroscopic appearance of a partial uterine septum.

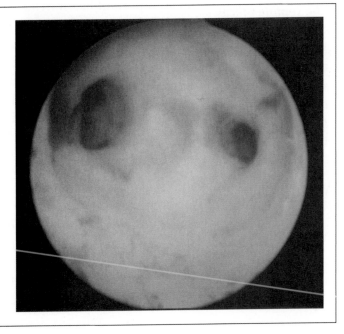

metroplasty for the septate uterus.[9] They noted that prior to metroplasty 88% of pregnancies resulted in miscarriage, whereas after surgical intervention the spontaneous abortion rate decreased 14%. Surgical intervention appears necessary in patients with two or three first or second trimester spontaneous abortions. It is more controversial in patients who have either not conceived or have only had a single miscarriage. Many argue that a single early pregnancy loss is a very common event in the population at large with subsequent term deliveries the most common outcome. However, others argue that hysteroscopic metroplasty should be performed early, particularly in older patients, given the relative simplicity of the procedure. Certainly, women undergoing hysteroscopy for any other indication should undergo surgical treatment if a septum is found since morbidity is extremely low once the procedure is already underway. In addition, those women who are to undergo assisted reproductive technologies should strongly consider having the uterine septum treated.

Several modalities can be used to incise the septum including the resectoscope using the electrosurgical loop, semirigid scissors inserted through the operating port of a hysteroscope, and fiberoptic laser. There are advantages and disadvantages to each of these techniques and the experience of the operator is the single most important factor in successful outcome. The most commonly used technique is the resectoscope, largely because it is available in most operating suites. As the septum appears to consist of largely fibromuscular tissue, it is usually relatively avascular and the incised segments retract into the endometrium anteriorly and posteriorly with incision. While a thicker septum may require some modification of the technique with a lateral thinning of the septum prior to apical incision, the ultimate technique and outcome is usually the same as with thinner septa.

KEY POINT

The septate uterus should be treated surgically in cases of recurrent spontaneous abortion and prior to the use of in vitro fertilization.

What's the Evidence?

Unfortunately, the only randomized control trials performed to date with regard to hysteroscopic resection of uterine septa have to do with surgical technique rather than reproductive outcome. All of the studies heretofore performed are observational studies and usually with small numbers. It is unlikely that with the current widespread acceptance of hysteroscopic metroplasty any randomized control trials comparing reproductive outcomes will be performed.

MÜLLERIAN AGENESIS The etiology of infertility in patients with Müllerian agenesis is obvious. While the etiology of this anomaly is currently uncertain, leading theories include the production of anti-Müllerian hormone *in utero* or inappropriate activation of the receptor for this hormone. The degree of the anomaly is quite variable and it is thought that approximately one-third of the cases are associated with urinary tract abnormalities. Genetically, these women have a normal 46,XX karyotype which distinguishes them from androgen insensitivity syndrome, the likeliest alternative in the differential diagnosis. The most common presenting complaint is that of primary amenorrhea after otherwise normal pubertal progression. Because these women have normal ovarian development, their secondary sexual characteristics are normal and ovulation does occur.[10] As with the uterine abnormalities, vaginal caliber can be variable. The classic presentation, however, is that of a severely shortened vagina. Treatment of this abnormality in order to achieve coital function can be nonsurgical as with Frank's dilator method. Using this method serial vaginal dilators are used to gradually increase the diameter and the depth of the vaginal barrel. In Ingram's modification of the Frank technique a custom manufactured bicycle seat is used to enable the constant application of perineal pressure using similar vaginal dilators. Since the patient can sit on the stool for longer periods of time without hand or finger fatigue as with the Frank method, progress tends to be more rapid and success more readily achieved using the Ingram technique. If the nonsurgical methods fail or the patient is not sufficiently motivated to use these, surgical procedures such as the McIndoe technique can be used. In this technique the vaginal cavity is expanded using an incision, a skin graft is rotated into the space created by the incision, and serial vaginal forms are then used to maintain vaginal patency. While the patient with Müllerian agenesis is obviously unable to carry a pregnancy herself, she can avail herself of a gestational carrier after oocyte retrieval and fertilization with her partner's sperm.

DIETHYLSTILBESTROL EXPOSED UTERUS

The DES exposed uterus is category VII in the AFS classification scheme. While the data were poor with regard to its efficacy in preventing early pregnancy loss, approximately 2–10 million women were exposed to the medication in early pregnancy from 1938 to 1971, when the prescription of DES to pregnant women was finally banned. It is estimated that approximately two-thirds or more of the women who were exposed *in utero* to DES have some type of uterine anomaly, most commonly the hypoplastic, T-shaped cavity. As with the other uterine abnormalities, there is a great deal of controversy with regard to reproductive function in these patients. A significant part of the problem is ascertainment bias in that many of the women who were exposed are unaware of their exposure and their mothers, who took the medication, are often uncertain as to whether they received DES. Therefore, they are not identified unless they have reproductive problems.

It is unlikely that DES causes infertility. In a review of the literature, Goldberg and Falconi determined that the overall pregnancy rate for DES exposed patients was 72% which is not different from the 79% in control groups available in many of these same studies.[11] The same review, however, determined that there was an increase in rates of pregnancy wastage and late obstetric complications. The rate of ectopic pregnancy was significantly higher in DES exposed patients, 5% compared to 0.5% in control populations. Spontaneous abortion was also significantly increased in DES exposed patients, 24% compared to 13% in controls. Finally, preterm delivery in DES exposed patients was twice that seen in control populations. Overall, term delivery and live birth in the exposed patients were approximately 76% compared to 92% in controls.

Given that DES exposure is also associated with developmental compromise of the cervix, the question has arisen as to whether cervical cerclage is beneficial in these patients. Unfortunately, a review of the literature reveals that there are no randomized controlled trials comparing the placement of cerclage with conservative management. Further, some have suggested that metroplasty would benefit these patients since uterine anomalies are associated with DES exposure and these patients have a significant increase in adverse obstetric outcomes. One of the specific anomalies associated with DES is myometrial hypertrophy which may be associated with a compromised endometrial cavity. Two studies have described treating this abnormality by hysteroscopically incising the endometrial cavity in an attempt to normalize its volume. Unfortunately, both of these studies were extremely small and uncontrolled, and therefore no definitive recommendation can be made with regard to the efficacy of the procedure. Heightened surveillance of the pregnancy is of course recommended for women who are DES exposed. However, no firm recommendations can be made for either cervical cerclage or metroplasty in order to improve outcomes.

Acquired Anomalies

ASHERMAN'S SYNDROME

While Asherman's syndrome occurs most commonly after dilation and curettage of the recently pregnant uterus, other forms of uterine surgery such as myomectomy may also cause this disorder. In underdeveloped regions, miliary endometrial tuberculosis is also responsible for a significant percentage of the cases. In tuberculous endometritis the adhesions are usually severe, frequently causing obliteration of the endometrial cavity.[12] There is controversy as to whether infection is a predisposing factor when curettage is performed, but it is clear that a D&C performed remote from delivery, such as might occur in retained products of conception, is associated with much higher incidence of intrauterine adhesions. The two most common symptoms leading to the diagnosis of Asherman's are infertility and hypo- or amenorrhea. The initial diagnosis of Asherman's is currently based on the hysterosalpingogram (HSG) with the characteristic severe angles, sharp contours, and irregular appearance (Fig. 3-3). The AFS classification scheme for intrauterine adhesions assigns a score on the basis of the extent to which the cavity is involved, the type of adhesions seen at the time of hysteroscopy, and the clinical menstrual pattern experienced by the patient. The mildest cases involve less than a third of the cavity with filmy adhesions and a normal menstrual pattern. Severe disease is diagnosed when greater than two-thirds of the cavity is involved, when the adhesions are dense, and when the patient is amenorrheic.[5]

Hysteroscopic resection is the primary treatment for Asherman's syndrome. Efficacious treatment also requires preventing readhesion and intrauterine devices and Foley catheters

Figure 3-3: Intrauterine adhesions with characteristic severe angles, sharp contours, and irregular appearance in a patient undergoing hysterosalpingogram.

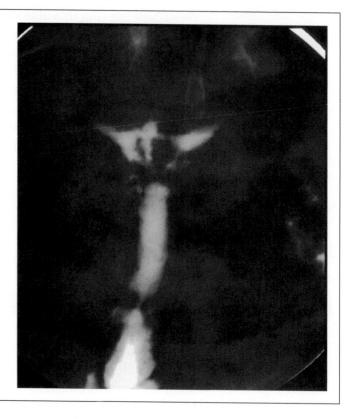

have been used to prevent readhesion of the cavity following surgery, along with exogenous estrogen to promote endometrial growth. Some authors avoid using the Foley catheter because of concern that pressure on the endometrium will prevent regrowth of the tissue. Unfortunately, the studies that have been performed have involved small numbers and have been uncontrolled and therefore the optimal approach is uncertain. In recent years, devices have appeared on the market that are meant to specifically stint the endometrial cavity and prevent readhesions. These devices are shaped like an idealized endometrial cavity and have a flatter and smoother profile that is intended to be an advantage over the Foley balloon and the intrauterine device, respectively. Their efficacy in preventing readhesion remains to be proven.

Hysteroscopic lysis of mild intrauterine adhesions is associated with pregnancy rates of greater than 90% and miscarriage rates of approximately 15%. Unfortunately, even if a normal cavity is achieved after one or several attempts to lyse adhesions in those individuals with severe scarring, subsequent pregnancy rates are clearly lower. In a retrospective review of patients with severe Asherman's syndrome from France, Capella-Allouc and colleagues noted that up to four hysteroscopic procedures were necessary to fully normalize the uterine cavity. In only about half of the patients was optimal restoration achieved after a single procedure. The pregnancy rate after normalization of the cavity was 42.8% with a live birth rate of 32.1%. Not unexpectedly, the majority of the pregnancies came in the younger women. In patients less than 35 years of age there was a 62.5% pregnancy rate compared with 16.7% in those women who were 35 years and older.[13] Of the pregnancies, there was a 20% second trimester loss rate although two-thirds of these patients subsequently conceived again and had term deliveries after a cerclage was performed. In the patients with live births, over half were by cesarean section, primarily for fetal distress. Two of the pregnancies were associated with placenta accreta, one of these requiring a cesarean hysterectomy and the second requiring a hypogastric artery ligation.

KEY POINT

Women with severe Asherman's syndrome may have severely compromised function and obstetric outcome even after optimal lysis of adhesions.

Patients undergoing hysteroscopic resection should be advised preoperatively that a multistage procedure may be required. Resultant pregnancies should be closely monitored—possibly in a tertiary care facility—and cervical cerclage considered.

UTERINE LEIOMYOMA

Uterine leiomyomata are present in approximately 20–25% of women over the age of 35. They present a potential source of infertility, particularly in women who delay childbearing for professional or other reasons. Historically, leiomyomata or fibroids as they are commonly called are also the source of significant controversy as regards causing infertility. Unfortunately, most of the literature in this area has involved series with small numbers and retrospective, uncontrolled data. In addition, many of the studies have failed to describe the location and size of the fibroids. Even when the location of the fibroid is identified, suboptimal techniques may have been used to localize the fibroids therefore leading to further weakness in the studies. Additional confusion is created by studies that fail to control for age of the infertile patient or other infertility factors in addition to the fibroids themselves.

Figure 3-4: Submucous fibroid identified at the time of saline sonohysterogram.

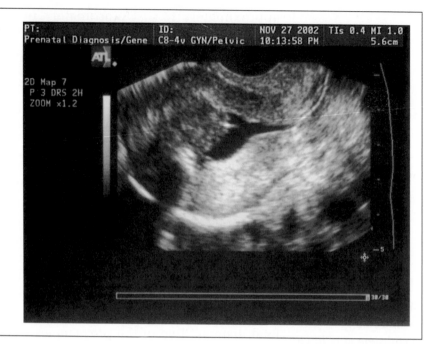

The least controversial location for a fibroid as a cause for infertility is the submucosal leiomyoma (Fig. 3-4). Fortunately, in this location the fibroid is relatively easy to resect hysteroscopically. With improvements in instruments and techniques, even relatively large submucosal fibroids can be resected quickly and safely, particularly if the fibroid protrudes >50% of its volume into the cavity.[14] Since few infertility specialists would recommend trying to achieve a pregnancy in a patient with a submucus fibroid, relatively little information is available with regard to the natural history of submucus fibroids and pregnancy. One study evaluated the outcomes of 106 assisted reproductive technology (ART) cycles in 88 patients with subserosal, intramural, and submucus fibroids and compared reproductive outcomes with 318 historical age-matched controls.[15] The study appears to support a lower pregnancy and implantation rate in patients with both submucus and intramural fibroids. In this series, 33 patients had subserosal fibroids, 46 had intramural fibroids, and 9 had submucus fibroids. None of the intramural fibroids appeared to impact the cavity, but the technique used to assess the location of the fibroids was transvaginal ultrasonography without the benefit of cavity distention using saline. The diagnosis of intramural fibroids is therefore suspect and the possibility of intracavitary intrusion cannot be completely eliminated. Each of the study cycles was matched according to patient age with three cycles of patients without fibroids who were treated contemporaneously in ART cycles. The pregnancy rate in the control group was 30.1% compared to a similar pregnancy rate of 34.1% in the subserosal fibroid group. Both the intramural and submucosal groups appeared to be compromised with regard to fertility with a 16.4 and 10% pregnancy rate per transfer, respectively. As expected, implantation rates were similarly compromised in the intramural and submucus group with a 6.4 and 4.3% rate in these two groups, respectively. Implantation rates in the control and subserosal group were almost identical at 15.8 and 15.7%, respectively. The findings were even more striking in the cohort of individuals with unexplained infertility. That is, with no clear fertility source identified, the pregnancy rate was 5.3% in the intramural group and 0% in the submucus group. This clearly suggests that in a subset of individuals where no other fertility factor appears to be present, fibroids have a substantial impact on fertility rates. Interestingly, in this study neither number of fibroids nor their size appeared to impact pregnancy or implantation rates.

Hysteroscopic resection of submucus fibroids would therefore be expected to improve pregnancy rates and outcome in this patient population. A retrospective review of patients undergoing hysteroscopic myomectomy between January 1990 and September 1998 was undertaken in order to evaluate this possibility.[16] The patient population of 59 patients included 35 patients (59%) who had fertility factors in addition to the fibroids. In the majority of the cases (75%) the fibroids were resected in a single surgical episode, but the remaining 25% required a second surgical procedure to completely resect the tumor. The pregnancy rate after the resection was 27% (16 of the 59 patients) with half of these pregnancies occurring spontaneously and the other 8 requiring assisted reproductive technologies to achieve. The best pregnancy rate was achieved in those patients with myomata as their only fertility factor, particularly if the fibroid was larger than 5 cm in diameter. The overall pregnancy rate was 41.6% in patients with the myomas as the only apparent cause compared with 26.3% in the patients with a single factor and a 6.3% pregnancy rate if two or more additional factors were present. In spite of the apparent success of the procedure, the authors suggest that the efficacy of submucus resection of fibroids is probably overstated. Age in particular appeared to play an additional role with six out of eight women that conceived over the age of 35 having a subsequent first trimester miscarriage even after the myomectomy procedure. The implication of this study is that the subgroup of submucous myoma patients who are younger, have larger myomas, and no other infertility factors have the best prognosis for improvement in fertility.

If there is any question that submucus fibroids are related to either infertility or recurrent miscarriage the literature is even more inconsistent with regard to intramural fibroids. Some manuscripts even suggest that subserosal fibroids that do not affect the uterine cavity can cause reproductive failure. One of the reasons that this may be the case is the fact that location is not specified in many of these papers and both subserosal and intramural fibroids are lumped together in the same category. Li and colleagues retrospectively reviewed their experience with myomectomy as it affected reproductive outcome in patients with both intramural and subserosal fibroids.[17] They analyzed a cohort of 51 women who were to undergo laparotomy and myomectomy using microsurgical techniques for both intramural and subserosal fibroids. All patients expressed a desire to achieve pregnancy after surgery, and patients with other infertility factors were excluded from the study. Using multiple regression analysis they found that the only factor that affected conception rate in this population was patient age. This suggested to the authors that fertility was not compromised by the presence of the fibroids. Further, the size, number, and location of fibroids were unrelated to conception rates. Women that were ≤35 years of age had 74% chance of conceiving after myomectomy whereas those ≥36 years had a 30% chance of conception. The regression model included history of fertility; therefore a history of failure to achieve pregnancy after 1 year of trying did not seem to have an influence on the chance of conception after myomectomy. Pregnancy loss rate, however, was substantially affected by the myomectomy. Patients in this cohort had a 60% chance of having a spontaneous abortion prior to the procedure. However, following the procedure the pregnancy loss rate was 24%; this difference was found to be statistically significant. The impact was most substantial in that subgroup of patients where recurrent loss was the indication for the surgery. Even with the procedure, pregnancy losses were substantial at 33% but were considerably lower than the 79% miscarriage rate prior to the procedure in this subgroup.

In order to try to isolate those cases with an intramural component to the fibroid, Hart and colleagues conducted a prospective controlled trial in a group of patients who were to undergo assisted reproductive technologies.[18] They excluded patients with fibroids >5 cm in diameter and they used a control group of women without fibroids at ultrasound who were undergoing *in vitro* fertilization at the same time. Saline sonohysterography or hysteroscopy was performed on patients whose fibroids appeared to impact the cavity on transvaginal ultrasound. Unfortunately, the patients with fibroids were noted to be significantly older thereby clouding any conclusions that the authors might draw from the review. Nevertheless, the population of patients without fibroids clearly had higher implantation rates, higher overall pregnancy rates, and higher ongoing pregnancy rates. In a logistic regression model performed with the same set of data, and after adjusting for the number of embryos and their quality, the only significant variables that were shown to impact implantation and pregnancy rates were the presence of intramural fibroids and age. In fact, the chances of having an ongoing pregnancy were essentially halved by the presence of intramural fibroids. As with many of the other fibroid studies, the need for a prospective, randomized control trial is clear.

Surrey and colleagues also looked at the intramural leiomyoma question in a group of patients undergoing *in vitro* fertilization.[19] The advantage of this study is that the authors used more stringent criteria to identify and exclude submucus fibroids. They stratified the groups by age and presence of fibroids. A subanalysis using a group of patients between the ages of 35 and 39 without fibroids was an attempt to control for the generally older age group of patients with fibroids present. In the younger population (<40), implantation rates were significantly lower in patients with fibroids when compared to the similarly aged group of patients without fibroids. The same results were found when comparing the subgroup of patients in the 35–39 years age range. In the older population of patients >40 years of age implantation rates did not appear to be significantly impacted. While there was a trend toward lower pregnancy and live birth rates in the fibroid population, this did not achieve statistical significance. Going along with the decreased implantation rate in the fibroid population, the rates of multiple implantations were significantly higher in patients who had no evidence of intramural fibroids.

It has been suggested that one of the reasons that intramural fibroids may impact fertility rates is compromise of vascular flow to the endometrial lining. In their study, Surrey and colleagues looked at the pulsatility index and did not find a relationship. Finally, there was no evidence that the size or volume of the intramural fibroids had an impact on implantation rates. While this study suggested a trend in impaired reproductive outcomes, the live births achieved at 49% was still highly respectable and these investigators suggested that while some minimal impact may be appreciated, it is not enough to risk the possible morbidity of a surgical procedure to remove the intramural fibroids. Indeed, in the older populations studied in this cohort there is no impact suggesting that surgical procedure in this population is even less justified.

As has been previously noted, a substantial number of the studies reviewing fibroids and infertility suffer from small numbers, lack of controls, retrospective design, and uncertain localization of the fibroids. In an effort to improve the issue of small numbers, Pritts conducted a metaanalysis of the available literature in order to assess the impact of fibroids on reproductive outcome and to determine whether resecting fibroids had any impact in improving said outcomes.[20] Using this combination of studies, she determined that only patients with submucosal fibroids and therefore compromised endometrial cavities had lower pregnancy and implantation rates. When compared to infertile controls, these women had a relative risk of pregnancy of 0.32 (95% confidence interval of 0.13–0.70) and implantation relative risk of 0.28 (95% confidence interval of 0.10–0.72) which demonstrates a robust compromise of reproductive function in those women with abnormal cavities. The relative risk of pregnancy in women with subserosal fibroids compared to infertile controls was 1.11 (95% confidence interval 0.06–1.72). Those individuals with only

KEY POINT

In the absence of randomized data, resection of submucous fibroids in infertile patients appears to be indicated.

intramural fibroids had a relative risk of pregnancy of 0.94 (95% confidence interval 0.73–1.20) and an implantation relative risk of 0.81 (95% confidence interval 0.60–1.09). The evidence appears to show that intramural and subserosal fibroids do not impact reproduction function whereas submucosal fibroids do. Consistent with this finding, Pritts combined the results of two studies evaluating the resection of submucus fibroids. In this small metaanalysis she determined that there was a notable increase in pregnancy rates after myomectomy versus a control group with infertility but without fibroids (relative risk of 1.72; 95% confidence interval 1.13–2.58). As has been previously stated, however, this review cited the need for randomized control trials. In cases of submucus fibroid where the evidence appears to be strongest, the data are subject to confounding due to their retrospective nature.

Despite the fact that subserosal and intramural fibroids appear not to be significantly associated with infertility, debate continues as to whether a laparoscopic approach to the fibroids has a beneficial effect on reproductive outcome. In an uncontrolled retrospective review of 91 patients, Dubuisson and colleagues noted that the laparoscope could be used to remove fibroids and achieve a subsequent pregnancy. In particular, they noted that in patients where the myoma was the only possible source of the infertility, pregnancy rates after laparoscopic myomectomy were 70.8% (17/25) patients.[21] In the review, they also noted that the rate of uterine rupture was only 1% in over 100 deliveries. The authors observed that the impact of myomectomy for patients with other infertility factors was substantially less with only 26 out of 66 patients (45.6%) achieving pregnancy.

One of the few randomized studies looking at fibroids and myomectomy compared laparoscopic versus abdominal myomectomy with regard to subsequent fertility and obstetric outcome.[22] In this study, 65 patients were randomized to laparotomy and 66 to laparoscopy. Operative time was slightly lower in the laparotomy group although this did not achieve statistical significance. The drop in hemoglobin postoperatively was greater in the abdominal laparotomy group as was the hospital stay. Subsequent pregnancy rates in both groups were comparable at 55.9 and 53.6% for the abdominal and laparoscopic approaches, respectively. Recurrence of the myomata occurred with comparable frequency in each group at 20.3% in the laparotomy group and 21.4% in the laparoscopy group. The percentage of preterm deliveries, vaginal deliveries, and cesarean sections were comparable in both groups. There were no uterine ruptures using either approach. It should be noted that no distinctions were made in this study with regard to the location of the fibroids. Presumably, if the approach was laparoscopic the majority should have been either subserosal or intramural but this is not addressed in the manuscript. It appears, however, that if the patient is to undergo myomectomy for fertility purposes, laparoscopy is a feasible approach if the experience of the operators is adequate.

In an effort to avoid the surgical complications associated with either abdominal or laparoscopic myomectomy, uterine fibroid embolization has been proposed as an alternative. Questions have arisen with regard to fertility following fibroid embolization. In a review of their experience, McLucas and colleagues identified 52 women younger than the age of 40 who indicated that they were interested in future fertility after the embolization procedure.[23] Of these 52 women, 14 subsequently had pregnancies (27.0%). Ten of these women (19.2%) had term deliveries, one of which was complicated by preterm labor, placenta previa, and abruptio placentae. All the other term deliveries were without complications. Patients considering uterine artery embolization should be counseled that the average radiation exposure for this procedure is approximately 14 rads which compares to 5 rads for a hysterosalpingogram. Patients should also note that hysterectomy as a complication of embolization is 5 per 1000 procedures. In their review, they also noted that 1 in 100 women appear to have compromised ovarian function after the procedure but this number may be as high as 40% in women over age 35. Causality was not explored and would be difficult to determine. While the authors note that pregnancy rates of 20% were respectable, this rate is certainly less than ideal compared to 50% or greater pregnancy rate noted in some of the other leiomyoma studies previously reviewed.

ENDOMETRIAL POLYPS   The data on endometrial polyps and their association with infertility are very scarce with regard to causality and improvement of reproductive outcome after resection. One of the original manuscripts on the subject was published in 1989 by Brooks and colleagues. In what was essentially a case series looking at resection of both fibroids and polyps for indications of menorrhagia and infertility, these investigators determined that of the 10 polypectomies that took place eight were for a diagnosis of menorrhagia and two were for infertility. One of the two infertility patients subsequently conceived after a follow-up period of 3 months.[24] A second more extensive study was published in 1999 by Varasteh and colleagues.[25] In this publication, the investigators looked at pregnancy rates after hysteroscopic polypectomy and myomectomy in exclusively infertile women. They theorized that submucosal polyps might be associated with infertility and pregnancy loss by adversely affecting the endometrial environment causing bleeding or presenting an abnormal site for implantation. The authors only included those women who would be attempting to achieve pregnancy after their polypectomy, and they included patients who had had both resectoscopic removal of polyps as well as those that were excised by endometrial forceps. In their population, 36 patients underwent myomectomy, 23 polypectomy, and 19 had a diagnostic study. Cumulative pregnancy rates after hysteroscopy were noted to be 19 out of 36 (52.8%) after myomectomy, 18 of 23 (78.3%) after polypectomy, and 8 of 19 (42.1%) in patients who had had negative studies. They further noted that the relative risk of clinical pregnancy after polypectomy was 3.89 (95% confidence interval 1.62–9.36) compared to those who had had a normal cavity evaluation. Live birth rates after the polypectomy were 15 of 23 (65.2%) compared with 7 of 19 (36.8%) in women with a normal cavity. The spontaneous abortion rate in the polypectomy group was 27.7% once a clinical pregnancy had been established compared with 37.5% for the normal group, a difference which did not reach statistical significance. Interestingly, only those patients with submucus myomas >2 cm in diameter achieved an improvement in pregnancy rate compared to individuals with a normal cavity. This study therefore suggested that both large myomas and polyps were associated with infertility and justified their removal by hysteroscopic means. The author suggested that randomized controlled trials would settle the issue definitively but doubted that such a trial would take place since it would be difficult to justify leaving a polyp *in utero* once they had been identified by hysteroscopic means.

Imaging in the Evaluation of Uterine Function and Infertility

Imaging is a critical part of any evaluation for either infertility or recurrent spontaneous abortion. Given this fact there are four types of studies that can be undertaken for evaluation. Traditionally, patients have undergone hysterosalpingogram to assess the uterine cavity but more recently transvaginal sonography and saline sonohysterography have been employed in an attempt to improve detection of abnormalities of the uterine cavity and myometrium. Magnetic resonance imaging (MRI) is frequently used to diagnose uterine malformations. While the hysteroscope is considered the gold standard for evaluation of the endometrial cavity, it is expensive and more invasive. If alternatives to hysteroscopy can be found or can allow the patient to undergo operative hysteroscopy and therefore obviate the diagnostic study, patient savings may be enhanced and discomfort reduced.

Classically, alternatives to hysteroscopy have been compared with endoscopic evaluation of the uterine cavity in attempt to assess the sensitivity, specificity, and positive and negative predictive values of the technique. Loverro and colleagues[26] evaluated 134 infertile women who were investigated both at transvaginal sonography and hysteroscopy for endometrial irregularities, echo patterns, and distortions of the endometrial echo. Immediately after transvaginal sonography, diagnostic hysteroscopy was performed and a correlation established between the two studies. Using hysteroscopy as the gold standard, transvaginal sonography was noted to have a sensitivity of 84.5% (49 out of 58), a specificity of 98.7% (74 out of 75), a positive predictive value of 98% (49 out of 50), and a negative predictive value of 89.2% (74 out of 83). The examiners also noted that in addition to the uterine findings, polycystic ovaries, benign ovarian cysts, and endometriomas were detected. Interestingly, the lowest sensitivity in the subgroups examined was for polyps where 79.2% sensitivity was noted. A similar protocol and findings were noted by Shalev and colleagues from Israel.[27] This group followed a population of 78 infertile women undergoing IVF and embryo transfer and oocyte donation. These women were all scheduled to undergo diagnostic hysteroscopy. Prior to this procedure they underwent transvaginal sonography in the follicular phase of the menstrual cycle. The investigators looked for lesions within the uterine cavity, presence of a hyperechoic complex, and an irregular endometrial lining. As opposed to the previous study, the sonographers were present at the time of surgery and were able to direct the operator to examine areas in the uterine cavity that appeared to be abnormal on the previously performed sonography. Again, using hysteroscopy as the gold standard, the sensitivity of transvaginal sonography was 100% and the specificity 96.3%. These investigators claimed to be able to identify intrauterine adhesions, particularly at the midcycle when the endometrial lining appeared to be trilaminar. In fact, the diagnosis of intrauterine adhesions by sonography had a sensitivity of 80%, a specificity of 100%, a positive predictive value of 100%, and a negative predictive value of 97%. In addition to these impressive findings, the investigators advocated against performing the transvaginal sonography in the early follicular phase noting that the endometrium is very thin and that polyps and myomas may be less visible than during the late follicular phase.

Sonohysterography is increasingly used in an attempt to enhance visualization of intracavitary abnormalities. A group of collaborators from University of Copenhagen compared transvaginal sonohysterography and hysteroscopy in the setting of infertility, miscarriage, and abnormal bleeding. The strength of this study was that it was blinded and therefore the ultrasonographer and the surgeon performing the hysteroscopy were unaware of each other's findings. In addition, standardized criteria were used to determine the presence of endometrial polyps and fibroids. Endometrial polyps were defined as smooth margined and homogeneous while submucus fibroids were defined as heterogeneous round structures arising in the myometrium. Sixty women underwent the procedures. Again, sensitivity, specificity, positive predictive value, and negative predictive value were very high at 90.9, 100, 100, and 90%, respectively. False positive findings were thought to be due to blood clots in the cavity whereas false negative results were secondary to overlooking very small polyps, usually <2 mm in diameter. In contrast to the previous investigators, sonohysterography was felt to be best performed for endometrial polyps during the follicular

As experience is gained, the sonohysterogram will likely replace the hysterosalpingogram for assessing cavitary defects.

phase and for submucus fibroids during the secretory phase of the cycle. This group concluded that with a normal uterine cavity at saline sonohysterography, no hysteroscopy is necessary for infertility patients.[28]

The hysterosalpingogram is generally the first procedure performed in infertility and recurrent spontaneous abortion patients. In a prospective study, 65 infertile women underwent hysterosalpingogram, transvaginal sonography, sonohysterography, and diagnostic hysteroscopy evaluations.[29] Again, using hysteroscopy as the gold standard, these investigators evaluated the accuracy of these procedures in determining the presence of the polypoid lesions, uterine malformations, intrauterine adhesions, and endometrial hyperplasia. Overall, sonohysterography was considered the most accurate test particularly in detection of polypoid lesions and endometrial hyperplasia. With regard to sensitivity, "polypoid" lesions, which included both polyps and submucus fibroids, the hysterosalpingogram performed most poorly with a 50% sensitivity and a positive predictive value of 28.6%. The transvaginal sonogram was intermediate in performance with a sensitivity of 75% and a positive predictive of also 75%. The sonohysterogram was in complete agreement with regard to the presence of these polypoid lesions with 100% sensitivity and 100% positive predictive value. The specificity and the negative predictive value were also 100% for the sonohysterogram. In addition, the sensitivity for hysterosalpingogram with regard to uterine malformations was 44.4% with a positive predictive value of 66.7%. Sonohysterogram was somewhat better with a sensitivity of 77.8% and a positive predictive value of 100%. In contrast to the previously cited study, transvaginal sonography did not detect any of the cases of intrauterine adhesions while sonohysterogram was 75% sensitive and had a 42.9% positive predictive value with regard to these abnormalities. The sonohysterogram was therefore most like the hysteroscope in detecting polypoid lesions in virtually all circumstances. In addition, endometrial hyperplasia was also detected at high rate of frequency with this technology. Adhesions were less easily found with a sonohysterogram but its sensitivity, specificity, positive predictive value, and negative predictive value were all comparable to the hysterosalpingogram in terms of accuracy.

In summary, the sonohysterogram appears to be gaining acceptance as the appropriate first line technology for evaluating the uterine cavity.

MRI has been suggested by many to be a valuable alternative to surgical evaluation of Müllerian anomalies, but its sensitivity and specificity have been questioned by others. In cases where complex anomalies are suspected, anatomic evaluation prior to surgery is also useful for purposes of planning the procedure. At a referral facility for complex reproductive tract disorders in London, Minto and colleagues evaluated MRI's performance prior to surgical evaluation and correction of complex Müllerian anomalies.[30] The radiologist was blinded to the individual histories of the nine young women evaluated but reviewed the films with the operating surgeon prior to the procedure. While the overall gross uterine anatomy was correct in all cases, the MRI incorrectly diagnosed a remnant horn as nonfused when in fact it was fused. Additionally, the imaging technique failed to identify the presence of a small nonfused rudimentary horn. Three normal ovaries were missed by the technique and a streak ovary was incorrectly identified as normal. Concordance was even less precise with regard to cervical and vaginal anomalies. In the six patients with abnormal vaginas, the MRI was correct in only three of the cases. Of the eight normal cervices in the group, one was identified as rudimentary and nonpatent. One case of cervical agenesis was identified as normal. MRI was responsible for identifying nongynecologic anomalies in five out of the nine patients, including four cases of bone and muscle anomalies and one case of renal agenesis.

The surgeons in this series modified their surgical approach in four out of the nine patients. In two cases, a hysteroscopic approach was abandoned in favor of abdominal metroplasty. One patient had her rudimentary horn excised rather than having metroplasty and another patient was noted to have a very thick septum and the hysteroscopic approach was augmented with abdominal visualization by laparoscopy. As a result of the case series, the authors concluded that ultrasound is initially most useful in delineating simple Müllerian anomalies, but MRI is more useful than either hysterosalpingography or diagnostic laparoscopy in preparation for definitive diagnosis and surgical intervention. Nevertheless, the technique is far from perfect and appears to complement surgical diagnosis rather than replace it.

Summary of Therapeutic Options

The typical patient presenting for evaluation of infertility will undergo a hysterosalpingogram since evaluation of tubal function is important and no other modality provides this information in such a cost-effective fashion. Since uterine abnormalities are also prevalent in this population, incidental cavitary findings will also occur. The preponderance of the evidence at this time is that the saline sonohysterogram is the appropriate next step in order to further delineate the location of the abnormality and to map the surgical approach that may need to take place. If an endometrial polyp or a submucous fibroid is present, there is reasonable evidence that resection of these common anomalies may need to take place, particularly if no other fertility factors are identified. A nuanced conversation will also need to take place with regard to age. Evidence suggests that in the otherwise unexplained infertile patient, younger patients are more likely to benefit from resection of anomalies. Using the same reasoning, however, the older infertility patient may be pressed to intervene sooner to eliminate these abnormalities before she becomes even older and therefore more compromised with regard to reproductive competence.

The couple with recurrent miscarriage is less concerned with tubal function since fertilization is obviously taking place. The hysterosalpingogram is currently the initial imaging modality of choice for these individuals but, as has been seen, the ability of this study to identify, measure, and localize lesions such as the septate uterus and intrauterine adhesions may be less than ideal. Again, the saline sonohysterogram appears to have advantages in this regard. As experience is gained with this study, more providers may move to ultrasound for anatomic evaluation of the uterus.

Improvements in pregnancy outcomes will come from further research into the factors that facilitate the process of implantation. A good example of this is the poor outcomes associated with "normalization" of the cavity in severe cases of intrauterine adhesions.

Only by taking the process from the molecular to the clinical will specific interventions be taken with commensurate success rates.

Discussion of Cases

CASE 1

You are evaluating a 35-year-old G1P1001 Black female with secondary infertility of 18 months duration. She describes increasingly heavy menstrual cycles with clots and severe dysmenorrhea. The patient had no difficulty conceiving at age 29 and delivered at term a viable female infant. Despite coital frequency every 1–2 days around the time of ovulation as detected by urinary luteinizing hormone (LH) predictor kits, she has been unable to conceive. The bimanual pelvic examination reveals a minimally enlarged uterus. Her partner has normal semen parameters and, while heavy, patient's menses come at a 28–30-day interval. The midluteal progesterone level is 16 ng/mL, which is determined to be consistent with normal ovulation. The patient's follicle-stimulating hormone (FSH) on day 3 of the cycle is 7 mIU/mL with an estradiol of 63 pg/mL. These values reassure you that the patient has normal ovarian reserve. At the time of hysterosalpingogram, the uterine cavity is noted to have multiple filling defects but the fallopian tubes appear to be patent.

What additional testing would you recommend?

- **Saline sonohysterogram**
- **Saline sonohysterogram shows a 1.8 cm × 2.3 cm filling defect that protrudes approximately half of its volume into the**

uterine cavity. The filling defect appears to arise in the anterior fundal myometrium, has a heterogeneous consistency, and an oval contour. In your experience these characteristics suggest to you that it is a fibroid.

How would you manage this patient?

This patient has secondary infertility with no other etiology than the submucosal fibroid identified as a potential cause. In addition to infertility, the patient is also noted to have worsening menorrhagia which may also be related to the leiomyoma. You counsel the patient that fibroids may be associated with infertility, particularly in those individuals where no other factor is identified. The patient's age is also a factor in that as she enters later reproductive life, surgical intervention has not been shown to be as effective in improving pregnancy outcome. The menorrhagia gives you another indication for surgical resection. In the absence of this symptom and other fertility factors you would still need to discuss hysteroscopic ablation or removal of the fibroid as treatment to improve fecundity. Certainly if the patient is considering moving on to more aggressive therapy with *in vitro* fertilization, she would be counseled to normalize the cavity in order to improve success rates.

CASE 2

A 29-year-old G4P0040 presents to your clinic despondent over the four first trimester spontaneous miscarriages that she has experienced over the past 24 months. Her primary care provider (PCP) has obtained a thyroid-stimulating hormone (TSH) level of 1.2 mIU/mL. Both the patient and her partner have normal karyotypes. A panel consisting of anticardiolipin antibodies, lupus anticoagulant, homocysteine, factor V Leiden, proteins C and S is found to be normal. Feeling that he has exceeded his level of expertise, the patient's PCP sends her to you for further evaluation.

What additional testing would you consider in this patient?

- An evaluation of the adequacy of progesterone support in the luteal phase. While controversial, classically this condition has been evaluated by obtaining an endometrial biopsy in the late luteal phase of the menstrual cycle. If the first biopsy is three or more days out of phase with the day of the cycle, a repeat biopsy is performed in the subsequent cycle. Two such abnormal biopsies confirm the diagnosis of luteal phase defect. Because of the cumbersome nature of this protocol and the inter- and intraobserver variability among pathologists, the endometrial biopsy has fallen out of favor with many providers.
- Investigation of the patient's uterine anatomy. In the past, this evaluation has been undertaken with a hysterosalpingogram (HSG). The HSG has been shown to be less reliable, however, than ultrasound-based imaging techniques. In addition, the distinction between a septate

and bicornuate uterus cannot be made on the basis of the HSG. There is also the issue of provider confidence in performing each modality. Several studies have shown that in competent hands, the saline sonohysterogram has better sensitivity, specificity, positive, and negative predictive values than the HSG in diagnosing uterine anomalies. However, even in expert hands, the saline sonohysterogram is better at detecting cavitary lesions than uterine anomalies and you should consider doing additional testing such as MRI or laparoscopy to confirm the presence of a single fundus in the case of a septate uterus. Laparoscopy has the additional advantage that it can be performed in conjunction with hysteroscopic treatment of uterine septum. It does add cost and potential morbidity to the procedure.

You offer the patient a laparoscopy and hysteroscopy. At the time of laparoscopy you confirm the presence of a single fundus. A single broad band of white tissue consistent with a septum is identified longitudinally down the uterine midline and extending two-third of the distance to the internal os. What would be your next step?

- Using the electrosurgical instrument, laser or hysteroscopic scissors, you could incise the septum. As the septum is incised, it has a tendency to retract into the myometrium. There is generally no need to place a stint since fibrosis is unlikely to occur and there is very little likelihood of subsequent intrauterine adhesion formation.

- **In the absence of other factors responsible for recurrent pregnancy loss, you can counsel the patient that she should** attempt to conceive and that the available literature suggests that there would be an improvement in viable delivery rate.

REFERENCES

1 Giudice LC. Potential biochemical markers of uterine receptivity. *Hum Reprod* 14(Suppl 2):3–16, 1999.

2 Meldrum DR. Female reproductive aging-ovarian and uterine factors. *Fertil Steril* 59(1):1–5, 1993.

3 Paulson RJ, Boostanfar R, Peyman S, et al. Pregnancy in the sixth decade of life: obstetric outcomes in women of advanced reproductive age. *JAMA* 288(18):2320–2323, 2002.

4 Lin PC, Bhatnagar KP, Nettleton GS, et al. Female genital anomalies affecting reproduction. *Fertil Steril* 78(5):899–915, 2002.

5 American Fertility Society. The American Fertility Society classifications of adnexal adhesions, distal tubal occlusion, tubal occlusion secondary to tubal ligation, tubal pregnancies, Müllerian anomalies and intrauterine adhesions. *Fertil Steril* 49(6):944–955, 1988.

6 Nahum GG. Uterine anomalies. How common are they, and what is their distribution among subtypes? *J Reprod Med* 43:877–887, 1998.

7 Raga F, Bauset C, Remohi J, et al. Reproductive outcome of congenital Müllerian anomalies. *Hum Reprod* 12(10):2277–2281, 1997.

8 Sims JA, Gibbons WE. Treatment of human infertility: the cervical and uterine factors. In: Adashi E, Rock J, Rosenwaks Z (eds.), *Reproductive Endocrinology, Surgery and Technology*. Philadelphia, PA: Lippincott-Raven, 1996, p. 2153.

9 Homer HA, Li TC, Cooke ID. The septate uterus: a review of management and reproductive outcome. *Fertil Steril* 73(1):1–14, 2000.

10 Folch M, Pigem I, Konje JC. Müllerian agenesis: etiology, diagnosis, and management. *Obstet Gynecol Survey* 55(10):644–649, 2000.

11 Goldberg JM, Falcone T. Effect of diethylstilbestrol on reproductive function. *Fertil Steril* 72(1):1–7, 1999.

12 Schenker JG. Etiology of and therapeutic approach to synechia uteri. *Eur J Obstet Gynecol Reprod Biol* 65:109–113, 1996.

13 Capella-Allouc S, Morsad F, Rongieres-Bertrand C, et al. Hysteroscopic treatment of severe Asherman's syndrome and subsequent fertility. *Hum Reprod* 14(5):1230–1233, 1999.

14 Gimpelson RJ. Hysteroscopic treatment of the patient with intracavitary pathology (myomectomy/polypectomy). *Obstet Gynecol Clin North Am* 27(2):327–337, 2000.

15 Healy DL. Impact of uterine fibroids on ART outcome. *Environ Health Perspect* 108(Suppl 5):845–847, 2000.

16 Fernandez H, Sefrioui O, Virelizier C, et al. Hysteroscopic resection of submucosal myomas in patients with infertility. *Hum Reprod* 16(7):1489–1492, 2001.

17 Li TC, Mortimer R, Cooke ID. Myomectomy: a retrospective study to examine reproductive performance before and after surgery. *Hum Reprod* 14(7):1735–1740, 1999.

18 Hart R, Khalaf Y, Cheng-Toh Y, et al. A prospective controlled study of the effect of intramural uterine fibroids on the outcome of assisted conception. *Hum Reprod* 16(11):2411–2417, 2001.

19 Surrey ES, Lietz AK, Schoolcraft WB. Impact of intramural leiomyomata in patients with a normal endometrial cavity on in-vitro fertilization-embryo transfer cycle outcome. *Fertil Steril* 75(2):405–410, 2001.

20 Pritts EA. Fibroids and infertility: a systematic review of the evidence. *Obstet Gynecol Surv* 56(8):483–491, 2001.

21 Dubuisson JB, Chapron C, Fauconnier A, et al. Laparoscopic myomectomy. *Ann N Y Acad Sci* 943:269–275, 2001.

22 Seracchioli R, Rossi S, Govoni E. Fertility and obstetric outcomes after laparoscopic myomectomy of large myomata: a randomized comparison with abdominal myomectomy. *Hum Reprod* 15(12):2663–2668, 2000.

23 McLucas B, Goodwin S, Adler L, et al. Pregnancy following uterine fibroid embolization. *Int J Gynecol Obstet* 74:1–7, 2001.

24 Brooks PG, Loffer FD, Serden SP. Resectoscopic removal of symptomatic intrauterine lesions. *J Reprod Med* 34(7):435–437, 1989.

25 Varasteh NN, Neuwirth RS, Levin B. Pregnancy rates after hysteroscopic polypectomy and myomectomy in infertile women. *Obstet Gynecol* 94:168–171, 1999.

26 Loverro G, Nappi L, Vicino M, et al. Uterine cavity assessment in infertile women: a comparison of transvaginal sonography and hysteroscopy. *Eur J Obstet Gynecol Reprod Biol* 100:67–71, 2001.

27 Shalev J, Meizner I, Bar-Hava I. Predictive value of transvaginal sonography performed before routine diagnostic hysteroscopy for evaluation of infertility. *Fertil Steril* 73(2):412–417, 2000.

28 Gronlund L, Hertz J, Palmgren Colov N. Transvaginal sonohysterography and hysteroscopy in the evaluation of female infertility, habitual abortion or metrorrhagia. *Acta Obstet Gynecol Scand* 78:415–418, 1999.

29 Reis Soares S, Barbosa dos Reis MM, Fernando Camargos A. Diagnostic accuracy of sonohysterography, transvaginal sonography and hysterosalpingography in patients with uterine cavity diseases. *Fertil Steril* 73(2):406–411, 2000.

30 Minto CL, Hollings N, Hall-Craggs M, et al. Magnetic resonance imaging in the assessment of complex Müllerian anomalies. *BJOG* 108:791–797, 2001.

Male Factor Infertility

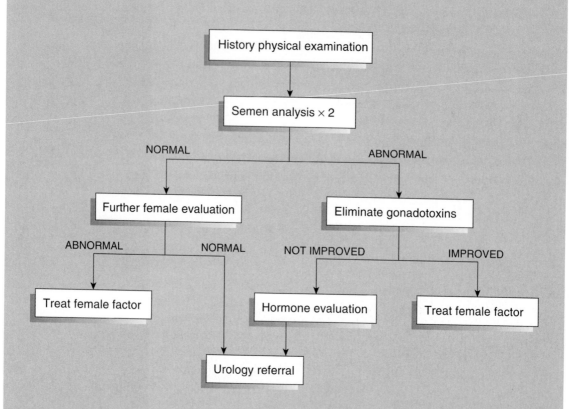

4 Male Factor Infertility

Paul J. Turek

One must show the greatest respect towards any thing that increases exponentially, no matter how small.

Garrett Hardin (1968)

Introduction

Among couples with infertility, roughly 40% have causal or associated male factors. In addition, 1–10% of male factor infertility is a direct result of an underlying, often treatable, but possibly life-threatening medical condition.[1] Therefore, evaluation of the male factor should proceed concurrently with the female. The male evaluation is conducted systematically to acquire relevant information from the history, physical examination, semen analysis, and hormone assessment. Treatments should include nonsurgical, surgical, and assisted reproductive options, with maternal reproductive potential a critical consideration in the decision.

Guiding Questions

MALE INFERTILITY EVALUATION

- Have social habits, drug use, and potential recreational and occupational exposures been reviewed with the male partner?
- Was proper collection technique discussed with the patient prior to the semen analyses?
- Are the two semen analyses consistent (i.e., do they vary <25%) or is a third test necessary?
- Has a urologist seen the patient and assessed him for varicocele, cancer, or absent vas deferens?

The Male History and Physical Examination

A thorough history reviews past and current attempts at paternity. Important medical problems to elucidate include recent fevers, systemic illnesses such as diabetes, cystic fibrosis, cancer, and infections. Prior surgery, including orchidopexy, herniorraphy, trauma, open, retroperitoneal, pelvic, or bladder and prostate procedures may be relevant to fertility. A family history of cryptorchidism, midline defects, or hypogonadism is also important. A developmental history of hypospadias, congenital anomalies, and diethylstilbesterol (DES) exposure may also be found. The use of medications (Table 4-1) should be reviewed. A social history may elucidate the habitual use of gonadotoxins: alcohol, tobacco, recreational drugs, and/or anabolic steroids. The use of spermicidal lubricants, and incorrect patterns and timings of intercourse may be noted from a sexual history. Lastly, an occupational history is important to determine exposure to ionizing radiation, chronic heat, benzene-based solvents, dyes, pesticides, herbicides, and heavy minerals (Table 4-1).

Childhood diseases may also affect fertility. A history of mumps can be significant if the infection occurs postpubertally. After age 11, unilateral orchitis is found with 30% of mumps

Table 4-1. **DRUGS/EXPOSURES WITH POTENTIAL ADVERSE EFFECTS ON MALE FERTILITY**

Alcohol	Lead
Alkylating agents	Lithium
(e.g., cyclophosphamide)	Monoamine oxidase inhibitors
Allopurinol	Marijuana
Antipsychotics	Medoxyprogesterone
Arsenic	Nicotine
Aspirin (large doses)	Nitrofurantoin
Caffeine	Phenytoin
Calcium channel blockers	Spironolactone
Cimetidine	Sulfasalazine
Cocaine	Testosterone
Colchicine	Tricyclic antidepressants
Dibromochloropropane	Valproic acid
(pesticides)	
Diethylstilbesterol	

infections and bilateral orchitis in 10% of cases. Mumps orchitis is thought to cause pressure necrosis of testis tissue; testis atrophy is usually obvious later in life. Cryptorchidism is also associated with decreased sperm production. This is true for both unilateral and bilateral cases. Longitudinal studies of affected boys have shown that abnormally low sperm counts can be found in 30% of men with unilateral cryptorchidism and 50% of men with bilateral undescended testes.

The physical examination assesses body habitus including obesity, gynecomastia, and secondary sex characteristics. The phallus may reveal evidence of hypospadias, chordee, plaques, or venereal lesions. The testes should be evaluated for size and consistency and contour irregularities suggestive of a mass. Remember that 80% of testis volume is determined by spermatogenic activity; hence, the finding of testis atrophy is likely due to decreased sperm production. Palpation of the epididymides should note any induration, fullness, or nodules indicative of infections or obstruction. Careful delineation of each vas deferens may reveal agenesis, atresia, or injury. The spermatic cords above the testes should be felt for asymmetry suggestive of a lipoma or varicocele. Lastly, a rectal examination is important in identifying large cysts, infections, or dilated seminal vesicles, all of which may be associated with infertility.

KEY POINT

Testicular examination is crucial, as infertile men are also more likely to have testis cancer. Also, meaningful varicoceles are diagnosed exclusively by physical examination.

Semen Evaluation

KEY POINT

Review information from prior semen analyses. Trends in semen quality over time can be an important clue to etiologic factors including recovery from gonadotoxin exposure.

Although not a true measure of fertility, the semen analysis, if abnormal, may suggest that the probability of achieving fertility is lower than normal. Two semen analyses, performed with 2–3 days of sexual abstinence, are required due to the large biological variability inherent in semen quality. Clean or sterile containers should be used. Condoms and lubricants need to be avoided. The specimen should be kept at body temperature during transport. Normal values can be found in Table 4-2[2]; however, there is recent debate concerning precisely which values are considered truly "normal."[3] Of the routine semen parameters, concentration and motility appear to correlate best with fertility. Recall that spermatogenesis takes 80 days to complete, so that semen quality on ejaculation is reflective of biological influences occurring 2–3 months prior.

Table 4-2.   SEMEN ANALYSIS—WHO MINIMAL STANDARDS OF ADEQUACY[a]

Ejaculate volume	1.5–5.5 cc
Sperm concentration	$>20 \times 10^6$ sperm/mL
Motility	>50%
Forward progression	2 (scale 1–4)
Morphology	>30% WHO (>14% Kruger)

[a]Also no agglutination (clumping), white cells, or increased viscosity.

The evaluation of the various shapes of sperm is termed morphologic assessment. Several descriptive systems exist to evaluate morphology, and within each classification system, sperm are designated normal or abnormal based on a list of criteria. It is believed that sperm morphology may correlate with a man's fertility potential. In general, sperm morphology is a sensitive indicator of testicular health because sperm morphology is determined within the testis. The main role of morphology in the male evaluation is to complement the semen analysis data and better estimate the chances of fertility.

Computer-aided semen analyses (CASA) couple videotechnology with digitalization and microchip information processing to categorize sperm features by set algorithms. Most commonly, CASA systems report sperm concentration, motility, and velocities (curvilinear, straight line) and can be used to assess sperm shape through nuclear features. Although the technology is promising, when manual semen analysis findings are compared to CASA on identical specimens, CASA tends to overestimate sperm counts by 30% in the presence of high levels of contaminating cells such as immature sperm or white blood cells. In addition, at high sperm concentrations, motility can be underestimated with CASA. These variables need to be considered if CASA systems are used to report semen analysis findings.

Results of Initial Male Evaluation

The initial male evaluation may be normal or abnormal. If normal, further consideration should be given to female factor evaluation, including a more thorough assessment of ovulation, female pelvic anatomy, and age-related fertility issues. If the initial male evaluation reveals abnormalities, then further evaluation or treatment of the male factor is indicated.[4] Gynecologists can have a significant impact in reducing male factor infertility by simply counseling the couple regarding coital timing, gonadotoxin exposure, and lifestyle changes. For example, coital lubricants should also be avoided if possible, including Surgilube, K-Y jelly, and saliva. If necessary, vegetable oils, olive oil, and petroleum jelly are the safest for sperm.

Further lifestyle questions are required. Androgenic steroids, often taken by bodybuilders to increase muscle mass, act as contraceptives with respect to fertility. Excess testosterone inhibits the pituitary-gonadal hormone axis and virtually shuts down sperm production. The effect of anabolic steroids is usually, but not necessarily, reversible on withdrawl of the medication. In addition, the routine use of hot tubs, hot baths, Jacuzzis, or saunas should be discouraged as these activities can elevate intratesticular temperature and impair sperm production. Sports such as bicycling are safe unless associated with significant urinary symptoms (prostatitis) or pelvic "numbness" that may eventually lead to erectile dysfunction. Since sperm production normally occurs at an extremely high rate of 1000 sperm/s, it is understandable that normal fertility depends on a healthy body.

KEY POINT

An overall healthy body is best for a reproductively healthy body.

Further Male Factor Evaluation

If lifestyle and exposure recommendations do not normalize semen parameters or fertility, then referral to a urologist is indicated. There are currently best practice policies outlined for the male infertility evaluation by urologists.[4] A more thorough male evaluation should include an assessment of the pituitary-gonadal axis with testosterone and follicle-stimulating hormone (FSH) levels. Hormone testing is indicated in infertile men with sperm densities $<10 \times 10^6$ sperm/mL, or with evidence of a medical endocrinopathy.[5] The chance of finding a clinically significant endocrinopathy presenting as infertility is approximately 2%.[5] The more common patterns of hormonal disorders observed in male infertility are found in Table 4-3.

In addition to hormonal evaluation there are other adjunctive tests available to diagnose the cause of male factor infertility. These are generally ordered by a specialist and include the following.

KEY POINT

Hormonal evaluation of the infertile male should be done for sperm density $<10 \times 10^6$ sperm/mL, if there is impaired sexual function (impotence, low libido), or with findings suggestive of an endocrinopathy (i.e., thyroid).

Table 4-3. CHARACTERISTIC ENDOCRINE PROFILES IN INFERTILE MEN

CONDITION	T	FSH	LH	PRL
Normal NL	NL	NL	NL	
Primary testis failure	Low	High	NL/High	NL
Hypogonadotropic hypogonadism	Low	Low	Low	NL
Hyperprolactinemia	Low	Low/NL	Low	High
Androgen resistance	High	High	High	NL

Abbreviations: T, testosterone; FSH, follicle-stimulating hormone; LH, luteinizing hormone; PRL, prolactin.

SEMINAL FRUCTOSE AND POSTEJACULATE URINALYSIS

Fructose is normally present in the ejaculate. If absent, seminal vesicle agenesis or obstruction may exist. A postejaculate urinalysis (PEU) is a microscopic inspection of the first voided urine after ejaculation for sperm. Retrograde ejaculation is diagnosed in this manner.

SEMEN LEUKOCYTE ANALYSIS

On a routine light microscopic semen analysis, "round" cells are often found in addition to sperm. These are either immature sperm forms (spermatocytes) or white blood cells (leukocytes). It is important to distinguish between these two cell types because the treatments differ. Specific assays are used to stain the ejaculate for leukocytes.

ANTISPERM ANTIBODY TEST

The presence of IgA and IgG antibodies on sperm has been implicated as a cause of infertility in 5–10% of men. Certain risk factors may predispose to the presence of sperm antibodies and include obstruction (vasectomy), trauma or torsion, infection (prostatitis), and chronic heat exposure.

SPERM PENETRATION ASSAY

A test of sperm function, the sperm penetration assay (SPA) measures the ability of human sperm to penetrate a specially prepared hamster egg in the laboratory setting. For a positive penetration result, sperm capacitation and acrosome reactivity must occur.

SPERM CHROMATIN STRUCTURE ASSAY

There may be a relationship between sperm DNA integrity and male fertility potential. A high percentage of denatured DNA in sperm has been correlated with reduced fertility *in vivo* and *in vitro*. Although it appears that <10% of infertile ejaculates contain high levels of denatured DNA, such assays may serve as useful discriminators of fertility potential independent of other semen parameters.[6]

SCROTAL DOPPLER ULTRASOUND

High frequency (7.5–10 mHz) ultrasound of the scrotum has become a mainstay in the evaluation of testicular and scrotal lesions.

TRANSRECTAL ULTRASOUND

High frequency (5–7mHz) transrectal ultrasound (TRUS) offers superb imaging of the prostate, seminal vesicles, and ejaculatory ducts. TRUS has virtually replaced the more invasive vasography in diagnosing obstructive lesions.

CT SCAN/MRI PELVIS

Since the advent of TRUS, these studies are only rarely indicated. One indication is the evaluation of the retroperitoneum in a patient with a solitary right varicocele.

GENETIC TESTING

Increasingly, genetic abnormalities have been shown to account for male infertility.[7] Deletion of regions on the Y chromosome (microdeletions) occur in about 6% of men with low sperm counts and 15% of men with azospermia. In addition, 2% of men with low counts and 15–20% of men with azospermia will harbor chromosomal abnormalities detected by cytogenetic analysis (karyotyping). These include conditons like Klinefelter's syndrome and translocations of nonsex chromosomes. Roughly 80% of azoospermic men with congenital absence of the vas deferens (CAVD) and one-third of men with unexplained states of obstruction will harbor cystic fibrosis gene mutations. Thus, genetic testing on infertile males is currently indicated for the following:

1. A semen analysis with sperm concentrations <10 million sperm/mL and the couple is considering *in vitro* fertilization (IVF) and intracytoplasmic sperm injection (ICSI) (Y microdeletions and karyotype).
2. There is no sperm in the ejaculate and the couple is considering testis sperm extraction with IVF and ICSI (Y microdeletions and karyotype).

KEY POINT

Adjunctive tests are indicated in the male evaluation if they: (a) delineate treatable, specific pathophysiology (i.e., varicocele) or (b) define life-threatening pathology.

3. A semen analysis shows no or low sperm concentration and there is at least one absent vas deferens on physical examination (cystic fibrosis gene mutations).
4. They have other syndromes or conditions suggested by personal or family histories.

Discussion of Cases

CASE 1

A 29-year-old man and his 28-year-old partner present with 1 year of infertility. Her evaluation revealed a prior terminated pregnancy at age 25, regular ovulatory cycles, no history of endometriosis, and a normal hysterosalpingogram. His history reveals no prior paternity or significant medical history. He has noted a recent waxing and waning discomfort in the left scrotum. His physical examination shows a large left varicocele and a tender left epididymis. His semen analyses show normal volumes, sperm concentrations of 60–70 million sperm/mL, and motilities ranging from 25 to 30%. Elevated round cells are noted in each semen analysis.

What other tests, if any, would you recommend at this point?

Certainly a referral to a urologist is in order to evaluate the pain and varicocele. The differential diagnosis of such pain could include epididymitis, prostatitis, or varicocele. More complete evaluation of the seminal "round" cells is also important with an Entz or monoclonal antibody stain to identify whether or not pyospermia is present.

What is your initial management?

A clinically symptomatic male partner should be treated for prostatitis or epididymitis, both of which might impair sperm motility through excessive leukocytes and reactive oxygen species in the ejaculate. After treatment, the semen analysis should be repeated. This "treat-and-reassess" approach should also be taken with suspected gonadotoxin exposures in the male, since most are indeed reversible.

CASE 2

A 35-year-old man and his 30-year-old partner have been married for 5 years and trying for 2 years to conceive. Her evaluation has revealed no prior pregnancies, regular ovulatory cycles, no history of endometriosis, a normal hysterosalpingogram, and a normal early cycle FSH and estradiol. His history is significant for a 1-year history of decreased libido, poor erections, and mild depression. Two properly performed semen analyses reveal low ejaculate volumes (1.4 mL) with low sperm concentrations (18 million sperm/mL) with low motility (35%).

What other tests, if any, would you recommend at this point?

Infertility could result from the poor semen quality, erectile dysfunction, or both. The patient should have a hormonal evaluation and should be referred to a urologist for complete evaluation of erectile dysfunction.

The hormone profile reveals the total testosterone is low at 175 ng/mL (normal 260–1000 ng/mL), the FSH is low at 1.2 mIU/mL (normal 2–8 mIU/mL).

What is the working diagnosis?

Hyperprolactinemia can account for (1) poor semen quality, (2) low libido, (3) erectile dysfunction, and (4) hypogonadotrophic hypogonadism. Therefore, a morning serum prolactin level should be ordered. It returns 125 ng/mL (normal 2–15 ng/mL). A sella tursica CT or MRI scan is needed along with referral to an endocrinologist for medical or surgical therapy.

REFERENCES

1 Honig SC, Lipshultz LI, Jarow JP. Significant medical pathology uncovered by a comprehensive male infertility evaluation. *Fertil Steril* 62:1028, 1994.

2 The Semen Analysis. *WHO Laboratory Manual for the Examination of Human Semen and Semen-Cervical Mucus Interaction.* Cambridge: Cambridge University Press, 1992, p. 20.

3 Guzick DS, Overstreet JW, Factor-Litvak P, et al. Sperm morphology, motility, and concentration in fertile and infertile men. *N Engl J Med* 345:1388, 2001.

4 Jarow JP, Sharlip ID, Belker AM, et al. Male Infertility Best Practice Policy Committee of the American Urological Association Inc. *J Urol* 167:2138, 2002.

5 Sigman M, Jarow JP. Medical evaluation of infertile men. *Urology* 50:659, 1997.

6 Zini A, Fischer MA, Sharir S, et al. Prevalence of abnormal sperm DNA denaturation in fertile and infertile men. *Urology* 60:1069, 2002.

7 Black L, Turek PJ. The genetics of male infertility. What every couple wants to know. *Fam Urol* 5:22, 2000.

Common Medical Conditions and Their impact on Reproductive Function

Mitchell P. Rosen
Marcelle I. Cedars

Introduction

The diagnosis of female reproductive dysfunction is primarily—and justifiably—focused on the female reproductive system: ovulatory dysfunction is responsible for fully 40% of female factor infertility, and tubal and pelvic pathology account for an additional 40%. When diagnostic efforts do not yield an etiologic explanation, "unexplained infertility" is acknowledged, and nonspecific fertility treatment is often initiated. However, with improved understanding of the reproductive impact of common medical comorbidities—and of their treatments—infertility can be better explained and better treated. Although data are usually limited, and specific etiologies are often hypothetical, awareness of the existing evidence is essential to providing the best possible care for patients desiring conception.

This chapter addresses the impact of common medical diseases on reproductive function (Table 5-1). Discussed for each comorbid condition are: (1) clinical evidence for an association

91

Table 5-1. **COMMON MEDICAL DISEASES IN WOMEN**

Psychiatric disease
Mood disorders

Neurologic disease
Epilepsy
Multiple sclerosis
Migraines

Cardiovascular disease
Pulmonary disease
Asthma

Endocrine disease
Diabetes
Thyroid disease (see Chap. 8)
Pituitary disorders (see Chap. 8)
PCOS (see Chap. 8)

Chronic liver disease
Transplant

Gastrointestinal disease
Hemochromatosis
Celiac disease
Inflammatory bowel disease

Chronic renal disease
Transplant

Autoimmune disease
Rheumotoid arthritis
Systemic lupus erythematosus

Infectious disease
Human immunodeficiency virus
Tuberculosis

with subfertility and/or adverse early pregnancy outcomes, (2) proposed etiologies and supporting evidence, (3) reproductive risks, and (4) benefits of common medical treatments, and recommendations for optimizing fertility treatment. A better understanding of the impact of medical disease on fecundity enables modification of fertility treatment, improving efficacy, and addressing disease-specific safety risks. Adjustment of medical treatment, or initiation of treatment for an undiagnosed condition, may obviate assisted reproduction altogether.

Guiding Questions

- Is the patient followed by a physician for a medical illness?
- Does the patient take any prescription medications?
- Does the patient take any over-the-counter (OTC) medications on a regular basis (including nonsteriodal anti-inflammatory drugs [NSAIDs] and antihistamines)?
- Does the patient take any herbal medications?
- Does the patient complain of undiagnosed gastrointestinal (GI) symptoms?

Psychiatric Disease

MOOD DISORDERS

Mood disorders are common in women of reproductive age. In the United States, it is reported that 20–30% of young women experience depression sometime in their lives, and the incidence is twofold that of men.[1] The prevalence of depression appears to be unrelated to ethnicity, income, or marital status.

Mood disorders (e.g., depression and anxiety) may present to the reproductive endocrinologist with a wide range of clinical manifestations (see Diagnostic Statiscal Manual of Mental Disorder, 4th edition [DSM-IV]), including menstrual abnormalities ranging from obvious dysfunction (e.g., anovulation) to more subtle defects (e.g., luteal phase deficiency). Whether the mood disorder is a cause or a consequence of the reproductive disturbance is not always clear. The incidence of clinical depression, decreased self-esteem, and sexual dysfunction do not appear to differ significantly between women undergoing infertility evaluation and those with no known fertility issues. Several studies have investigated a possible causal relationship between psychopathology and infertility with conflicting results.

It is clear that the converse is true: the psychologic impact of the infertility diagnosis can be profound. Several studies have demonstrated a strong relationship between patients experiencing infertility and psychologic distress, especially after unsuccessful infertility treatment.[2–6] Although symptoms may not meet DSM-IV criteria for axis I disease, there is suggestion that some subfertile patients experience maladaptive responses which may, in turn, impact fertility.[7,8]

Several studies have investigated the incidence of stress during fertility treatment, and the impact of psychologic intervention on outcomes.[9,10] One study attempted to separate procedural stress from baseline stress, and measure the independent impact on treatment outcomes (e.g., number of oocytes retrieved, pregnancy rates, live birth rates). Baseline stress was found to influence all outcomes measured, while procedural stress affected only the number of oocytes retrieved.[11] Others have suggested that psychologic intervention in couples experiencing psychologic distress improves treatment outcomes.[9] Once pregnant, women who conceive via assisted reproduction do not seem to differ psychologically from those who conceive naturally.[12]

The most common medications used to treat mood disorders, selective serotonin reuptake inhibitors (SSRIs), are not believed to affect reproductive function. However, SSRIs can moderately increase serum prolactin,[13,14] which is characteristically associated with altered gonadotropin-releasing hormone (GnRH) pulsatility, blunted luteinizing hormone (LH) surge, and luteal phase defects. While there is currently no clinical evidence that fertility or menstrual cyclicity is affected by SSRI treatment, subtle defects may be difficult to elucidate. It is therefore reasonable to consider changing to an alternative (non-SSRI) antidepressant medication, or adding a normalizing dopamine agonist, for a patient with unexplained infertility and elevated prolactin. SSRIs, unlike other psychotropic drugs associated with adverse fetal affects, do not appear to increase rates of spontaneous abortion or congenital malformations, even if used early in pregnancy.[15,16]

The evaluation of the infertile patient should include psychiatric assessment to identify patients who may benefit from intervention. In particular, formal psychologic evaluation should be offered in cases of prior psychiatric illness, change in mental status, substance abuse, marital distress, and use of a third party in reproduction (donor/surrogate).

KEY POINT

Stress is a frequent comorbidity of infertility and mental status should be evaluated, in all patients, and treated appropriately.

Neurologic Disease

Epilepsy, multiple sclerosis (MS), and migraine headaches are among the more common neurologic conditions affecting women of reproductive age.

Seizures can be classified as partial or generalized; they can develop secondary to a distinct etiology (e.g., malignant, metabolic, infectious, or genetic), or may be idiopathic. Epilepsy affects nearly 1.0% of the U.S. population and has no gender preference.[17] Estimates suggest that approximately 1.1 million women of childbearing age have epilepsy.[18]

Reproductive endocrine disorders occur more frequently in women with epilepsy, particularly those with temporal lobe epilepsy (TLE), a partial seizure disorder. Several studies have demonstrated that these women experience anovulation with higher frequency than the general population.[19-21] Investigators suggest that there is a relationship between the lateralization of epileptic discharge and the endocrine dysfunction.[19-23] In one group of epileptic women, 56% had menstrual dysfunction, with a variant of polycystic ovarian syndrome (PCOS) seen in 20% of patients and hypothalamic amenorrhea (HA) observed in another 12%.[21] The women with left-sided temporal eliptiform discharges were more likely to develop PCOS while those with right-sided foci more commonly had hypothalamic amenorrhea (see Fig. 5-1). Further, women with left

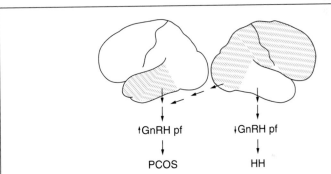

Figure 5-1: Proposed neuroendocrine model of some reproductive endocrine disorders in women with epilepsy and the relationship among EEG focus and laterality, pulsatile secretion of GnRH, and reproductive endocrine disorder. Left temporal and right nontemporal epileptiform discharges may increase gonadotropin-releasing hormone pulse frequency (GnRH pf) and thereby promote the development of polycystic ovarian syndrome (PCOS). Right temporal epileptiform discharges may decrease GnRH pf, resulting in hypogonadotropic hypogonadism (HH). (*Source:* Herzog AG. A relationship between particular reproductive endocrine disorders and the laterality of epileptiform discharges in women with epilepsy. *Neurology* 43(10):1907–1910, 1993.)

temporal lobe epilepsy showed a trend toward higher LH pulse frequencies compared to women with right temporal foci[23] (see PCOS).

One possible explanation for this observation is anatomic: the amygdala is a common site of involvement in TLE, and its direct anatomic connection to the hypothalamic nuclei may alter the regulation of GnRH. This explanation has been supported by studies demonstrating that stimulation or ablation of the amygdala can alter LH and follicle-stimulating hormone (FSH) pulsatility.[21] Other studies demonstrate lateral asymmetries exist in the temporal lobes and within the hypothalamus.[24,25] Interestingly, it has been shown that the GnRH content in the right mediobasal hypothalamic nuclei is greater than that in the left.[24]

The association between generalized epilepsy and reproductive function is undetermined; however, a recent study demonstrated that fertility rates in women aged 25–39 years with treated epilepsy are significantly less than those in the general population (0.75 CI 0.68–0.83).[26] The etiology is unclear, but may include social factors such as lower rates of marriage, fear of transmitting epilepsy to offspring or teratogenic potential of medications (e.g., valproate). However, there may also be a biological explanation. Menstrual disorders in women with generalized epilepsy are common (50%), and there is evidence for a higher incidence of premature ovarian failure[27] (which decreases time of reproductive potential). Furthermore, gonadotropin disturbances have been seen in women with generalized seizures.[28] However, a pathway from generalized eliptiform discharges to the hypothalamus has not been determined.

Others have found a relationship between antiepileptic drug therapy (AED) and reproductive endocrine disorders, especially PCOS. In particular, valproate use is associated with a high incidence of menstrual irregularities, obesity, hyperinsulinemia, hyperandrogenism, and polycystic ovaries.[29–31] These findings were independent of type of seizure disorder. Women not using AED did not have menstrual disturbances, and the frequency of PCOS in women receiving AED besides valproic acid was no different than the general population. When the affected women were switched to lamotrigine, menstrual function improved and polycystic-appearing ovaries (PCAO) resolved in most women. Differences in AED regimens may be partially explained by alterations in metabolism of sex steroid hormones: valproic acid inhibits cytochrome P450 enzymes, increasing the concentration of androgens. This is in distinction to other AED which may increase SHBG or cytochrome P450 activity and *decrease* bioavailability of hormones.

In a recent study,[28] reproductive function, particularly ovulatory failure, was evaluated in women with epilepsy. Women with idiopathic generalized epilepsy (IGE) were significantly more likely to experience ovulatory failure (27.1%) compared to those with localized related epilepsy (LRE, includes all partial seizures) (14.3%) or controls (10.9%). This increased risk was independent of antiepileptic therapy (AED). Interestingly, current or past use (within 3 years) of valproic acid was associated with anovulation (38%) and may be additive to the direct effect of the seizure disorder.[28] It has also been shown that women with IGE and with recent use of valproic acid had a significantly increased incidence of polycystic ovaries (41% versus 15%) while those with LRE did not.[28] The authors commented that the differences in anovulation and PCAO seen in women with LRE compared to TLE may be explained by the LRE group including those patients with extratemporal discharges.

Other studies have found no association between epilepsy and reproductive disorders.[32,33] A case series with 101 women with epilepsy found the incidence of polycystic ovaries to be no different than in the general population, even when stratified into partial versus generalized seizure disorders.[34] Interpretation of these small, conflicting studies is further complicated by inconsistent definition of PCOS. A recent cross-disciplinary survey illustrated that physicians are not sufficiently aware of the reproductive health consequences in women with epilepsy.[35] Even though there is no consensus regarding the etiology of menstrual dysfunction, it is imperative to be aware of the association not only with reproductive disorders, but also with sexual dysfunction, osteoporosis, and the potential for major birth defects in the offspring.

KEY POINT

Temporal lobe epilepsy appears to have a negative effect on hypothalamic function and may therefore impact fertility.

MULTIPLE SCLEROSIS

Multiple sclerosis is an autoimmune disorder characterized by demyelination of neurons in the central nervous system (CNS). It is the most common chronic neurologic disease in young adults, with a peak age of onset between 20 and 40 years old. The prevalence of MS varies with sex, race, and geographic location; it is most common among White women. In a recent U.S. survey (the Nurses Health Study), the prevalence of MS was 3.9 per 1000 women.[36]

Few studies have directly addressed the impact of MS on reproductive function. The largest case series (14 patients with regular menstrual cycles and without diagnosed infertility) showed significant increases in serum prolactin, FSH, LH, and total and free testosterone in women with MS.[37] The authors theorized that the etiology of these hormonal alterations may be altered dopaminergic tone. Dopamine inhibits the release of prolactin, and decreased dopaminergic tone may disturb reproductive function via hyperprolactinemia-mediated suppression of the hypothalamic-pituitary axis. However, as dopamine may directly inhibit gonadotropin secretion, the decreased dopamine observed in these patients (as inferred from serum prolactin levels) may offer partial protection from the effects of hyperprolactinemia. This relationship is subtle and incompletely understood. While it is plausible that the hypothalamic-pituitary axis and gonadotropin pulsatility may be altered by CNS demyelination, there is currently no clinical evidence that MS reduces fertility. However, clinical evidence for an association between MS and hyperandrogenism[38] deserves further study.

Therapy for MS may impact fertility. Current regimens for relapsing MS include immunomodulatory agents (e.g., interferon-beta [INF-beta] or glatiramer acetate) and antineoplastic agents (e.g., mitoxantrone or cyclophosphamide). A recent review of the limited data suggests that INF-beta can cause menstrual disturbances, and possibly has a dose-dependent abortive effect.[38] It is therefore recommended that INF therapy be discontinued if pregnancy is desired. However, as no teratogenic effects have been observed, inadvertent fetal exposure is not an indication for termination. Similarly, there are little data on the effects of mitoxantrone on fertility, although one case report suggests an association with premature ovarian failure.[39] It is well-established that other chemotherapies, such as cyclophosphamide, are chemotoxic to the ovary and can cause premature ovarian failure.[40]

Multiple sclerosis does not influence pregnancy course or birth outcomes. A recent study showed that the rate of pregnancy complications, low birth weight, and malformations were no higher among women with MS.[41] In addition, pregnancy does not seem to have deleterious affects on the overall course of disease and may, in fact, reduce relapse rates,[42] although exacerbation rates may be increased in the 3 months postpartum. This trend may be explained by hormonal influence on the immune system: estrogen and progesterone are thought to decrease production of Th1 cytokines and increase the production of Th2 cytokines, promoting an anti-inflammatory milieu.[43] One retrospective study followed this hypothesis (in nonpregnant patients) and demonstrated that a subset of patients had increased exacerbations just prior to menses.[44] The authors theorized that the loss of the anti-inflammatory effect of estrogen and progesterone at this point in the menstrual cycle triggered relapse.

When pregnancy and the puerperium are considered together, the number of relapses of maternal disease is unchanged, and offspring appear to have no increased risk of morbidity.[45] Thus, it is considered safe to achieve pregnancy with the diagnosis of MS, although it is important to assess current medications and offer counseling with a perinatologist prior to fertility treatment.

MIGRAINES

Migraine headaches are common in women and a relationship between attacks and sex steroids has been proposed.[46,47] Despite this possible hormonal relationship, migraineurs do not appear to have a higher prevalence of infertility. However, certain medications used to manage migraines have been either associated with subfertility or an increased incidence of congenital abnormalities; therefore a medication assessment is necessary prior to fertility treatment.

Although the data are limited and conflicting, there have been isolated case reports which associate ergotamines with congenital abnormalities and preterm labor[48-51]; therefore ergots are not recommended in pregnancy. Historically, the triptans are also considered contraindicated in pregnancy, but ongoing registries have not documented an increase in the prevalence of major birth defects or adverse pregnancy outcomes with inadvertent exposure to sumatriptan during organogenesis and later pregnancy.[52,53] However, the current information is not enough to eliminate small increases in birth defects. Therefore, preconceptional counseling is suggested in any patient who is using triptans regularly.

While migraine-specific medications (e.g., triptans and beta-blockers) do not appear to interfere with reproductive function or increase the rate of spontaneous abortion,[54] nonspecific medications such as NSAIDs can result in reversible female infertility.[55-58] These drugs can impair prostaglandin-mediated ovulation and implantation, and should be discontinued prior to administering fertility treatment (see Chap. 1).

KEY POINT

Patients taking NSAIDs for migraine headaches should discontinue treatment prior to attempting fertility.

Cardiovascular Disease

Common cardiovascular diseases affecting women of reproductive age include valvular heart disease (e.g., mitral valve prolapse), hypertension, and hyperlipidemia; less common are atherosclerosis and cardiomyopathy. There are currently no data to support an association between common cardiovascular diseases among women and infertility or spontaneous abortion.

Antihypertensive therapy has not been associated with the inability to conceive. However, certain medications (notably methyldopa, verapamil, and ACE inhibitors) are associated with elevated serum prolactin levels, and there are several documented cases that described the associated clinical manifestations of hyperprolactinemia (i.e., breast discharge).[59,60] Although these medications have not been reported to reduce reproductive potential, prolactin alterations are certainly capable of interfering with reproduction, and the lack of data should not eliminate concern for women on these medications.

Despite observing minimal impact on fertility, there is controversy on whether antihypertensive usage should be continued in pregnancy. Blood pressure (BP) decreases during the first half of pregnancy, and treatment of mild-to-moderate chronic hypertension during pregnancy does not alter the associated adverse outcomes of preexisting hypertension on pregnancy.[61-63] Furthermore, although the data are limited, it is noteworthy to know which antihypertensives have been associated with adverse affects on the fetus (see Table 5-2).[63]

There are few publications that have investigated the impact of hyperlipidemia on pregnancy outcomes. Animal data suggest there are associated adverse outcomes; mainly a fourfold increase in abortion, a twofold increase in neonatal mortality, and low birth weight.[64] Additionally, there are limited data on whether anti-hypercholestrolemic therapies impact fertility or fetal outcomes. Despite the lack of sufficient data, statins have been associated with teratogenicity and therefore, are contraindicated in pregnancy.

Prior to administering fertility treatment in any patient with cardiovascular disease, a medication assessment is required and preconception counseling with a perinatologist is recommended. Although, these cardiovascular diseases do not directly cause reproductive dysfunction, it is recommended to measure a serum

Table 5-2. **ANTIHYPERTENSIVE THERAPY OF CHRONIC HYPERTENSION IN PREGNANCY**

DRUG	**DOSAGE**	**ADDITIONAL COMMENTS**
Methyldopa	500–3000 mg in 2–4 divided doses	Considered to be drug of choice because of extensive experience
Labetalol	200–1200 mg in 2–3 divided doses	Similar in efficacy and safety to methyldopa
Beta-blockers	Variable	Possibility of fetal bradycardia, lower birth weight (when used early in pregnancy)
Calcium channel blockers	Variable	Scant data for use in pregnancy
Clonidine	0.1–0.8 mg in 2–4 divided doses	Limited data
Thiazide diuretics	Variable	May be associated with diminished volume expansion in pregnancy: may be necessary in salt-sensitive hypertensives at lower doses
Angiotensin-converting enzyme inhibitors	Contraindicated	Contraindicated in pregnancy: neonatal anuric renal failure
Angiotensin receptor antagonists	Contraindicated	Contraindicated in pregnancy: neonatal anuria renal failure

SOURCE: August P, Falkner B. Hypertension in pregnancy and in children. In: Antman E (ed.), *Cardiovascular Therapeutics: A Modified Companion to Braunwald's Heart Disease.* Philadelphia, PA: W.B. Saunders, Chap. 38, 2001.

prolactin in any woman presenting with unexplained infertility or a shortened luteal phase, especially if the patient is being treated with methyldopa or verapamil. If the prolactin is moderately elevated, a change in medications can be considered.

Pulmonary Disease

ASTHMA   Asthma is among the most common chronic medical conditions, with a prevalence of 14 million persons (7 million women) in the

United States.[65] Childhood asthma is more common in boys, but no gender preference is seen in adulthood.

Asthma is likely not associated with infertility. There are limited data on whether therapy (e.g., beta-agonists, anti-inflammatories) has an impact on reproductive function. In a case-control study, ovulatory infertility was increased twofold in patients who started asthma therapy prior to age 21.[66] However, no other studies have confirmed this association; therefore more data are needed before considering asthma therapy as a cause of infertility. Furthermore, asthma medications (including steroids) have not been associated with early pregnancy loss.[67]

While no effect on conception has been identified, there are limited data suggesting that steroid use may add a small increased risk for oral clefts.[68] However, the effects of uncontrolled asthma on the fetus may be more detrimental. Patients with moderate asthma, or those who use steroids regularly, should be offered preconception counseling with a perinatologist prior to fertility treatment.

Endocrine Disease

DIABETES

Diabetes mellitus (DM) is a chronic disease characterized by altered glucose homeostasis and abnormalities in carbohydrate, protein, and fat metabolism. An association with subfertility has been demonstrated. But while the pathophysiologies of the microvascular, macrovascular, and neurologic sequelae of DM are well-characterized, the mechanism of reproductive dysfunction remains unclear.

Type I diabetes mellitus (TIDM) is a disease of insulin deficiency secondary to immune-mediated pancreatic islet beta cell destruction. The onset of the disease occurs most often during adolescence. The prevalence of TIDM in the general population is approximately 0.3%. Type II diabetes mellitus (TIIDM) is an etiologically distinct disorder initiated not by insulin deficiency, but by insulin resistance.[69] As the disease progresses, islet cells are increasingly unable to meet peripheral demands for insulin. The prevalence of TIIDM at age 20–44 is approximately 3%, and increases with age.[70]

Diabetes can have dramatic effects on multiple systems, including the reproductive endocrine axis. If the onset of TIDM precedes menarche, menarche is often delayed and patients are more likely to develop menstrual disturbances.[71-73] Onset after menarche is also associated with a two- to threefold increase in the incidence of menstrual irregularities compared to controls.[71,72] Within the TIDM population, menstrual dysfunction is more prevalent in women with poor glycemic control.[72] Some have reported that TIDM women with low body mass index (BMI) are more likely to have menstrual irregularities, and to have PCAO.[74] The latter finding suggests that the etiology of PCAO in insulin-deficient TIDM may be different than that in type II diabetes, in which insulin *resistance* has been hypothesized to play a causal role in a similar abnormality of the ovary. Alternatively, the etiologies may be similar, with insulin resistance being a consequence of a common pathophysiology leading to PCOA in both types of diabetes. The mechanism of TIDM-mediated reproductive endocrine disturbance is not well known, although most observations point to hypothalamic dysfunction. It has been shown, for example, that women with insulin-dependent diabetes have relatively low serum concentrations of LH.[75] It is also well documented that women with nutritional restriction (e.g., anorexia nervosa) have decreased gonadotropins as a result of disruption in hypothalamic pulsatile secretion of GnRH[76–78]; this may be relevant as diabetes can be modeled as intracellular starvation. In addition, anovulatory diabetic women have depressed prolactin levels when compared to anovulatory nondiabetic women,[79] suggesting that enhanced dopaminergic tone may contribute to the depression of pituitary function at or above the pituitary level. Although the data suggest that the menstrual abnormalities observed in TIDM women are a result of a depressed hypothalamic drive, the underlying basis is still unclear and more studies are needed to determine if the reproductive disturbance is a direct effect of diabetes, or a function of general nutritional deprivation.

While these menstrual abnormalities suggest that reproductive potential is impaired, there are little data explicitly evaluating fertility rates in TIDM women. One study supported an association of subfertility withTIDM, with the degree of subfertility correlated with daily insulin dose.[80] Furthermore, if pregnancy is achieved in women with *poor* glycemic control, early pregnancy complications are frequently experienced.[81] There is also limited evidence that TIDM may be associated with a higher incidence of premature menopause, which would also impact lifetime reproductive potential.[82]

There are limited data on the impact of type II diabetes on reproductive function. This may be attributable to a limited population since the incidence of type II DM is most often post-menopausal (although a growing population of childhood-onset type II diabetes has emerged in the past decade.[83] Type II diabetes has many similarities to PCOS, sharing risk factors (e.g., obesity), proposed etiology (insulin resistance), and hereditary patterns (parents of women with PCOS have a higher incidence in type II diabetes).[84] The impact of type II diabetes on reproduction can be modeled simply as an increased risk for PCOS; although more study is needed to achieve a complete understanding.

Although somewhat controversial, the majority of evidence suggests women with preexisting diabetes are more likely than controls to have early pregnancy wastage.[85–88] The etiology is not well known, but several studies have demonstrated an association between poor glycemic control and spontaneous abortions.[89–91] Moreover, the evidence suggests that the magnitude of risk for spontaneous abortion is correlated with glycosylated hemoglobin levels. The exact threshold of glycemia that is associated with increased pregnancy loss is not completely known; but it may be apparent with slight abnormalities in glucose control. A recent prospective study showed that type I diabetics with a HbA1C >7.5 have a four-fold increase in pregnancy loss over diabetics with good glycemic control.[81]

KEY POINT

Both type I and type II diabetes may impact fertility and pregnancy health. Optimal control should be obtained prior to fertility management.

Poor glycemic control is also associated with other adverse pregnancy outcomes, including congenital malformations. While the exact mechanism has not been clearly established, the pathogenesis leading to these outcomes may be similar. A postulated mechanism is shown in Fig. 5-2.[92] Nonphysiologic concentrations of glucose induce a downregulation of embryonic glucose receptors, causing intraembryonic hypoglycemia. This triggers the apoptotic pathway, leading to either fetal malformations or spontaneous abortion.

Diabetes is a prevalent chronic disease affecting reproductive potential. Glycemic control should be optimized prior to fertility treatment; few women with TIDM will resolve their menstrual disturbance with improved control.[93] The improvement in glycemic control is more likely to impact the pregnancy outcome, as pregnancy loss, congenital malformations, and maternal complications will be decreased.

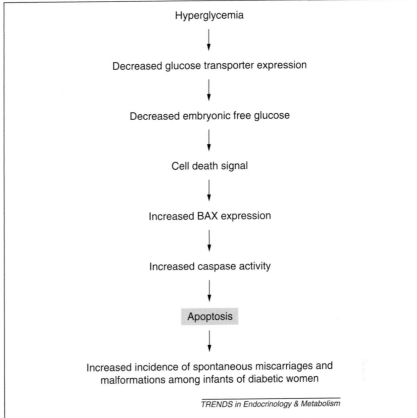

Hyperglycemia

↓

Decreased glucose transporter expression

↓

Decreased embryonic free glucose

↓

Cell death signal

↓

Increased BAX expression

↓

Increased caspase activity

↓

Apoptosis

↓

Increased incidence of spontaneous miscarriages and
malformations among infants of diabetic women

TRENDS in Endocrinology & Metabolism

Figure 5-2: Hypothetical etiology of diabetic embryopathy as a
preimplantation embryonic event. Maternal hyperglycemia results in down
regulation of the facilitative glucose transporter at the blastocyst stage. The
resultant decrease in glucose acts as a cell death signal, triggering an
increase in the expression of the proapoptotic protein BAX, which leads to
activation of caspases, DNA fragmentation, and morphological charges
consistent with apoptosis. This paradigm been shown to occur in animal
models, and is in part responsible for the increase in pregnancy loss and
congenital malformation seen among diabetic animals. This paradigm might
also occur in diabetic women. (*Source*: Moley KH. Hyperglycemia and
apoptosis: mechanisms for congenital malformations and pregnancy loss in
diabetic women. *Trends Endocrinol Metab* 12(2):78–82, 2001.)

Gastrointestinal Disease

Several intestinal disorders commonly affect women of reproductive age, including chronic liver disease (hepatitis, alcoholism),
malabsorptive diseases (hemochromatosis, celiac disease [CD]),

and inflammatory bowel disorders (Crohn's disease, ulcerative colitis).

CHRONIC
LIVER DISEASE

In many parts of the world, chronic liver disease is most commonly caused by viruses. Hepatitis B has affected more than 2 billion people; there are currently 350 million chronic carriers[94] and approximately 50–75% develop chronic liver disease. While occurrence is low in Europe and the United States (which together account for less than 2% of cases),[95] hepatitis B remains a major health issue which can affect reproductive potential. Hepatitis C has affected more than 170 million people worldwide and 3.9 million in the United States (1.8% of the U.S. population); over 70% have chronic disease.[96] Cirrhosis (end-stage liver disease) will develop in over 20% of people chronically infected with hepatitis B or C.[95,96]

Alcoholism is responsible for the majority of chronic liver disease in many countries—with effective vaccination programs for hepatitis and an increase in extensive alcohol consumption. Approximately 10–15% of chronic alcoholics develop chronic liver disease. Women are known to be more susceptible to chronic disease than men,[97] perhaps because the lower levels of gastric alcohol dehydrogenase observed in women increase the effective dose seen by the liver.[98] The incidence of chronic liver disease and cirrhosis increases with comorbidities such as viral hepatitis.[99,100]

Menstrual irregularities are common in patients with chronic liver disease, and can be its first clinical manifestation.[101] By inference, reproductive potential is likely to be compromised. The mechanism of disruption may differ depending on the etiology, but almost certainly involves dysfunction of the hypothalamic-pituitary axis. For example, there is evidence that women with chronic alcoholic liver disease have a central defect: they have decreased serum levels of gonadotropins and have a depressed response to gonadotropin-releasing hormone.[102] The exact mechanism is unknown, but the malnutrition experienced in many of these women likely contributes to the alteration in hypothalamic drive. In addition, a direct toxic effect on the ovary may be important in patients with excessive alcohol intake: women of reproductive age who died of alcohol-induced cirrhosis were found to have decreased follicular development and absent corpora lutea.[101] This is likely because the ovaries contain alcohol dehydrogenase, and intraovarian ethanol metabolism may change redox conditions and alter the metabolism of sex steroids. The pathophysiology of menstrual dysfunction in liver disease, unrelated to alcohol, has not been well characterized. The data suggest there is no single mechanism: women can present with low or normal serum levels of gonadotropins and have corresponding biochemical differences.[103] Women who presented with hypogonadotropic amenorrhea had low serum levels of sex steroids and had clinical manifestations of malnutrition. While women with normal gonadotropins appeared to have a normal nutritional status and had elevated sex steroids. The origin of the increased estrogen and androgen is controversial; it is likely due to portosystemic shunting of androgens—with subsequent peripheral conversion to estrogen.[101] Alternatively, it can be due to altered metabolic clearance but good evidence is lacking.[103] In advanced liver disease, hyperprolactinemia was observed, although was not consistent; therefore it probably does not significantly contribute to the etiology of menstrual disturbances in women with chronic liver disease.

Menstrual irregularities generally resolve after liver transplant.[101,104,105] In one study normal menstrual function resumed, on average, 3 months following liver transplantation.[104] Although transplant patients are often on multiple immunosuppressive agents (e.g., corticosteroids, azathioprine, cyclosporine, FK-506), there are currently no data indicating that these medications impair fertility, and pregnancy outcomes appear favorable. Graft function is not generally compromised, as long as the graft and immunosuppressive agents are stable: the National Transplantation Pregnancy Registry (NTPR) recommends a 1–2-year period after transplantation to allow for this stabilization.

Pregnancy outcomes in this population appear favorable,[106] although the use of corticosteroids during organogenesis has been associated with an increase risk of cleft lip formation.[68] Although data are limited, other immunosuppressive agents used in these patients have not been associated with increased rates of congenital malformations.[101] Therefore, it is not necessary to discourage pregnancy in these patients, but preconceptional consultation with a perinatologist is important since several of these medications are associated with adverse pregnancy outcomes (e.g., intrauterine growth restriction [IUGR], hypertension, and glucose intolerance). In addition to immunosuppressive agents, posttransplant patients often require lifelong anticoagulation, and low molecular weight heparin should be substituted for coumadin (given the latter's well-established teratogenecity). If applicable, gonadotropins should be administered subcutaneously to decrease the theoretical risk of muscular hematoma, and heparin should be discontinued at least 24 h prior to any surgical intervention (and restarted 24 h after the procedure).

There are little data on infertility treatment in patients with liver transplants. However, if liver transplant patients can tolerate pregnancy, fertility treatment should not be withheld. There is one case report describing a woman who underwent superovulation, egg retrieval, and transfer without complication.[107] The pregnancy was complicated by the development of preeclampsia, and preterm premature rupture of membranes at 34 weeks. The authors concluded that fertility treatment appears safe in liver transplant patients; but pregnancy is at high risk and a multidisciplinary approach is needed (including perinatology, hematology, genetics, and transplant specialists).

HEMOCHROMATOSIS

Hemochromatosis is a disease of iron overload in which deposition in the liver, heart, pituitary, and other endocrine organs causes cell death, fibrosis, and functional damage. There are two types: primary, or hereditary, hemochromatosis (HHC) and secondary hemochromatosis. Secondary hemochromatosis is most often associated with blood transfusions for chronic hemolytic anemias.

Hereditary hemochromatosis results from dysregulation of intestinal iron absorption. The most common genetic mutation is located in the HFE gene on chromosome 6; transmission is autosomal recessive. The prevalence of HHC is approximately 1 in 200 and varies by geographic location, with a carrier frequency as high as 10%.[108,109] However, there is a gender difference in phenotypic expression. This is likely because women have a protective increased negative iron balance secondary to menstruation, pregnancy, and lactation. This is further supported by an observation that adult HHC tends to manifest earlier in women with premature menopause.[109,110]

A rare subtype of HHC—juvenile or type 2 hereditary hemochromatosis presents earlier in life. This disorder is similarly an autosomal recessive condition, but is distinct from HFE-linked disease: it is linked to chromosome 1.[111] The onset of disease is almost always before 30 years of age and there is no gender difference in

Table 5-3. **CHARACTERISTICS OF HFE (ADULT-ONSET) AND TYPE 2 (JUVENILE-ONSET) HEMOCHROMATOSIS**

	HFE (N = 93)	*Type 2 (N = 26)*	*P*
Age (years)	44·8 ± 10·7	23·3 ± 6·2	<0.0001
TS (%)	87·7 ± 11·5	88·6 ± 9·7	NS
SF (µg/L)	2830 ± 2239	3146 ± 1270	NS
Hypogonadism	18·4%	96·1%	<0.0001
Cardiopathy	6·5%	34·6%	<0.0001
Reduced glucose tolerance	26·9%	57·7%	0·003
Cirrhosis	51·6%	42·1%	NS
Arthropathy	12%	26·9%	NS
IR (g)	14·2 ± 8·9	14·0 ± 5·2*	NS
IR/age	0·32 ± 0·2	0·65 ± 0·3*	<0.001

Abbreviations: TS, transferrin saturation; SF, serum ferritin; IR, iron removed; NS, not significant ($P > 0.05$).
*Data available in 14 patients.
SOURCE: De Gobbi M, Roetto A, Piperno A, et al. Natural history of juvenile haemochromatosis. *Br J Haematol* 117:973–979, 2002. (modified)

phenotypic expression.[112,113] Juvenile hemochromatosis presents initially as postpubertal hypogonadism (secondary amenorrhea in women) in almost all patients with type 2 HHC (Table 5-3).[114] If undiagnosed, it often presents again later as life-threatening cardiomyopathy. In a small case series, the mean time from the first clinical signs of disease to diagnosis was approximately 10 years[113]; the diagnosis is unfortunately often made during hospitalization for heart failure and possible transplantation.

Hemochromatosis, primary or secondary, affects reproductive function largely via iron deposition in the hypothalamic-pituitary region, notably the anterior pituitary gland. Several reports describe patients with hemochromatosis and hypogonadotropic hypogonadism (HH),[115–117] for whom stimulation with GnRH does not appropriately increase gonadotropin levels.[118–120] Histologic data confirm that iron deposition can occur in the anterior pituitary, particularly the gonadotropes.[115] Furthermore, hemochromatosis can affect any of the hypothalamic-pituitary axes and result in a hormonal insufficiency.[115,119] Magnetic resonance imaging of patients with secondary hemochromatosis suggests that the etiology of hypogonadism in these patients is similar to that in primary HHC.[121–122] Although the evidence suggests a pituitary disturbance, one case report described a patient with HHC that displayed a combined hypothalamic-pituitary defect, and another report showed iron deposition in the testis.[118,123] There is no evidence that iron can deposit in the ovary.

There are little data on reproductive potential after the disease has been stabilized with therapy. One case series demonstrated restoration of gonadal function with therapy in men.[116,124] Data in women are even more limited, with no evidence that hypogonadotropic hypogonadism can be resolved or reproductive function can be restored without fertility therapy. Two cases of gonadotropin stimulation in this population have been reported: both resulted in follicular development, and one resulted in a twin pregnancy without complications.[117,125]

In summary, it is important to perform provocative pituitary testing to assess pituitary reserve prior to fertility therapy in any woman with a history of hemochromatosis. This is necessary since hemochromatosis can penetrate all cell types of the pituitary. In addition a consultation with a geneticist, hematologist, and perinatologist is strongly encouraged. Fertility therapy most likely will include exogenous gonadotropins since the gonadotropes are unlikely to secrete gonadotropins. In addition, although juvenile hemochromatosis is a rare disorder, it must be considered in the differential diagnosis of any young woman presenting with secondary amenorrhea and infertility, as the diagnosis is easily established, the treatment is highly effective, and the disease is life threatening if allowed to progress.

CELIAC DISEASE (GLUTEN-SENSITIVE ENTEROPATHY)

Celiac disease is an autoimmune malabsorption disorder characterized by inflammatory injury of the small intestinal mucosa with exposure to gluten-containing cereals, wheat, barley, rye, and possibly oats.[126,127] The diagnosis is likely if antitissue transglutaminase antibodies or antiendomysial antibodies are present, and is confirmed with histologic evaluation of the small intestinal mucosa.[127] The prevalence is difficult to measure because "silent" celiac disease (extraintestinal symptoms only) is so common,[128] but it is estimated that CD affects 1 in 200 in populations of European descent.[127,129–131] The estimated prevalence of CD in North America is 1–120 to 1–300; there appears to be no gender preference, and the disease can present in childhood or adulthood.[127]

CD is associated with endocrine dysfunction not only autoimmune-mediated (i.e., diabetes (IDDM) and thyroid disease), but also with a range of female reproductive disorders. Women with CD have delayed menarche and early menopause[132–135] and a higher prevalence of amenorrhea.[132] Furthermore, several studies have shown that the prevalence of silent celiac disease is higher among infertile women[136–138]; it is estimated that celiac disease affects 4–8% of women diagnosed with unexplained infertility.[136,137] In fact, CD may initially present as a reproductive endocrine disorder and possibly infertility.[139]

Several studies have demonstrated an association between early pregnancy loss and *untreated* celiac disease.[130,132,133,140–142] The estimated relative risk of miscarriage in women with untreated celiac disease may be nine times more than those treated.[140] Furthermore, the prevalence of silent celiac disease may be higher in patients who present with recurrent spontaneous abortion.[143,144] This finding is particularly interesting because the majority of these patients are classified as "unexplained" with no effective treatment.

Celiac disease is clearly associated with adverse pregnancy outcomes. Multiple case studies have demonstrated an increased incidence of IUGR and low birth weight in infants born to untreated mothers with celiac disease[143]; the relative risk may be 3–6 times higher than those treated with gluten-free diet. Recently, a large retrospective cohort study confirmed these findings—they showed a threefold increased risk of IUGR with untreated celiac disease[145] and the pregnancy outcomes were unrelated to disease severity. Although the data are limited, certain congenital defects (e.g., neural tube defects) may occur more frequently in celiac disease, secondary to folic acid malabsorption.[146,147] However, more data are needed before celiac disease is considered a *cause* of birth defects related to folic acid deficiency.

The etiology of reproductive impairment in CD is unknown. A possible mechanism may be malnutrition, especially in those women who have overt malabsorption. An association between reproductive dysfunction and nutritional deficiencies is well-established.[128] Although none of the study patients with subclinical disease and infertility were clinically undernourished, isolated deficiencies are possible.

Clinical evidence, although limited, suggests that treatment of CD improves fertility and pregnancy outcomes. There are reported cases of women with unexplained infertility who were diagnosed with CD, placed on a gluten-free diet, and conceived.[148,149] Women with higher miscarriage rates secondary to CD who subsequently underwent a gluten-free diet had miscarriage rates similar to controls;[133] rates of low birth weight and stillbirths may also be decreased.[145]

Celiac disease is increasingly appreciated as a prevalent disease with variable presentations, and often without gastrointestinal symptoms. Although the evidence is not conclusive, there is awareness that celiac disease is associated with reproductive endocrine disorders. Until more data are available, practitioners that provide care for reproductive age women should carefully elicit classic symptoms for CD (i.e., diarrhea, flatulence, steatorrhea) in any woman with unexplained amenorrhea or infertility, or repeat spontaneous abortions. Once there is a suspicion, celiac antibodies should be measured, and if present, confirmation with small bowel biopsy should be performed. As a reproductive disturbance can be the initial presentation of celiac disease, it may provide an opportunity to initiate effective treatment for a (otherwise asymptomatic) disorder adversely affecting a woman's health.

INFLAMMATORY BOWEL DISEASE

Ulcerative colitis and Crohn's disease are chronic, idiopathic inflammatory diseases of the gastrointestinal tract. Despite distinct pathologic characteristics, they are commonly grouped together as inflammatory bowel disease (IBD) because of shared clinical and epidemiologic features. The prevalence of IBD varies widely (1.6–24.5 per 100,000) based on geographic location. It is much higher in the United States and Europe than in Africa or Asia.[150] Inflammatory bowel disease affects both sexes equally, and the peak age of onset is between 15 and 25 years of age. The etiology is most likely multifactorial.[150]

It appears that women with IBD are subfertile,[151,152] but data on reproductive function in this population are limited. Delayed puberty (Stephens, Weber) and a higher incidence of menstrual disturbances (Weber) have been observed.[153,154] These findings suggest a direct effect of IBD on reproductive function, possibly secondary to the impact of malnutrition on GnRH drive and the hypothalamic-pituitary axis. However, it now appears that the majority of IBD-related subfertility is indirect, resulting not only from changes in patient behavior, but also from the sequelae of surgery. Multiple case studies have suggested that reproductive potential in IBD is reduced only *after* surgical intervention (e.g., proctocolectomy with ileal pouch-anal anastamosis). Olsen et al. performed a systematic 5-year follow-up study of 290 patients and illustrated that the fecundity of patients with medically managed ulcerative colitis was similar to that of a reference population, but that of postsurgical patients was significantly reduced (by 80%) (see Fig. 5-3).[155]

Hysterosalpingograms indicate that subfecundity in postsurgical IBD is attributable to adhesion formation and tubal factor infertility.[155–157] However, it should be recognized that the fertility impact of surgery is dependent on the anatomic site; not all abdominal surgery causes infertility. For example, the fecundity of patients with familial adenomatous polyposis is reduced with ileal pouch-anal anastamosis, but not with subtotal colectomy.[158]

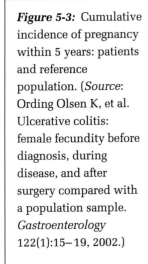

Figure 5-3: Cumulative incidence of pregnancy within 5 years: patients and reference population. (*Source*: Ording Olsen K, et al. Ulcerative colitis: female fecundity before diagnosis, during disease, and after surgery compared with a population sample. *Gastroenterology* 122(1):15–19, 2002.)

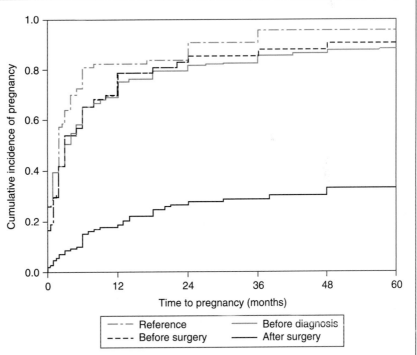

Further, a large cohort of women who had undergone appendectomy in childhood showed no increased incidence of infertility.[159]

IBD may be associated with adverse early pregnancy outcomes. The data suggest that women with Crohn's disease, but not ulcerative colitis, have an increased risk of miscarriage.[152] Moreover, the risk of miscarriage may be increased when disease is active.[160] The etiology is not completely known. Medications used to treat IBD (e.g., sulfasalazine, sulfapyridine, newer 5-aminosalicyclic acids) have not been shown to increase rates of spontaneous abortion or birth defects. Some of these agents inhibit the absorption of folic acid, and increased teratogenecity has not been seen when folic acid is supplemented.[161] Immunosuppressive agents (e.g., azathioprine, 6-mercaptopurine) have shown no impact on early pregnancy outcomes.

KEY POINT

Pelvic adhesive disease following surgical therapy for inflammatory bowel disease is the greatest fertility risk for women with these conditions.

In summary, inflammatory bowel disease impacts the fecundity of women of reproductive age, especially those who have undergone surgical intervention. As for any patient who has undergone abdominal surgery, it is important to obtain a hysterosalpingogram prior to administering fertility treatment (see Chap. 2). Medications used to treat IBD should be continued (and folic acid supplemented), as fertility and early pregnancy outcomes are unlikely to be adversely affected, and are probably improved if disease is better controlled. In women with menstrual disturbances, other causes should be excluded prior to attribution to IBD. Because the risk of infertility is higher in patients with IBD who have undergone surgery, potential reproductive impacts should be discussed with all women considering surgical treatment preoperatively.

Renal Disease

END-STAGE RENAL DISEASE

Chronic renal disease is most commonly secondary to systemic diseases (diabetes, hypertension, connective tissue disorders), but can also have a primary renal cause, including glomerulonephritis, tubulointerstitial, vascular and congenital etiologies. Patients with chronic renal disease can progress along a final common pathway to end-stage renal disease (ESRD), a uremic state defined by a requirement for chronic dialysis or renal transplantation, many without a definitive diagnosis. Although early chronic renal diseases are associated with endocrine abnormalities, these diseases lead to a similar endpoint. For simplicity, this discussion focuses on the impact of ESRD, itself, on reproduction.

End-stage renal disease has significant impact on our society: according to the United States Renal Data System, the prevalence of ESRD in 1996 was 283,932 persons.[162] The incidence increases with age and occurs more frequently in men. However, it affects all age groups and both sexes: over 73,000 of those affected were between the ages of 20 and 44 and approximately 46% were female.[162] Although these patients often develop other conditions (e.g., vascular disease, left ventricular hypertrophy) that can lead to mortality, life expectancy is improved with dialysis and/or transplantation, and complete rehabilitation is the goal. Therefore, reproductive potential remains an important issue for many ESRD patients.

An association between ESRD and reproductive dysfunction is well-established[163–165]; functional derangements include menstrual disturbances, anovulation, and infertility. The degree of dysfunction correlates with the severity of renal deterioration and often persists with treatment: up to 90% of women on dialysis have menstrual abnormalities ranging from menorrhagia to amenorrhea.[166,167] When renal disease is severe, conception and pregnancy rates are impaired: surveys have shown that only 1–7% of women on dialysis become pregnant.[168–170] In contrast to dialysis, renal transplantation offers potential for improvement of menstrual function[105,171–173] and restoration of fertility.

The etiology of ESRD-related menstrual disturbances is unclear, but the current consensus supports hypothalamic-pituitary dysfunction secondary to uremia.[164] FSH levels are typically normal, arguing against a direct ovarian effect. LH levels rise early in ESRD and progress with deteriorating renal function.[164,168,174] Some of this LH elevation has been attributed to decreased metabolic clearance, primarily due to diminished renal filtration since the renal system, at least in men, is responsible for over 40% of LH clearance.[164,175] However, aberrant LH pulsatility is also observed in uremic patients, implying abnormal hypothalamic regulation of GnRH secretion. Furthermore, studies have illustrated that LH responses to exogenous GnRH are inappropriate in patients with ESRD, which supports pituitary dysfunction.[164] In addition, women with chronic renal disease have decreased libido,[176,177] and this may contribute to subfertility in this population.

Elevated serum prolactin levels are common in chronic renal insufficiency and in dialysis patients.[164,178] Historically, changes in prolactin have been attributed to impaired renal filtration, but as prolactin is not significantly dependent on renal function for clearance,[179] increased secretion of prolactin is more likely. Hyperprolactinemia may be an independent factor contributing to menstrual abnormalities, but it is more likely a surrogate for hypo-thalamic-pituitary dysfunction secondary to altered central dopaminergic tone. Prolactin remains elevated in dialysis patients, for whom menstrual dysfunction generally persists, and often resolves after renal transplant, with resumption of menses.

Pregnancy outcomes with ESRD patients are suboptimal with an increased incidence of pregnancy loss observed at all gestational ages. In the Registry of Pregnancy in Dialysis Patients, the incidence of spontaneous abortions overall is 32%, with only 54% of pregnancies reaching the second trimester resulting in a live birth.[180] This outcome is unaffected by method (hemodialysis versus peritoneal dialysis). However, the initiation of dialysis treatment after conception improves pregnancy outcomes. Although maternal mortality rate is not increased over baseline, observations have shown many other pregnancy complications exist for both the mother and fetus. But reports over the past decade indicate that pregnancy outcomes are improving in patients receiving hemodialysis because of advances in dialysis therapy and improvements in obstetrical and neonatal care.[180,181]

Pregnancy after renal transplantation can be successful, but it is considered a high-risk pregnancy.[182] Despite improvements in menstrual function after kidney transplant (versus patients treated with dialysis), similar adverse pregnancy outcomes are observed, with increased rates of abortions, stillbirths, and preterm deliveries. At this time, there are no data on how various immunosuppressive agents such as azathioprine, cyclosporine, and prednisone impact reproductive function, but detrimental effects on pregnancy outcomes have not been observed.[183,184]

There are several cases in the literature that describe controlled ovarian stimulation in renal transplant patients; all resulted in multiple births.[107,185–187] One case was complicated by ovarian hyperstimulation syndrome (OHSS).[186] In this case, on the day of human chorionic gonadotropin (hCG) administration the patient had polycystic-appearing ovaries with 23 follicles and a serum estrodiol level of 4086 pg/mL. She had typical symptoms of OHSS, and a significant rise in serum urea and creatinine, but interestingly, her hematocrit remained within the normal range and she did not develop any evidence of third spacing. It was theorized that postrenal obstruction, secondary to enlarged ovaries, was the cause of her deteriorating renal function. It is not known whether these patients are more susceptible to OHSS. Although the data are scant, it is certainly plausible that renal transplants may have increased susceptibility to obstructive processes, and aggressive ovarian stimulation may carry increased risks. There are no data on fertility treatment in patients receiving dialysis.

The quality of life for women with ESRD has seen marked improvement, and more patients are now attempting to conceive. Since pregnancy outcomes are improving, there is no need to discourage pregnancy in patients who desire fertility treatment, although informed consent is necessary and preconception counseling with a perinatologist should be offered. The modality of fertility treatment should be tailored to the cause of subfertility, although a conservative approach is recommended.

Autoimmune Diseases

There is substantial evidence for an increased risk of spontaneous abortion with autoimmune disease, notably antiphospholipid syndrome (APS) (see Chap. 19). However, the association with other autoimmune disease is less compelling. Furthermore, the causal relationship between autoimmunity and infertility is more controversial, and data are often contradictory. Although the mechanism of how autoimmune disease might affect reproductive function has not been fully elucidated, there is suggestion that the antibodies themselves are a major contributing factor. This association has led to the measurement of antibodies in cases of unexplained infertility or pregnancy loss, even in the absence of clinical signs of disease. The quality of data supporting this practice is questionable, and will not be discussed in this section. The following will focus on the two most common autoimmune diseases, rheumatoid arthritis (RA) and systemic lupus erythematosus (SLE), and briefly discuss the impact of reproductive function using the available literature.

RHEUMATOID ARTHRITIS

Rheumatoid arthritis is a chronic, multisystem inflammatory disease. Although there are a variety of systemic manifestations, the characteristic feature is primarily destruction of the peripheral joints. The development of RA is not completely known; the evidence suggests that the mechanism is due to a combination of genetic (HLA-DRB1 association), and environmental exposure.[188] The prevalence of RA varies from one population to another; in Whites of Europe and North America the prevalence is approximately 1% and the disease is at least twice as common in women than in men.[189] Although the incidence of RA, in general, increases with age, it is relatively prevalent in (~2%) women during the reproductive years.

The literature about whether RA impacts reproductive function is quite limited and controversial. Initially, several studies suggested that nulliparity was present more in women with RA; other observations suggested that pregnancy delayed the onset of RA. Therefore, it was postulated that nulliparity was a risk factor for RA. This observation, although not proving a cause and effect relationship, may be interpreted as an affect of undiagnosed RA.[190] However, follow-up studies did not confirm that parity was associated with RA, and for that reason it remained questionable that RA was associated with infertility.[191] In 1993, resurgence arose questioning whether recent onset RA was associated with fertility; a case-control study directly showed that fecundability (>12 months without pregnancy with unprotected intercourse) was reduced in women with recent onset RA compared to controls.[192] Although the results were significant, bias may have been introduced since the study sample and controls were not matched for baseline characteristics. However, Pope and others recently performed the most complete study to date.[193] They matched the study population with controls for age and marital status and showed that an association between RA and nulliparity, infertility (6 months without pregnancy with unprotected intercourse), and miscarriage does not exist (Table 5-4).[193]

Although there is no consensus that RA has a direct effect on fertility, several reports implicate common therapeutic agents for RA, especially NSAIDs.

NSAIDs are a common cause of reversible infertility.[56,57,194,195] The pharmacologic target for NSAIDs is cycloxygenase (COX). They exert their effect by blocking the synthesis of prostaglandins.[58] The

***Table 5-4.* ODDS RATIOS FOR REPRODUCTIVE OUTCOMES FOR THE WOMEN WITH RHEUMATOID ARTHRITIS AND CONTROLS**

	OR	95% CONFIDENCE INTERVAL	P
Nulliparity	1.4	(0.5–3.9)	0.6
Having been gravid	1.3	(0.5–3.3)	0.5
Infertility (ever)	0.7	(0.3–1.7)	0.4
Infertility and wanted child	0.7	(0.2–2.2)	0.4
OCP			
Ever use	0.6	(0.1–3.1)	0.9
≥5 years' use	1.7	(0.7–3.8)	0.4
Miscarriages	0.8	(0.3–2.5)	0.7
Abortions	0.9	(0.2–4.0)	0.9
Toxemia	0.9	(0.2–3.4)	0.9

Abbreviations: OCP, oral contraceptive pill; nulliparity, no live births; gravid, any pregnancy ever; infertility, regular sexual intercourse for at least 5 months without using contraception without becoming pregnant.

NOTE: The results were unchanged when controlling for level of education and age at first pregnancy for OCP use, miscarriages, abortions, and toxemia. Ratios matched for age and marital status.

SOURCE: Pope JE, Bellamy N, Stevens A. The lack of associations between rheumatoid arthritis and both nulliparity and infertility. *Semin Arthritis Rheum* 28(5):342–350, 1999.

evidence linking NSAIDs to infertility was initially proposed in animal studies showing that ovulation (follicular rupture) was largely dependent on prostaglandin production via COX-2 (see Fig. 5-4).[56,196–198] This was supported by several human studies that showed that a lutueinized unruptured follicles (LUF) can be induced with administration of NSAIDs.[199,200] Evidence for the reversible nature of infertility associated with NSAID use was provided by several case series that described patients originally diagnosed with unexplained infertility that were on long-term NSAIDs, subsequently conceived within a short interval after cessation of treatment.[57,58,193]

There are no data to suggest that fertility treatment exacerbates RA, and this is unlikely as other high estrogenic states (e.g., oral contraceptives and pregnancy) are known to improve symptoms. Rheumatoid arthritis has not been associated with any particular maternal complications, and there are only scarce data suggesting association with adverse fetal outcomes (e.g., IUGR and premature birth).

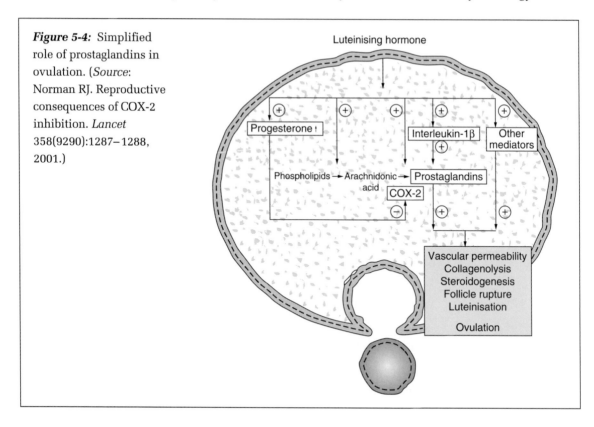

Figure 5-4: Simplified role of prostaglandins in ovulation. (*Source:* Norman RJ. Reproductive consequences of COX-2 inhibition. *Lancet* 358(9290):1287–1288, 2001.)

KEY POINT

While RA, itself, does not increase infertility, a thorough screen of therapeutics with potential adverse effects should be sought.

Prior to fertility treatment, a medication assessment is recommended. NSAIDs should be discontinued. In addition, women with RA may be taking disease-modifying antirheumatic drugs (DMARDs), immunosuppressive agents which are potentially harmful to the fetus (e.g., methotrexate, gold compounds, antimalarials, sulfasalazine leflunomide, cyclosporine, antitumor necrosis factor agents, and cytotoxic drugs). Preconception counseling with a high-risk obstetrical specialist is recommended prior to engaging in fertility therapy.

SYSTEMIC LUPUS ERYTHEMATOSUS

Systemic lupus erythematosus is a complex autoimmune disorder affecting multiple organs, including kidneys, hematologic, joints, and so forth. The etiology like other autoimmune diseases is not clear, but is thought to be multifactorial (i.e., genetic and environmental). The prevalence of SLE is approximately 0.05%; it is higher among Blacks and Asians than Whites[201] and it predominately affects women of childbearing age, with a female to male ratio of 9:1.[202] The clinical manifestations are intermittent and vary from mild to severe. But with treatment of SLE, survival improves and more women are able to remain in remission.

The literature suggests that SLE does not directly impact the ability to conceive.[203] However, certain sequelae of the disease (e.g., lupus nephritis) or common therapies (e.g., cyclophosphamide) can cause reproductive dysfunction. This dysfunction may be temporary, as in the case of renal insufficiency during a lupus flare, but can also be permanent: ovarian failure is a common result of cyclophosphamide therapy (11–59%) and is age-dependent.[204–206] Nonetheless, shorter courses or a lower dose of cyclophosphamide may decrease the chance of ovarian failure especially in older reproductive aged women who have a higher risk of ovarian failure.[206]

On the other hand, the literature does support that SLE is affiliated with early pregnancy loss. The rate of spontaneous abortion in women with SLE is reported to be as high as 35%, substantially higher than the general population.[207] Although the exact mechanism is not clear, certain predictive factors—active renal disease[208] and the presence of antiphospholipid antibodies[207] have been identified. The association with antiphospholipid antibodies is not surprising since primary antiphospholipid syndrome itself is a known disease of recurrent pregnancy loss. Patients with SLE have a predisposition to develop a secondary form of APS, which is clinically indistinguishable from the primary form.

SLE is also associated with adverse pregnancy outcomes.[208–211] The most notable adverse maternal outcome is an increased risk of preeclampsia; disease-specific risk factors include lupus nephritis and the presence of antiphospholipid antibodies. Exacerbation of lupus in pregnancy is controversial, but it is clear that flares can occur in any trimester and in the puerperium period. If the disease is in remission prior to conception, there is a decreased likelihood of exacerbation. Furthermore, SLE is associated with adverse fetal outcomes, including stillbirth, IUGR, and premature birth. These risks are increased in patients with active renal disease or antiphospholipid antibodies.[207]

Although SLE is not believed to have a direct effect on fecundity, women with SLE are frequently in a position where fertility treatment is desired. Some patients delay childbearing in order to achieve disease remission, and others plan to start therapy for their disease process with an agent that can cause ovarian failure (e.g., cyclophosphamide) and desire cryopreservation.

However, there is some concern about the safety of ovulation induction and the resulting high estrogenic state in women with SLE.[212] It is thought that estrogen is involved in the pathogenesis of SLE, with indirect evidence supplied by the predominance of SLE in women during the reproductive years, and in case reports of SLE exacerbations in other high estrogenic states (e.g., combination oral contraceptive therapy and pregnancy).[213,214] In addition, there are several reports that indicate ovulation induction is associated with (mostly mild) lupus flares, thrombophlebetis (in women with antiphospholipid antibodies), and OHSS (in patients with lupus nephritis).[215–217] The largest case series to date (19 patients, over half with primary APS) concluded that ovulation induction does not cause exacerbations, but study subjects with antiphospholipid antibodies received prophylactic therapy.[218] In order to reduce the potential adverse affects of ovulation induction, some clinicians suggest prophylactic therapy: anti-inflammatory agents for all SLE patients, and heparin and/or aspirin for patients with antiphospholipid antibodies (even without a prior history of thrombosis). This practice was initially extrapolated from several studies showing improved pregnancy outcomes with prophylactic therapy in patients with APS[219,220] (see Chap. 19). Prospective studies are needed to support the use of prophylactic therapy in patients with SLE in the absence of APS.

KEY POINT

The associated increased risk for fertility- and pregnancy-related issues, associated with SLE, are in those women with renal disease and/or evidence of antiphospholipid syndrome.

Although data are limited, fertility therapy is generally considered safe for women with SLE, but patients must be fully evaluated to identify potential risk factors, including renal disease or antiphospholipid antibodies. It is prudent to await remission prior to fertility treatment to improve pregnancy outcomes. If antiphospholipid antibodies are present in a woman with SLE, anticoagulant therapy, even in the absence of prior events (e.g., thrombotic, miscarriage), is reasonable despite the lack of data at this time. Preconception counseling prior to fertility therapy with a high-risk obstetrical specialist should be offered to discuss not only adverse pregnancy outcomes, but also medications and their potential for adverse fetal effects.

Infectious Disease

HIV

It is estimated that 850,000–950,000 people are currently living with the human immunodeficiency virus (HIV) in the United States.[221] Approximately 86% are of reproductive age, with women comprising 20% of this group.[222]

Subfertility in women infected with HIV is well-documented.[223,224] While this is attributable, in part, to social and behavioral factors, a recent survey suggests that fertility is reduced independent of contraception use.[225] One possible explanation is a higher prevalence of tubal factor infertility, as the incidence of other sexually transmitted diseases (e.g., chlamydia, gonorrhea) is higher among women infected with HIV. There is also evidence for endocrine dysregulation in a subset of HIV-positive patients.

Some studies argue that HIV does not significantly contribute to menstrual disturbances,[226,227] while others suggest that women with HIV experience anovulation with greater frequency than controls. A recent study showed a 20% prevalence of amenorrhea in women with HIV.[228] Other investigators have illustrated that women with HIV were more likely to experience amenorrhea (or oligomenorrhea) and have less moliminal symptoms than controls, after adjusting for age, CD4 count, and cigarette smoking.[229] This observation suggests that the reproductive disturbance in these women is independent of the severity in disease. However, other studies contend that menstrual disturbances are more likely in patients with higher viral loads and lower CD4 counts, and argue that immunosuppressed women are less likely to ovulate.[230,231]

When amenorrheic women were compared to eumenorrheic women in an HIV-positive population, fasting hyperinsulinemia and insulin-to-glucose ratios were found to be significantly higher in the amenorrheic group.[232] While the mechanism is likely multifactorial, there is a subset for whom a lipodystrophy syndrome—with changes in fat distribution (i.e., increased truncal obesity and reduced subcutaneous fat) and metabolic derangements—is thought to be responsible.[232] Some investigators have argued that this syndrome may be an effect of antiretroviral medications such as protease inhibitors, which are known to cause insulin resistance,[233] but elevated insulin and insulin-to-glucose ratios are observed even in women not receiving protease inhibitor therapy.[232]

Interestingly, women without evidence of this lipodystrophy syndrome are equally likely to experience menstrual disturbances and hyperinsulinemia. In these cases, there were no differences in weight, truncal or total body fat, or free and total testosterone. In the study demonstrating a 20% prevalence of amenorrhea in women with HIV, amenorrhea was found to be independent of BMI.[228] These observations support the existence of additional independent contributions of HIV infection to reproductive dysfunction.

Women infected with HIV can also develop an anovulatory syndrome similar to PCOS. Many women, especially those with wasting syndrome, are androgen-deficient,[234] but a subset of women with lipodystrophy syndrome have been shown to have increased serum androgen levels (particularly total and free testosterone) compared to a matched control population.[235] These women have significantly increased LH/FSH ratios and decreased SHBG levels, consistent with what has been observed in a subset of women with PCOS (see Chap. 8). To date the ovarian morphology has not been well studied, but two recent case reports have described polycystic-appearing ovaries in this population.[236,237]

In 1994, the Ethics Committee of the American Society of Reproductive Medicine expressed significant concerns about offering assisted reproductive techniques to HIV-positive patients, including the risk of transmission to partner or offspring, and the likelihood of hardship for children due to the shortened life span of infected parents. However, the last decade has seen considerable improvements in treatment: the transmission of HIV with optimal care (combination antiretroviral therapy and/or an elective cesarean section) is now less than 2% (International Perinatal HIV Group) and life expectancy (and quality of life) have dramatically improved.[238] In light of these advances, the Ethics Committee now recommends that infertility treatment may be offered to patients infected with HIV, but must include appropriate evaluation, counseling, and follow-up.[222]

Infertility treatment can also affect transmission rates in discordant couples. It is a difficult decision to conceive naturally in discordant couples because of the risk for seroconversion

KEY POINT

*Assisted
reproduction may
decrease
transmission of HIV
to partners and
offspring.*

and vertical transmission. If a man is HIV positive and a female partner is HIV negative, the woman has approximately a 0.1–0.2% risk of seroconverting with an act of unprotected intercourse.[239–241] With repeated timed intercourse, the rate of transmission may increase, posing serious risks to the woman and child. Since, the HIV virus is located in semen and has not been shown to infect spermatozoa, sperm washing techniques such as the density gradient are very effective at removing HIV, and with the addition of polymerase chain reaction (PCR) verification, the risk of transmission from seropositive male partners to mothers and children is virtually eliminated.[242,243] However, studies evaluating the safety of intrauterine insemination (IUI) are still in progress and couples need to be cautioned about the potential risk. If the woman is HIV positive and the man is HIV negative, seroconversion of the male partner can be reduced with an IUI. If both partners are infected with HIV, and there is no concern for transmission between partners, it is important to assess the health of each person, and to offer preconception counseling regarding effective ways of reducing vertical transmission.

TUBERCULOSIS

Approximately 2 billion people—one-third of the world's population—are infected with tuberculosis (TB), and an estimated 2 million persons die each year from the disease.[244] Eight million new cases of TB were reported in 1997, with over 50% of these occurring in Southeast Asia.[245] Despite the persistence of this global burden, there has been a dramatic decline in TB infections in the United States since 1992 (15,078 cases in 2002, a decline of 43.5% from 1992). A resurgence of TB prior to 1992—attributable to the HIV epidemic, immigration, and deterioration in infrastructure—has since been reversed with stronger policies to control ongoing transmission. However, not all ethnic groups benefit equally from control measures: Blacks, Hispanics, and foreign-born persons have the highest TB rate in the United States.[244] Tuberculosis contributes directly to infertility by infecting the female reproductive tract. Genital tuberculosis (GT) can occasionally be the primary site of infection if a male partner is infected and transmission is sexual, but GT is almost always preceded by infection in other organs, usually the lungs.[246] It is estimated that pulmonary TB disseminates to the genital tract in 5–15% of cases (Rock). The

Table 5-5. INCIDENCE OF GENITAL TUBERCULOSIS

AUTHORS	YEAR	COUNTRY	INCIDENCE (%)
Schaffer	1976	United States	1
Padubridi	1980	India	4
Margelis K, et al.	1992	South Africa	6.2
De Vynck WE, et al.	1990	South Africa	8.7
Emenobolu J, et al.	1993	North Nigeria	16.7
Tripathy and Tripathy	2001	India	3

SOURCE: Tripathy SN. Infertility and pregnancy outcome in female genital tuberculosis. *Int J Gynaecol Obstet* 76(2): 159–163, 2002.

fallopian tubes are the most common site of initial involvement, with subsequent direct extension to the endometrium (50–90% of cases), ovaries (20–30%), and cervix (5–15%).[247,248] Infection can lead to adhesion formation, tubal blockage, or tuboovarian masses, all of which can contribute to infertility.[249] The prevalence of GT in infertile patients varies widely with geography (from less than 1 to 16%). The reported incidence in the United States is approximately 1% (see Table 5-5).[250]

Infertility is, in fact, the most frequent (75%) presenting complaint in women with GT.[248] Other presenting symptoms include abdominal or pelvic pain, abnormal bleeding (less than 20%) or peritonitis, and tuboovarian abscesses (rare). Since symptomatic manifestations are rare, and clinical suspicion is usually low, GT is a challenging diagnosis in the setting of infertility. It is important to identify patients at high risk, including foreign immigrants (especially from Asia) and patients with a history of pulmonary TB. Hysterosalpingogram characteristics include a "lead pipe" appearance of the fallopian tubes, calcification of the adnexa, bilateral cornual block, and shriveled or obliterated uterine cavity.[250] Definitive diagnosis of GT is made with positive cultures of mycobacteria from the genital tract, but the use of histopathologic criteria—granulomas and Langhan's giant cells on tissue biopsy—is also well-accepted.[247] Menstrual secretions can also be cultured for mycobacteria in approximately 70% of cases.[251]

KEY POINT

A high index of suspicion for genital TB should guide management in recent immigrants from Southeast Asia.

Treatment of GT infertility begins with antituberculosis therapy. Historically, pregnancy outcomes after treatment (medical and surgical) have been generally poor, and the risks of ectopic pregnancy and spontaneous abortion are increased.[252–254] Pregnancy rates can now be significantly improved with *in vitro* fertilization (IVF) (16–25% per transfer),[249,254] but success remains dependent on normal endometrial function. One study demonstrated a 42.9% pregnancy rate in patients with GT and trophic endometrium, and 0% in patients with atrophic endometrium.[247] An initial investigation of the endometrium, given the high rate of uterine extension, is warranted prior to initiating IVF in patients with GT.

What's the Evidence?

- Several studies have investigated a possible causal relationship between psychopathology and infertility. Results are conflicting. There is a strong relationship between the experience of psychologic distress and infertility, particularly following unsuccessful treatment.[2–6] Studies during IVF have shown that baseline stress was found to influence all outcomes measured while procedural stress affected on the number of oocytes retrieved with IVF.[11] Psychologic intervention may improve treatment outcome.[9]

- Epilepsy is associated with a higher frequency of anovulation than is seen in the general population.[19–21] Even women with treated epilepsy appear to be at increased risk for infertility[26] and premature ovarian failure.[27] Treatment for epilepsy may also increase risk of ovulatory dysfunction.[29–31]

- INF-beta treatment, for multiple sclerosis, may cause menstrual disorders and increase risk of abortion.[38]

- The dose of insulin used by patients with type I diabetes appears to correlate with the degree of subfertility.[80] Poor glycemic control, with either type I or type II diabetes, is associated with increased risk for pregnancy loss.[89–91]

- Several studies have shown that the prevalence of silent celiac disease is higher among infertile women.[136–138] It has been further estimated that 4–6% of women with unexplained infertility have undiagnosed celiac disease.[136,137]

- Several case studies have provided evidence that the usage of NSAIDs causes a reversible form of unexplained infertility.[57,58,193]

Discussion of Cases

CASE 1

History   A 27-year-old female and her partner come to your office for an infertility evaluation. The patient reports menarche at age 13 followed by regular, cyclic, predictable menses. Over the last 2–3 years, she has noticed a progressive lessening of menstrual flow and increased interval between cycles. Over the last year, she has had no menses. The patient has some constipation, but no other GI symptoms. She denies vasomotor symptoms, galactorrhea, or any change in hair growth. She does report a back injury, 3 years prior to presentation, for which she has been on chronic treatment. The patient takes daily narcotics for pain relief.

Physical Examination   On examination, the patient is 65 cm and weighs 115 lb. Her BP and pulse are normal. She has no evidence of hair growth or skin changes and breast development is normal. On pelvic examination, the vagina is pale and flat and no cervical mucus is seen. Bimanual examination is normal.

What laboratory testing would you request?
FSH, estradiol, prolactin, thyroid-stimulating hormone (TSH)

The patient appears to be hypoestrogenic having amenorrhea and evidence of estrogen deficiency on examination. Estrogen deficiency can be caused by either a failure of the ovary or a failure of the central nervous system to "signal" the ovary to produce follicles and estrogen.

Results:
FSH: 1.2 mIU/mL
Estradiol: 22 pg/mL
Prolactin: 7 ng/mL
TSH: 3.2 mIU/L

These findings are consistent with hypogonadotropic hypogonadism.

What are possible causes of this abnormality?

Possible causes of hypogonadotropic hypogonadism are congenital (Kallman's syndrome), central tumor, and functional (stress, exercise, low body weight). This patient had normal puberty and regular cycles prior to the amenorrhea and thus does not have congenital hypogonadism. Tumors that suppress gonadotropins tend to be large and would be expected to suppress prolactin and TSH as well. As these values are normal, this is also unlikely. Therefore, the patient most likely has a functional cause of her amenorrhea.

Closer questioning of this patient does not reveal any excessive exercise (in fact, the patient's pain prohibits most strenuous activity) or any evidence of an eating disorder. And, while her weight is low, it does not meet criteria likely to induce amenorrhea. What other causes might there be for her condition?

The patient may well have stress due to the chronic pain, but may also have gonadotropin suppression from her chronic opiate usage. It turns out the patient is currently treated with Dilaudid 4–8 mg at least four times daily. It is recommended the patient wean off her narcotics as you suspect hypothalamic suppres-

sion due to the chronic opiate usage. Over a 6-month period of time, the patient is able to considerably lessen her usage of narcotics (although she has not stopped completely). Her cycles gradually return.

Are there any other precautions or considerations regarding a change in her medication?

You should assure she is not moving to NSAIDs as these may allow resumption of menses, but interfere with either follicle rupture or implantation.

Once the patient has significantly decreased her narcotics and stopped NSIADs, she conceives within two cycles.

CASE 2

History A 35-year-old nulligravid female presents for an infertility evaluation with her husband. They have been extensively evaluated without a cause of infertility being identified. The female partner has had documentation of ovulation, including an endometrial biopsy that was normal. She has also had normal cycle day 3 testing of ovarian reserve. She has also had a laparoscopy showing normal pelvic anatomy. Her husband has had a normal semen analysis.

The patient's medical history is negative. She currently takes no medications or OTC products. You take a careful review of systems and find the patient has some nonspecific GI

symptoms including flatus and occasional diarrhea. She also has some abdominal bloating on occasion. Interestingly, although, she has no family history of osteoporosis, she was told at a health fair, where she had a heel ultrasound, that she may have low bone density.

What test might be indicated in this patient?

Antitissue transglutaminase antibodies. Testing is positive. You place the patient on a gluten-free diet. Surprisingly, her GI symptoms improve dramatically and within 4 months, the patient has conceived.

REFERENCES

1 Kuehner C. Gender differences in unipolar depression: an update of epidemiological findings and possible explanations. *Acta Psychiatr Scand* 108(3):163–174, 2003.

2 Stoleru S, et al. Psychological characteristics of infertile patients: discriminating etiological factors from reactive changes. *J Psychosom Obstet Gynaecol* 17(2):103–118, 1996.

3   Stoleru S, et al. Psychological factors in the aetiology of infertility: a prospective cohort study. *Hum Reprod* 8(7):1039–1046, 1993.

4   Mazure CM, Greenfeld DA. Psychological studies of in vitro fertilization/embryo transfer participants. *J In Vitro Fert Embryo Transf* 6(4):242–256, 1989.

5   Lee TY, Sun GH, Chao SC. The effect of an infertility diagnosis on treatment–related stresses. *Arch Androl* 46(1):67–71, 2001.

6   Moller A. Infertility is not only a medical phenomenon but a life crisis. *Lakartidningen* 86(37):3037–3041, 1989.

7   Fassino S, et al. Anxiety, depression and anger suppression in infertile couples: a controlled study. *Hum Reprod* 17(11):2986–2994, 2002.

8   Fassino S, et al. Temperament and character in couples with fertility disorders: a double-blind, controlled study. *Fertil Steril* 77(6): 1233–1240, 2002.

9   Domar AD, et al. Impact of group psychological interventions on pregnancy rates in infertile women. *Fertil Steril* 73(4):805–811, 2000.

10   McNaughton-Cassill ME, et al. Development of brief stress management support groups for couples undergoing in vitro fertilization treatment. *Fertil Steril* 74(1):87–93, 2000.

11   Klonoff-Cohen H, et al. A prospective study of stress among women undergoing in vitro fertilization or gamete intrafallopian transfer. *Fertil Steril* 76(4):675–687, 2001.

12   Klock SC, Greenfeld DA. Psychological status of in vitro fertilization patients during pregnancy: a longitudinal study. *Fertil Steril* 73(6):1159–1164, 2000.

13   Cowen PJ, Sargent PA. Changes in plasma prolactin during SSRI treatment: evidence for a delayed increase in 5-HT neurotransmission. *J Psychopharmacol* 11(4):345–348, 1997.

14   Peterson MC. Reversible galactorrhea and prolactin elevation related to fluoxetine use. *Mayo Clin Proc* 76(2):215–216, 2001.

15   Kulin NA, et al. Pregnancy outcome following maternal use of the new selective serotonin reuptake inhibitors: a prospective controlled multicenter study. *JAMA* 279(8):609–610, 1998.

16   Hendrick V, et al. Birth outcomes after prenatal exposure to antidepressant medication. *Am J Obstet Gynecol* 188(3):812–815, 2003.

17   Hauser WA, Annegers JF, Rocca WA. Descriptive epidemiology of epilepsy: contributions of population-based studies from Rochester, Minnesota. *Mayo Clin Proc* 71(6):576–586, 1996.

18   Yerby MS. Pregnancy, teratogenesis, and epilepsy. *Neurol Clin* 12(4):749–771, 1994.

19 Herzog AG. A relationship between particular reproductive endocrine disorders and the laterality of epileptiform discharges in women with epilepsy. *Neurology* 43(10):1907–1910, 1993.

20 Bauer J, et al. Reproductive dysfunction in women with epilepsy: recommendations for evaluation and management. *J Neurol Neurosurg Psychiatr* 73(2):121–125, 2002.

21 Herzog AG, et al. Reproductive endocrine disorders in women with partial seizures of temporal lobe origin. *Arch Neurol* 43(4):341–346, 1986.

22 Herzog AG, et al. Temporal lobe epilepsy: an extrahypothalamic pathogenesis for polycystic ovarian syndrome? *Neurology* 34(10):1389–1393, 1984.

23 Drislane FW, et al. Altered pulsatile secretion of luteinizing hormone in women with epilepsy. *Neurology* 44(2):306–310, 1994.

24 Gerendai I, Halasz B. Neuroendocrine asymmetry. *Front Neuroendocrinol* 18(3):354–381, 1997.

25 Nordeen EJ, Yahr P. Hemispheric asymmetries in the behavioral and hormonal effects of sexually differentiating mammalian brain. *Science* 218(4570):391–394, 1982.

26 Wallace H, Shorvon S, Tallis R. Age-specific incidence and prevalence rates of treated epilepsy in an unselected population of 2,052,922 and age-specific fertility rates of women with epilepsy. *Lancet* 352(9145):1970–1973, 1998.

27 Klein P, Serje A, Pezzullo JC. Premature ovarian failure in women with epilepsy. *Epilepsia* 42(12):1584–1589, 2001.

28 Morrell MJ, et al. Predictors of ovulatory failure in women with epilepsy. *Ann Neurol* 52(6):704–711, 2002.

29 Isojarvi JI, et al. Obesity and endocrine disorders in women taking valproate for epilepsy. *Ann Neurol* 39(5):579–584, 1996.

30 Isojarvi JI, et al. Valproate, lamotrigine, and insulin-mediated risks in women with epilepsy. *Ann Neurol* 43(4):446–451, 1998.

31 Isojarvi JI, et al. Polycystic ovaries and hyperandrogenism in women taking valproate for epilepsy. *N Engl J Med* 329(19):1383–1388, 1993.

32 Olafsson E, Hauser WA, Gudmundsson G. Fertility in patients with epilepsy: a population-based study. *Neurology* 51(1):71–73, 1998.

33 Murialdo G, et al. Effects of valproate, phenobarbital, and carbamazepine on sex steroid setup in women with epilepsy. *Clin Neuropharmacol* 21(1):52–58, 1998.

34 Murialdo G, et al. Menstrual cycle and ovary alterations in women with epilepsy on antiepileptic therapy. *J Endocrinol Invest* 20(9):519–526, 1997.

35 Morrell MJ, et al. Health issues for women with epilepsy: a descriptive survey to assess knowledge and awareness among healthcare providers. *J Womens Health Gend Based Med* 9(9):959–965, 2000.

36 Hernan MA, Olek MJ, Ascherio A. Geographic variation of MS incidence in two prospective studies of US women. *Neurology* 53(8): 1711–1718, 1999.

37 Grinsted L, et al. Serum sex hormone and gonadotropin concentrations in premenopausal women with multiple sclerosis. *J Intern Med* 226(4):241–244, 1989.

38 Walther EU, Hohlfeld R. Multiple sclerosis: side effects of interferon beta therapy and their management. *Neurology* 53(8):1622–1627, 1999.

39 Shenkenberg TD, Von Hoff DD. Possible mitoxantrone-induced amenorrhea. *Cancer Treat Rep* 70(5):659–661, 1986.

40 Blumenfeld Z. Preservation of fertility and ovarian function and minimalization of chemotherapy associated gonadotoxicity and premature ovarian failure: the role of inhibin-A and -B as markers. *Mol Cell Endocrinol* 187(1–2):93–105, 2002.

41 Mueller BA, Zhang J, Critchlow CW. Birth outcomes and need for hospitalization after delivery among women with multiple sclerosis. *Am J Obstet Gynecol* 186(3):446–452, 2002.

42 Lorenzi AR, Ford HL. Multiple sclerosis and pregnancy. *Postgrad Med J* 78(922):460–464, 2002.

43 Piccinni MP, Maggi E, Romagnani S. Role of hormone-controlled T-cell cytokines in the maintenance of pregnancy. *Biochem Soc Trans* 28(2):212–215, 2000.

44 Zorgdrager A, De Keyser J. The premenstrual period and exacerbations in multiple sclerosis. *Eur Neurol* 48(4):204–206, 2002.

45 Worthington J, et al. Pregnancy and multiple sclerosis: a 3-year prospective study. *J Neurol* 241(4):228–233, 1994.

46 Kornstein SG, Parker AJ. Menstrual migraines: etiology, treatment, and relationship to premenstrual syndrome. *Curr Opin Obstet Gynecol* 9(3):154–159, 1997.

47 Mannix LK. Management of menstrual migraine. *Neurology* 9(4):207–213, 2003.

48 Au KL, Woo JS, Wong VC. Intrauterine death from ergotamine overdosage. *Eur J Obstet Gynecol Reprod Biol* 19(5):313–315, 1985.

49 Raymond GV. Teratogen update: ergot and ergotamine. *Teratology* 51(5):344–347, 1995.

50 de Groot AN, et al. Ergotamine-induced fetal stress: review of side effects of ergot alkaloids during pregnancy. *Eur J Obstet Gynecol Reprod Biol* 51(1):73–77, 1993.

51 Lippert TH, Bohm HR. The risk of dihydroergotamine treatment in pregnancy. *Geburtshilfe Frauenheilkd* 42(12):866–867, 1982.

52 Loder E. Safety of sumatriptan in pregnancy: a review of the data so far. *CNS Drugs* 17(1):1–7, 2003.

53 Fox AW, et al. Evidence-based assessment of pregnancy outcome after sumatriptan exposure. *Headache* 42(1):8–15, 2002.

54 Shuhaiber S, et al. Pregnancy outcome following first trimester exposure to sumatriptan. *Neurology* 51(2):581–583, 1998.

55 Duffy DM, Stouffer RL. Follicular administration of a cyclooxygenase inhibitor can prevent oocyte release without alteration of normal luteal function in rhesus monkeys. *Hum Reprod* 17(11): 2825–2831, 2002.

56 Stone S, Khamashta MA, Nelson-Piercy C. Nonsteroidal anti-inflammatory drugs and reversible female infertility: is there a link? *Drug Saf* 25(8):545–551, 2002.

57 Mendonca LL, et al. Non-steroidal anti-inflammatory drugs as a possible cause for reversible infertility. *Rheumatology* (Oxford) 39(8):880–882, 2000.

58 Smith G, et al. Reversible ovulatory failure associated with the development of luteinized unruptured follicles in women with inflammatory arthritis taking non-steroidal anti-inflammatory drugs. *Br J Rheumatol* 35(5):458–462, 1996.

59 Arze RS, et al. Amenorrhoea, galactorrhoea, and hyperprolactinaemia induced by methyldopa. *Br Med J (Clin Res Ed)* 283(6285): 194, 1981.

60 Gluskin LE, Strasberg B, Shah JH. Verapamil-induced hyperprolactinemia and galactorrhea. *Ann Intern Med* 95(1):66–67, 1981.

61 Rey E, Couturier A. The prognosis of pregnancy in women with chronic hypertension. *Am J Obstet Gynecol* 171(2):410–416, 1994.

62 Magee LA. Drugs in pregnancy. Antihypertensives. *Best Pract Res Clin Obstet Gynaecol* 15(6):827–845, 2001.

63 Rosenthal T, Oparil S. The effect of antihypertensive drugs on the fetus. *J Hum Hypertens* 16(5):293–298, 2002.

64 De Assis SM, Seguro AC, Helou CM. Effects of maternal hypercholesterolemia on pregnancy and development of offspring. *Pediatr Nephrol* 18(4):328–334, 2003.

65 Mannino DM, et al. Surveillance for asthma—United States, 1980–1999. *MMWR Surveill Summ* 51(1):1–13, 2002.

66 Grodstein F, et al. Self-reported use of pharmaceuticals and primary ovulatory infertility. *Epidemiology* 4(2):151–156, 1993.

67   Martinez-Rueda JO, et al. Factors associated with fetal losses in severe systemic lupus erythematosus. *Lupus* 5(2):113–119, 1996.

68   Carmichael SL, Shaw GM. Maternal corticosteroid use and risk of selected congenital anomalies. *Am J Med Genet* 86(3):242–244, 1999.

69   Olefsky JM. Insulin resistance and the pathogenesis of non-insulin dependent diabetes mellitus: cellular and molecular mechanisms. *Adv Exp Med Biol* 334:129–150, 1993.

70   Roman SH, Harris MI. Management of diabetes mellitus from a public health perspective. *Endocrinol Metab Clin North Am* 26(3):443–474, 1997.

71   Yeshaya A, et al. Menstrual characteristics of women suffering from insulin-dependent diabetes mellitus. *Int J Fertil Menopausal Stud* 40(5):269–273, 1995.

72   Kjaer K, et al. Epidemiology of menarche and menstrual disturbances in an unselected group of women with insulin-dependent diabetes mellitus compared to controls. *J Clin Endocrinol Metab* 75(2):524–529, 1992.

73   Strotmeyer ES, et al. Menstrual cycle differences between women with type 1 diabetes and women without diabetes. *Diabetes Care* 26(4):1016–1021, 2003.

74   Adcock CJ, et al. Menstrual irregularities are more common in adolescents with type 1 diabetes: association with poor glycaemic control and weight gain. *Diabet Med* 11(5):465–470, 1994.

75   Djursing H. Hypothalamic-pituitary-gonadal function in insulin treated diabetic women with and without amenorrhea. *Dan Med Bull* 34(3):139–147, 1987.

76   Laughlin GA, Dominguez CE, Yen SS. Nutritional and endocrine-metabolic aberrations in women with functional hypothalamic amenorrhea. *J Clin Endocrinol Metab* 83(1):25–32, 1998.

77   Marshall JC, Eagleson CA, McCartney CR. Hypothalamic dysfunction. *Mol Cell Endocrinol* 183(1–2):29–32, 2001.

78   Warren MP. Health issues for women athletes: exercise-induced amenorrhea. *J Clin Endocrinol Metab* 84(6):1892–1896, 1999.

79   Djursing H, et al. Depressed prolactin levels in diabetic women with anovulation. *Acta Obstet Gynecol Scand* 61(5):403–406, 1982.

80   Briese V, Muller H. Diabetes mellitus—an epidemiologic study of fertility, contraception and sterility. *Geburtshilfe Frauenheilkd* 55(5):270–274, 1995.

81   Temple R, et al. Association between outcome of pregnancy and glycaemic control in early pregnancy in type 1 diabetes: population based study. *BMJ* 325(7375):1275–1276, 2002.

82 Dorman JS, et al. Menopause in type 1 diabetic women: is it premature? *Diabetes* 50(8):1857–1862, 2001.

83 Sir-Petermann T. Angel B, Maliqueo M, Carvajal F, Santos JL, Perez-Bravo F. Prevalence of Type II diabetes mellitus and insulin resistance in parents of women with polycystic ovary syndrome. *Diabetologia* 45(7):959–964, 2002.

84 Kaufman FR Type 2 diabetes mellitus in children and youth: a new epidemic. *J Pediatr Endocrinol Metab.* 15 Suppl 2:737–744, 2002.

85 Brydon P, et al. Pregnancy outcome in women with type 2 diabetes mellitus needs to be addressed. *Int J Clin Pract* 54(7):418–419, 2000.

86 Lorenzen T, et al. A population-based survey of frequencies of self-reported spontaneous and induced abortions in Danish women with Type 1 diabetes mellitus. Danish IDDM Epidemiology and Genetics Group. *Diabet Med* 16(6):472–476, 1999.

87 Dorman JS, et al. Temporal trends in spontaneous abortion associated with Type 1 diabetes. *Diabetes Res Clin Pract* 43(1):41–47, 1999.

88 Mills JL, et al. Incidence of spontaneous abortion among normal women and insulin-dependent diabetic women whose pregnancies were identified within 21 days of conception. *N Engl J Med* 319(25):1617–1623, 1988.

89 Hanson U, Persson B, Thunell S. Relationship between haemoglobin A1C in early type 1 (insulin-dependent) diabetic pregnancy and the occurrence of spontaneous abortion and fetal malformation in Sweden. *Diabetologia* 33(2):100–104, 1990.

90 Langer O, Conway DL. Level of glycemia and perinatal outcome in pregestational diabetes. *J Matern Fetal Med* 9(1):35–41, 2000.

91 Razna I, et al. Influence of pre-conception pregnancy planning in women with diabetes mellitus I on the number of spontaneous abortions and major congenital malformations in their children. *Ginekol Pol* 70(10):744–752, 1999.

92 Moley KH. Hyperglycemia and apoptosis: mechanisms for congenital malformations and pregnancy loss in diabetic women. *Trends Endocrinol Metab* 12(2):78–82, 2001.

93 O'Hare JA, Eichold BH 2nd, Vignati L. Hypogonadotropic secondary amenorrhea in diabetes: effects of central opiate blockade and improved metabolic control. *Am J Med* 83(6):1080–1084, 1987.

94 Kane M. Global programme for control of hepatitis B infection. *Vaccine* 13(Suppl 1):S47–S49, 1995.

95 Poovorawan Y, Chatchatee P, Chongsrisawat V. Epidemiology and prophylaxis of viral hepatitis: a global perspective. *J Gastroenterol Hepatol* 17(Suppl):S155–S166, 2002.

96 Kim WR. The burden of hepatitis C in the United States. *Hepatology* 36(5 Suppl 1):S30–S34, 2002.

97 Maddrey WC. Alcohol-induced liver disease. *Clin Liver Dis* 4(1):115–131, vii, 2000.

98 Lieber CS. Susceptibility to alcohol-related liver injury. *Alcohol Alcohol Suppl* 2:315–326, 1994.

99 Yoshihara H, Noda K, Kamada T. Interrelationship between alcohol intake, hepatitis C, liver cirrhosis, and hepatocellular carcinoma. *Recent Dev Alcohol* 14:457–469, 1998.

100 Degos F. Hepatitis C and alcohol. *J Hepatol* 31(Suppl 1):113–118, 1999.

101 Laifer SA, Guido RS. Reproductive function and outcome of pregnancy after liver transplantation in women. *Mayo Clin Proc* 70(4):388–394, 1995.

102 Van Thiel DH, Gavaler JS, Schade RR. Liver disease and the hypothalamic pituitary gonadal axis. *Semin Liver Dis* 5(1):35–45, 1985.

103 Cundy TF, et al. Amenorrhoea in women with non-alcoholic chronic liver disease. *Gut* 32(2):202–206, 1991.

104 Parolin MB, et al. Normalization of menstrual cycles and pregnancy after liver transplantation. *Arq Gastroenterol* 37(1):3–6, 2000.

105 Cundy TF, O'Grady JG, Williams R. Recovery of menstruation and pregnancy after liver transplantation. *Gut* 31(3):337–338, 1990.

106 Armenti VT, et al. Pregnancy after liver transplantation. *Liver Transpl* 6(6):671–685, 2000.

107 Case AM, et al. Successful twin pregnancy in a dual-transplant couple resulting from in-vitro fertilization and intracytoplasmic sperm injection: case report. *Hum Reprod* 15(3):626–628, 2000.

108 Hanson EH, Imperatore G, Burke W. HFE gene and hereditary hemochromatosis: a HuGE review. Human genome epidemiology. *Am J Epidemiol* 154(3):193–206, 2001.

109 Burke W, et al. Hereditary hemochromatosis: gene discovery and its implications for population-based screening. *JAMA* 280(2):172–178, 1998.

110 Moirand R, et al. Clinical features of genetic hemochromatosis in women compared with men. *Ann Intern Med* 127(2):105–110, 1997.

111 Roetto A, et al. Juvenile hemochromatosis locus maps to chromosome 1q. *Am J Hum Genet* 64(5):1388–1393, 1999.

112 Camaschella C, Roetto A, De Gobbi M. Juvenile hemochromatosis. *Semin Hematol* 39(4):242–248, 2002.

113 Kelly AL, et al. Hereditary juvenile haemochromatosis: a genetically heterogeneous life-threatening iron-storage disease. *QJM* 91(9):607–618, 1998.

114 De Gobbi M, et al. Natural history of juvenile haemochromatosis. *Br J Haematol* 117(4):973–979, 2002.

115 Pedersen-Bjergaard U, Thorsteinsson B, Kirkegaard BC. Pituitary function in hemochromatosis. *Ugeskr Laeger* 158(13):1818–1822, 1996.

116 Kelly TM, et al. Hypogonadism in hemochromatosis: reversal with iron depletion. *Ann Intern Med* 101(5):629–632, 1984.

117 Meyer WR, et al. Secondary hypogonadism in hemochromatosis. *Fertil Steril* 54(4):740–742, 1990.

118 Siminoski K, D'Costa M, Walfish PG. Hypogonadotropic hypogonadism in idiopathic hemochromatosis: evidence for combined hypothalamic and pituitary involvement. *J Endocrinol Invest* 13(10):849–853, 1990.

119 Oerter KE, et al. Multiple hormone deficiencies in children with hemochromatosis. *J Clin Endocrinol Metab* 76(2):357–361, 1993.

120 Duranteau L, et al. Non-responsiveness of serum gonadotropins and testosterone to pulsatile GnRH in hemochromatosis suggesting a pituitary defect. *Acta Endocrinol* (Copenh) 128(4):351–354, 1993.

121 Sparacia G, et al. Magnetic resonance imaging of the pituitary gland in patients with secondary hypogonadism due to transfusional hemochromatosis. *MAGMA* 8(2):87–90, 1999.

122 Sparacia G, et al. Transfusional hemochromatosis: quantitative relation of MR imaging pituitary signal intensity reduction to hypogonadotropic hypogonadism. *Radiology* 215(3):818–823, 2000.

123 Vogt HJ, et al. Idiopathic hemochromatosis in a 45-year-old infertile man. *Andrologia* 19(5):532–538, 1987.

124 Hamer OW, et al. Successful treatment of erectile dysfunction and infertility by venesection in a patient with primary haemochromatosis. *Eur J Gastroenterol Hepatol* 13(8):985–988, 2001.

125 Farina G, et al. Successful pregnancy following gonadotropin therapy in a young female with juvenile idiopathic hemochromatosis and secondary hypogonadotropic hypogonadism. *Haematologica* 80(4):335–337, 1995.

126 Collin P, et al. Endocrinological disorders and celiac disease. *Endocr Rev* 23(4):464–483, 2002.

127 Farrell RJ, Kelly CP. Celiac sprue. *N Engl J Med* 346(3):180–188, 2002.

128 Rostami K, et al. High prevalence of celiac disease in apparently healthy blood donors suggests a high prevalence of undiagnosed celiac disease in the Dutch population. *Scand J Gastroenterol* 34(3):276–279, 1999.

129 Lebenthal E, Branski D. Celiac disease: an emerging global problem. *J Pediatr Gastroenterol Nutr* 35(4):472–474, 2002.

130 Ferguson A. Celiac disease, an eminently treatable condition, may be underdiagnosed in the United States. *Am J Gastroenterol* 92(8):1252–1254, 1997.

131 Hin H, et al. Coeliac disease in primary care: case finding study. *BMJ* 318(7177):164–167, 1999.

132 Smecuol E, et al. Gynaecological and obstetric disorders in coeliac disease: frequent clinical onset during pregnancy or the puerperium. *Eur J Gastroenterol Hepatol* 8(1):63–89, 1996.

133 Sher KS, Mayberry JF. Female fertility, obstetric and gynaecological history in coeliac disease: a case control study. *Acta Paediatr Suppl* 412:76–77, 1996.

134 Rujner J, Metera M, Grajkowska W. Delayed puberty in an 18-year-old female patient with late diagnosis of celiac disease. *Pol Tyg Lek* 45(38–39):790–791, 1990.

135 Rujner J. Age at menarche in girls with celiac disease. *Ginekol Pol* 70(5):359–362, 1999.

136 Meloni GF, et al. The prevalence of coeliac disease in infertility. *Hum Reprod* 14(11):2759–2761, 1999.

137 Collin P, et al. Infertility and coeliac disease. *Gut* 39(3):382–384, 1996.

138 Vancikova Z, et al. The serologic screening for celiac disease in the general population (blood donors) and in some high-risk groups of adults (patients with autoimmune diseases, osteoporosis and infertility) in the Czech Republic. *Folia Microbiol (Praha)* 47(6):753–758, 2002.

139 Rostami K, et al. Coeliac disease and reproductive disorders: a neglected association. *Eur J Obstet Gynecol Reprod Biol* 96(2):146–149, 2001.

140 Ciacci C, et al. Celiac disease and pregnancy outcome. *Am J Gastroenterol* 91(4):718–722, 1996.

141 Sher KS, et al. Infertility, obstetric and gynaecological problems in coeliac sprue. *Dig Dis* 12(3):186–190, 1994.

142 Foschi F, et al. Celiac disease and spontaneous abortion. *Minerva Ginecol* 54(2):151–159, 2002.

143 Gasbarrini A, et al. Recurrent spontaneous abortion and intrauterine fetal growth retardation as symptoms of coeliac disease. *Lancet* 356(9227):399–400, 2000.

144 Martinelli P, et al. Coeliac disease and unfavourable outcome of pregnancy. *Gut* 46(3):332–335, 2000.

145 Norgard B, et al. Birth outcomes of women with celiac disease: a nationwide historical cohort study. *Am J Gastroenterol* 94(9): 2435–2440, 1999.

146 Dickey W, et al. Screening for coeliac disease as a possible maternal risk factor for neural tube defect. *Clin Genet* 49(2):107–108, 1996.

147 Hozyasz KK. Coeliac disease and birth defects in offspring. *Gut* 49(5):738, 2001.

148 Ferguson R, Holmes GK, Cooke WT. Coeliac disease, fertility, and pregnancy. *Scand J Gastroenterol* 17(1):65–68, 1982.

149 McCann JP, Nicholls DP, Verzin JA. Adult coeliac disease presenting with infertility. *Ulster Med J* 57(1):88–89, 1988.

150 Karlinger K, et al. The epidemiology and the pathogenesis of inflammatory bowel disease. *Eur J Radiol* 35(3):154–167, 2000.

151 Mayberry JF, Weterman IT. European survey of fertility and pregnancy in women with Crohn's disease: a case control study by European collaborative group. *Gut* 27(7):821–825, 1986.

152 Moody GA, et al. The effects of chronic ill health and treatment with sulphasalazine on fertility amongst men and women with inflammatory bowel disease in Leicestershire. *Int J Colorectal Dis* 12(4):220–224, 1997.

153 Stephens M, Batres LA, Ng D, Baldassano R. Growth failure in the child with inflammatory bowel disease. *Semin Gastrointest Dis* 12(4):253–262, October 2001.

154 Weber AM, Ziegler C, Belinson JL, Mitchinson AR, Widrich T, Fazio V. Gynecologic history of women with inflammatory bowel disease. *Obstet Gynecol* 86(5):843–847, November 1995.

155 Arkuran C, McComb P. Crohn's disease and tubityal infertil: the effect of adhesion formation. *Clin Exp Obstet Gynecol* 27(1):12–13, 2000.

156 Ording Olsen K, et al. Ulcerative colitis: female fecundity before diagnosis, during disease, and after surgery compared with a population sample. *Gastroenterology* 122(1):15–19, 2002.

157 Oresland T, et al. Gynaecological and sexual function related to anatomical changes in the female pelvis after restorative proctocolectomy. *Int J Colorectal Dis* 9(2):77–81, 1994.

158   Olsen KO, et al. Female fecundity before and after operation for familial adenomatous polyposis. *Br J Surg* 90(2):227–231, 2003.

159 Andersson R, Lambe M, Bergstrom R. Fertility patterns after appendicectomy: historical cohort study. *BMJ* 318(7189):963–967, 1999.

160 Hudson M, et al. Fertility and pregnancy in inflammatory bowel disease. *Int J Gynaecol Obstet* 58(2):229–237, 1997.

161 Hernandez-Diaz S, et al. Folic acid antagonists during pregnancy and the risk of birth defects. *N Engl J Med* 343(22):1608–1614, 2000.

162 Incidence and prevalence of ESRD. United States Renal Data System. *Am J Kidney Dis* 32(2 Suppl 1):S38–S49, 1998.

163 Handelsman DJ. Hypothalamic-pituitary gonadal dysfunction in renal failure, dialysis and renal transplantation. *Endocr Rev* 6(2):151–182, 1985.

164 Handelsman DJ, Dong Q. Hypothalamo-pituitary gonadal axis in chronic renal failure. *Endocrinol Metab Clin North Am* 22(1):145–161, 1993.

165 Handelsman DJ, Spaliviero JA, Turtle JR. Hypothalamic-pituitary function in experimental uremic hypogonadism. *Endocrinology* 117(5):1984–1995, 1985.

166 Lim VS. Reproductive function in patients with renal insufficiency. *Am J Kidney Dis* 9(4):363–367, 1987.

167 Zingraff J, et al. Pituitary and ovarian dysfunctions in women on haemodialysis. *Nephron* 30(2):149–153, 1982.

168 Schmidt RJ, Holley JL. Fertility and contraception in end-stage renal disease. *Adv Ren Replace Ther* 5(1):38–44, 1998.

169 Hou S. Pregnancy in chronic renal insufficiency and end-stage renal disease. *Am J Kidney Dis* 33(2):235–252, 1999.

170 Romao JE Jr, et al. Pregnancy in women on chronic dialysis. A single-center experience with 17 cases. *Nephron* 78(4):416–422, 1998.

171 Kim JH, et al. Kidney transplantation and menstrual changes. *Transplant Proc* 30(7):3057–3059, 1998.

172 Hou S. Pregnancy in organ transplant recipients. *Med Clin North Am* 73(3):667–683, 1989.

173 Merkatz IR, et al. Resumption of female reproductive function following renal transplantation. *JAMA* 216(11):1749–1754, 1971.

174 Lim VS, et al. Ovarian function in chronic renal failure: evidence suggesting hypothalamic anovulation. *Ann Intern Med* 93(1):21–27, 1980.

175 Pepperell RJ, Kretser DM, Burger HG. Studies on the metabolic clearance rate and production rate of human luteinizing hormone and on the initial half-time of its subunits in man. *J Clin Invest* 56(1):118–126, 1975.

176 Palmer BF. Sexual dysfunction in uremia. *J Am Soc Nephrol* 10(6):1381–1388, 1999.

177 Palmer BF. Sexual dysfunction in men and women with chronic kidney disease and end-stage kidney disease. *Adv Ren Replace Ther* 10(1):48–60, 2003.

178 Gomez F, et al. Endocrine abnormalities in patients undergoing long-term hemodialysis. The role of prolactin. *Am J Med* 68(4):522–530, 1980.

179 Leavey SF, Weitzel WF. Endocrine abnormalities in chronic renal failure. *Endocrinol Metab Clin North Am* 31(1):107–119, 2002.

180 Okundaye I, Abrinko P, Hou S. Registry of pregnancy in dialysis patients. *Am J Kidney Dis* 31(5):766–773, 1998.

181 Chao AS, et al. Pregnancy in women who undergo long-term hemodialysis. *Am J Obstet Gynecol* 187(1):152–156, 2002.

182 Pickrell MD, Sawers R, Michael J. Pregnancy after renal transplantation: severe intrauterine growth retardation during treatment with cyclosporin A. *Br Med J (Clin Res Ed)* 296(6625):825, 1988.

183 Tardivo I, et al. Pregnancy after kidney transplantation. Review of the international literature and presentation of personal case reports. *Minerva Urol Nefrol,* 54(2):119–126, 2002.

184 Michael J. The management of renal disease in pregnancy. *Clin Obstet Gynaecol* 13(2):319–334, 1986.

185 Furman B, et al. Multiple pregnancies in women after renal transplantation. Case report that rises a management dilemma. *Eur J Obstet Gynecol Reprod Biol* 84(1):107–110, 1999.

186 Khalaf Y, et al. Ovarian hyperstimulation syndrome and its effect on renal function in a renal transplant patient undergoing IVF treatment: case report. *Hum Reprod* 15(6):1275–1277, 2000.

187 Lockwood GM, Ledger WL, Barlow DH. Successful pregnancy outcome in a renal transplant patient following in-vitro fertilization. *Hum Reprod* 10(6):1528–1530, 1995.

188 Ollier WE, Harrison B, Symmons D. What is the natural history of rheumatoid arthritis? *Best Pract Res Clin Rheumatol* 15(1):27–48, 2001.

189 Symmons DP. Epidemiology of rheumatoid arthritis: determinants of onset, persistence and outcome. *Best Pract Res Clin Rheumatol* 16(5):707–722, 2002.

190 Spector TD, Roman E, Silman AJ. The pill, parity, and rheumatoid arthritis. *Arthritis Rheum* 33(6):782–789, 1990.

191 Heliovaara M, et al. Parity and risk of rheumatoid arthritis in Finnish women. *Br J Rheumatol* 34(7):625–628, 1995.

192 Nelson JL, et al. Fecundity before disease onset in women with rheumatoid arthritis. *Arthritis Rheum* 36(1):7–14, 1993.

193 Pope JE, Bellamy N, Stevens A. The lack of associations between rheumatoid arthritis and both nulliparity and infertility. *Semin Arthritis Rheum* 28(5):342–350, 1999.

194 Calmels C, et al. A new case of NSAID-induced infertility. *Rev Rhum Engl Ed* 66(3):167–168, 1999.

195   Akil M, Amos RS, Stewart P. Infertility may sometimes be associated with NSAID consumption. *Br J Rheumatol* 35(1):76–78, 1996.

196   Norman RJ. Reproductive consequences of COX-2 inhibition. *Lancet* 358(9290):1287–1288, 2001.

197   Walker RF, Schwartz LW, Manson JM. Ovarian effects of an anti-inflammatory-immunomodulatory drug in the rat. *Toxicol Appl Pharmacol* 94(2):266–275, 1988.

198   Lim H, et al. Multiple female reproductive failures in cyclooxygenase 2-deficient mice. *Cell* 91(2):197–208, 1997.

199   Athanasiou S, et al. Effects of indomethacin on follicular structure, vascularity, and function over the periovulatory period in women. *Fertil Steril* 65(3):556–560, 1996.

200   Pall M, Friden BE, Brannstrom M. Induction of delayed follicular rupture in the human by the selective COX-2 inhibitor rofecoxib: a randomized double-blind study. *Hum Reprod* 16(7):1323–1328, 2001.

201   Petri M. Epidemiology of systemic lupus erythematosus. *Best Pract Res Clin Rheumatol* 16(5):847–858, 2002.

202   Masi AT, Kaslow RA. Sex effects in systemic lupus erythematosus: a clue to pathogenesis. *Arthritis Rheum* 21(4):480–484, 1978.

203   Le Thi Huong D, Wechsler B, Piette JC. Ovulation induction therapy and systemic lupus erythematosus. *Ann Med Interne* (Paris) 154(1):45–50, 2003.

204   Blumenfeld Z, et al. Preservation of fertility and ovarian function and minimizing gonadotoxicity in young women with systemic lupus erythematosus treated by chemotherapy. *Lupus* 9(6):401–405, 2000.

205   Mok CC, ong RW, Lau CS. Ovarian failure and flares of systemic lupus erythematosus. *Arthritis Rheum* 42(6):1274–1280, 1999.

206   Mok CC, Lau CS, Wong RW. Risk factors for ovarian failure in patients with systemic lupus erythematosus receiving cyclophosphamide therapy. *Arthritis Rheum* 41(5):831–837, 1998.

207   Mok CC, Wong RW. Pregnancy in systemic lupus erythematosus. *Postgrad Med J* 77(905):157–165, 2001.

208   Rahman P, Gladman DD, Urowitz MB. Clinical predictors of fetal outcome in systemic lupus erythematosus. *J Rheumatol* 25(8): 1526–1530, 1998.

209   Petri M. Long-term outcomes in lupus. *Am J Manag Care* 7(16 Suppl):S480–S485, 2001.

210   Yasmeen S, et al. Pregnancy outcomes in women with systemic lupus erythematosus. *J Matern Fetal Med* 10(2):91–96, 2001.

211 Kiss E, et al. Pregnancy in women with systemic lupus erythematosus. *Eur J Obstet Gynecol Reprod Biol* 101(2):129–134, 2002.

212 Bruce IN, Laskin CA. Sex hormones in systemic lupus erythematosus: a controversy for modern times. *J Rheumatol* 24(8):1461–1463, 1997.

213 Jungers P, et al. Influence of oral contraceptive therapy on the activity of systemic lupus erythematosus. *Arthritis Rheum* 25(6): 618–623, 1982.

214 Sanchez-Guerrero J, et al. Past use of oral contraceptives and the risk of developing systemic lupus erythematosus. *Arthritis Rheum* 40(5):804–808, 1997.

215 Ben-Chetrit A, Ben-Chetrit E. Systemic lupus erythematosus induced by ovulation induction treatment. *Arthritis Rheum* 37(11):1614–1617, 1994.

216 Huong du LT, et al. Importance of planning ovulation induction therapy in systemic lupus erythematosus and antiphospholipid syndrome: a single center retrospective study of 21 cases and 114 cycles. *Semin Arthritis Rheum* 32(3):174–188, 2002.

217 Geva E, et al. Autoimmune disorders: another possible cause for in vitro fertilization and embryo transfer failure. *Hum Reprod* 10(10):2560–2563, 1995.

218 Guballa N, et al. Ovulation induction and in vitro fertilization in systemic lupus erythematosus and antiphospholipid syndrome. *Arthritis Rheum* 43(3):550–556, 2000.

219 Cowchock S. Treatment of antiphospholipid syndrome in pregnancy. *Lupus* 7(Suppl 2):S95–S97, 1998.

220 Rai R, et al. Randomised controlled trial of aspirin and aspirin plus heparin in pregnant women with recurrent miscarriage associated with phospholipid antibodies (or antiphospholipid antibodies). *BMJ* 314(7076):253–257, 1997.

221 Tamaki M, et al. Successful singleton pregnancy outcome resulting from in vitro fertilization after renal transplantation. *Transplantation* 75(7):1082–1083, 2003.

222 Human immunodeficiency virus and infertility treatment. *Fertil Steril* 77(2):218–222, 2002.

223 Gregson S, Zaba B, Garnett GP. Low fertility in women with HIV and the impact of the epidemic on orphanhood and early childhood mortality in sub-Saharan Africa. *AIDS* 13(Suppl A):S249–S257, 1999.

224 Glynn JR, et al. Decreased fertility among HIV-1-infected women attending antenatal clinics in three African cities. *J Acquir Immune Defic Syndr* 25(4):345–352, 2000.

225 Hunter SC, et al. The association between HIV and fertility in a cohort study in rural Tanzania. *J Biosoc Sci* 35(2):189–199, 2003.

226 Ellerbrock TV, et al. Characteristics of menstruation in women infected with human immunodeficiency virus. *Obstet Gynecol* 87(6):1030–1034, 1996.

227 Shah R, Bradbeer C. Women and HIV—revisited ten years on. *Int J STD AIDS* 11(5):277–283, 2000.

228 Grinspoon S, et al. Body composition and endocrine function in women with acquired immunodeficiency syndrome wasting. *J Clin Endocrinol Metab* 82(5):1332–1337, 1997.

229 Chirgwin KD, et al. Menstrual function in human immunodeficiency virus-infected women without acquired immunodeficiency syndrome. *J Acquir Immune Defic Syndr Hum Retrovirol* 12(5): 489–494, 1996.

230 Clark RA, et al. Frequency of anovulation and early menopause among women enrolled in selected adult AIDS clinical trials group studies. *J Infect Dis* 184(10):1325–1327, 2001.

231 Harlow SD, et al. Effect of HIV infection on menstrual cycle length. *J Acquir Immune Defic Syndr* 24(1):68–75, 2000.

232 Hadigan C, et al. Fasting hyperinsulinemia and changes in regional body composition in human immunodeficiency virus-infected women. *J Clin Endocrinol Metab* 84(6):1932–1937, 1999.

233 Walli R, et al. Treatment with protease inhibitors associated with peripheral insulin resistance and impaired oral glucose tolerance in HIV-1-infected patients. *AIDS* 12(15):F167–F173, 1998.

234 Grinspoon S, et al. Mechanisms of androgen deficiency in human immunodeficiency virus-infected women with the wasting syndrome. *J Clin Endocrinol Metab* 86(9):4120–4126, 2001.

235 Hadigan C, et al. Hyperandrogenemia in human immunodeficiency virus-infected women with the lipodystrophy syndrome. *J Clin Endocrinol Metab* 85(10):3544–3550, 2000.

236 Wilson JD, Dunham RJ, Balen AH. HIV protease inhibitors, the lipodystrophy syndrome and polycystic ovary syndrome—is there a link? *Sex Transm Infect* 75(4):268–269, 1999.

237 Vigano A, et al. Hyperinsulinemia induced by highly active antiretroviral therapy in an adolescent with polycystic ovary syndrome who was infected with human immunodeficiency virus. *Fertil Steril* 79(2):422–423, 2003.

238 Egger M, et al. Impact of new antiretroviral combination therapies in HIV infected patients in Switzerland: prospective multicentre study. Swiss HIV Cohort Study. *BMJ* 315(7117):1194–1199, 1997.

239 Mandelbrot L, et al. Natural conception in HIV-negative women with HIV-infected partners. *Lancet* 349(9055):850–851, 1997.

240 Mastro TD, Kitayaporn D. HIV type 1 transmission probabilities: estimates from epidemiological studies. *AIDS Res Hum Retroviruses* 14(Suppl 3):S223–S227, 1998.

241 Mastro TD, de Vincenzi I. Probabilities of sexual HIV-1 transmission. *AIDS* 10(Suppl A):S75–S82, 1996.

242 Semprini AE, et al. Insemination of HIV-negative women with processed semen of HIV-positive partners. *Lancet* 340(8831): 1317–1319, 1992.

243 Marina S, et al. Pregnancy following intracytoplasmic sperm injection from an HIV-1-seropositive man. *Hum Reprod* 13(11):3247–3249, 1998.

244 Trends in tuberculosis morbidity—United States, 1992–2002. *MMWR Morb Mortal Wkly Rep* 52(11):217–220, 222, 2003.

245 Dye C, et al. Consensus statement. Global burden of tuberculosis: estimated incidence, prevalence, and mortality by country. WHO Global Surveillance and Monitoring Project. *JAMA* 282(7):677–686, 1999.

246 Sutherland AM, Glen ES, MacFarlane JR. Transmission of genitourinary tuberculosis. *Health Bull (Edinb)* 40(2):87–91, 1982.

247 Marcus SF, et al. Tuberculous infertility and in vitro fertilization. *Am J Obstet Gynecol* 171(6):1593–1596, 1994.

248 Namavar Jahromi B, Parsanezhad PE, Ghane-Shirazi R. Female genital tuberculosis and infertility. *Int J Gynaecol Obstet* 75(3):269–272, 2001.

249 Parikh FR, et al. Genital tuberculosis—a major pelvic factor causing infertility in Indian women. *Fertil Steril* 67(3):497–500, 1997.

250 Tripathy SN. Infertility and pregnancy outcome in female genital tuberculosis. *Int J Gynaecol Obstet* 76(2):159–163, 2002.

251 Oosthuizen AP, Wessels PH, Hefer JN. Tuberculosis of the female genital tract in patients attending an infertility clinic. *S Afr Med J* 77(11):562–564, 1990.

252 Sutherland AM. The treatment of tuberculosis of the female genital tract with streptomycin, PAS and isoniazid. *Tubercle* 57(2):137–144, 1976.

253 Schaefer G. Female genital tuberculosis. *Clin Obstet Gynecol* 19(1):223–239, 1976.

254 Frydman R, et al. In vitro fertilization in tuberculous infertility. *J In Vitro Fert Embryo Transf*, 2(4):184–189, 1985.

6 Environmental Factors Affecting Fertility

Bill L. Lasley
Susan E. Shideler

Introduction

Concern about reproductive health has become a serious public issue. During the past 40 years, increasing numbers of women have delayed attempts to conceive children until their third or fourth decade of life. These women are among the first to recognize that reproductive health is not guaranteed. However, reproductive health is also not guaranteed even to women attempting pregnancy in their early- to midtwenties. In this age group alone, infertility rose from 4 to 10% between 1965 and 1982, while an additional 2 million couples were involuntarily childless.[1]

Of infants born between 1965 and 1982, 3–7% had some type of malformation, the majority of which could be attributed to a gene mutation.[1] Lawson et al.[2] report that spontaneous abortions or stillbirths occur in 10–20% of recognized pregnancies and early fetal losses occur at a similar percentage prior to the recognition of pregnancy. The number of these detected losses that are a result of an environmental hazard is unknown. The high number of assumed spontaneous pregnancy losses obscures the relatively small increases that might occur as a result of a recognized environmental exposure. What are the hazards, how do we identify them, and how do we establish safety standards?

According to Lasley and Overstreet,[3] exposure to environmental hazards and resultant infertility may be periodic: a relative condition, as opposed to being an absolute condition. Couples or their physicians may never recognize infertility as a problem when pregnancy is achieved after several years or when they have smaller families than planned. There are several reasons why this is the case.

KEY POINT

Identifying a negative effect from the environment is difficult due to the frequency of subfertility which occurs normally in humans.

Most of the dynamics of reproductive function are concealed. Spermatogenesis, ovulation, fertilization, implantation, and early fetal loss are not recognizable to the person experiencing them or to the casual observer. Infertility is not an immediate health risk, emergency, or a clinical issue unless pregnancy is desired. Failures in reproductive function alone do not reduce an individual's ability to survive although adverse effects on ovarian function can have serious downstream health effects. Reproductive health disturbances, then, may go undetected and it is likely that available statistics underestimate the magnitude of the problem. Infertility is not an infrequent condition in the human population. It occurs normally in the adolescent and aged. When pregnancy achievement is not a goal, infertility is usually not treated and is often undiagnosed. Several forms of female infertility have no known pathogenesis and no one knows if any of these are induced or enhanced by environmental hazards. Exposures known to be safe for men may not be for women as the reality of *gender-specific actions* are well documented by Enan and Cowers.[4] Physicians are, therefore, on the front line and must be able to not only detect the adverse effects of environmental hazards to reproductive health but also be able to explain to overly suspicious patents that not all aspects of reproductive failure are a result of toxicants, environmental hazards, or endocrine disruptors. It is unlikely that any infertility patient has not, at one time, been exposed to a putative endocrine disruptor, pesticide, or other putative reproductive toxicant and is equally likely to be concerned about such an exposure.

Guiding Questions

- Does either member of the couple smoke cigarettes?
- Does either member of the couple work outside the home?
- What type of job do they do?

- Is one member of the household primarily responsible for cleaning within the home?
- Are there any toxins at the workplace or at home (including solvents, pesticides, metals, and so on)?

Identifying Causes of Reproductive Failure

What are the real causative agents and what are the operating mechanisms responsible for the apparent rise in human infertility? Presently, only a few causes of reproductive and developmental diseases are fully understood at the mechanistic level, and almost all information comes from experimental evidence from laboratory rodents. There is a rapid expansion of the list of chemicals known to have adverse effects on the fertility of laboratory animals (Table 6-1). Unfortunately, the listing of putative toxicants expands more rapidly than the scientific identification of these putative toxicants.

Each year thousands of new chemicals enter the home and workplace without being tested appropriately for reproductive toxicity. The fact that approximately 65% of men and women in the workforce are of reproductive age, and the fact that there has been a 28% increase in the number of children born to working mothers from 1976 to 1998, suggest that occupational exposures to toxicants potentially affecting reproductive function have increased.[2] Not only are new potential reproductive toxicants added to industry every year, but the increase in home exposures increase at nearly the same rate. While toxic solvents (benzene, toluene, and ethylene glycol) and specific metals are recognized and defined as reproductive hazards, new categories of endocrine disruptors are being identified that have complex and multiple actions on reproduction and development.

Animal experiments and *in vitro* studies now show that compounds once thought to simply "mimic" steroid hormones (by competing with endogenous steroids for receptor binding and signal transduction pathways) are now thought to act through multiple, and sometimes new, pathways. New concepts are being introduced into the literature that include membrane receptors for steroidal estrogens and their xenobiotic mimics as well as "cross-talk" between cytosolic signal transduction cascades upstream of nuclear events leading to multiple gene suppression or activation.

Table 6-1. ASSOCIATED EFFECTS OF CHEMICALS[a]

CHEMICAL	ASSOCIATION	CHEMICAL	ASSOCIATION	CHEMICAL	ASSOCIATION
Alcohol	In pregnancy: (human) newborn abnormalities. In men: impotence and sperm abnormalities	Ethylene dibromide	In animals: chickens have impaired follicular growth and egg size; rat estrous cycles are impeded at high doses. In men: decreased sperm density and percent of normal forms	Nicotine	In rabbits and rats: impaired fetal growth. In mice: cleft palate and skeletal defects
Arsenic	In pregnancy: (human) decreased birthweight, increases spontaneous abortion. In rats: teratogenic	Ethylene glycol monomethyl ether	EGEE in humans: birth defects. In female animals: infertility. In male animals: testicular damage. In rats, mice, and rabbits: teratogenic	Polybrominated biphenyls	In humans: decreased body fat in children. In animals: (rat) liver carcinomas offspring; (pig) abnormalities in thyroid and liver offspring; (monkeys) disrupted menstrual cycles
Cadmium	In pregnancy: (animals) fetal death and malformations. In males: testicular toxicity, altered libido, and infertility	Ethylene glycol monomethyl ether	EGME in animals: (females) infertility; (males) testicular damage in mice, rats, and rabbits	Polychlorinated biphenyls	In women: dark pigmentation of offspring, shorter gestation, lower birthweight, altered menstrual cycles
Carbon disulfide	In women: altered menstrual cycles. In men: altered	Ethylene oxide	In humans: increased spontaneous abortion. In	2,4,5-Trichlorophenoxyacetic acid	In humans: seasonal increase in neural tube

Substance	Effects
	... libido, increased abnormal sperm
Carbon monoxide	In humans: intrauterine fetal death and neurologic deficits in surviving infants
Chlordecone	Developmental effects: (animals) malformations, stillbirths, and abortions. Females: (rats) constant estrus and damaged ovaries. In men: reduced sperm count and motility
Chloroprene	In men: sexual impotence and loss of libido
	rats: increased fetal abnormalities and mortality. In male rats: reduced testicular weight
Gossypol	Sterility in men, dogs, monkeys, rats, and hamsters
Hexachlorobenzene	In women: still-births, pink sores on infants, muscle atrophy. In children: death if exposed within 1 year of birth. In animals: (female rats) decreased litter size and birth weight; (female monkeys) histopathologic changes in ovaries
Lead	In women: increased spontaneous abortion, menstrual disorders, and
	defects and mis-carriages
2,3,7,8-Tetrachlorodibenzo-p-dioxin (TCDD)	In animals: (mice) kidney damage, cleft palate; (rats) internal organ hemorrhage; (females) changes in estrous cyclicity
Tobacco smoke	In women: retarded fetal growth, spontaneous abortion, bleeding during pregnancy, sudden infant death syndrome, long-term infant physical growth lag. In men: decreased sperm counts and normal forms
Toluene	In women: CNS dysfunction, craniofacial and limb abnormalities,

(continued)

Table 6-1. **ASSOCIATED EFFECTS OF CHEMICALS[a] (CONTINUED)**

CHEMICAL	ASSOCIATION	CHEMICAL	ASSOCIATION	CHEMICAL	ASSOCIATION
			infertility. In men: disturbances in sperm-related factors		and developmental delay in offspring; uterine pain
DDT	Prenatal exposure: (human females) altered ovarian function, altered development of the reproductive system. In adult women: menstrual irregularities	Lithium	In women: cardiac defects in offspring	Vinyl chloride	In women: ovarian dysfunction, benign uterine growths, prolapsed genital organs, declined sexual function. In men: decreased sexual function and increased spontaneous abortion in wives
DBCP	In females: (animals) altered ovarian function and decreased fertility. In men: decreased sperm count and fertility	Mercury	In women: during pregnancy, severe brain damage in children and spontaneous abortion; menstrual disorders outside of pregnancy. In men: altered libido, sperm production, and decreased fertility	Vitamin A	In women: urinary tract abnormalities and CNS defects in offspring

DES	Mirex	Warfarin
In utero: (human) increased vaginal and cervical carcinoma in female offspring. In males: increased frequency of abnormal reproductive tracts. In animals: (females) ovarian cystadenomas and ovarian lesions	In female mice: low fertility. In female rats: inhibition of ovulation	In pregnancy: (humans) still-births and malformations of the CNS, eye, and jaw if newborns

[a]After the United States General Accounting Office, Report to the Chairman, Committee on Governmental Affairs, U.S. Senate, Reproductive and Developmental Toxicants, Regulatory Actions Provide Uncertain Protection. GAO/PEMD-92-3, Appendix III: Selected Adverse Reproductive and Developmental Outcomes of the 30 Chemicals, October 1991.

KEY POINT

Exposure to environmental toxicants is frequent. Identifying a causal relationship between exposure and an effect on reproduction is more difficult.

While increasing numbers of women will be exposed to chemicals at work, even more women are likely to be exposed to other chemicals in the home and more likely to be exposed in the home under conditions that do not protect them as adequately as in industrial settings. Many, perhaps most, putative reproductive toxicants are synthetic polyaromatics and/or phenols that are common in household products and that are easily volatized, particularly with heat. Daily activities that include cooking, cleaning, infant care, and use of cosmetics result in a nearly constant exposure to a wide range of potential hazards. Thus, women's repeated episodic exposure to an array of household and cosmetic products can theoretically promote the gradual deposition of toxicants in body fat that can be released continuously or episodically with weight loss. Some of these toxicants have been shown to interfere with normal hormone function, to induce abnormal function in target cells, or to even be cytotoxic in animal experiments. A few toxins, like dioxin, are not only lipophilic but have prolonged half-lives and can continue to exert adverse effects years following a single, acute exposure. A comprehensive discussion of environmental exposures that relate to women's health issues is found in a recent review by Silbergeld and Flaws.[5]

IDENTIFYING THE INTERACTION BETWEEN REPRODUCTIVE FAILURE AND THE ENVIRONMENT

There are inherent difficulties in the assessment of interactions between environmental hazards and human reproductive function for both researchers and physicians. These difficulties include, but are not limited to, an accepted relatively high rate of spontaneous infertility in humans, the concealed nature of many reproductive processes and/or events, and the temporal dynamics of reproductive physiology (particularly in women). In addition, the species-specific nature of reproductive processes, when using animal models for experimentation, and the ethics involved in human research pose further difficulties. Except for rare occurrences when environmental exposures are recognized during the expression of adverse effects, information relating to the identification of specific toxicants and their sites and mechanisms of action must be detected through experimentation using animal models. In no other discipline is the use of animal models more problematic than it is in female reproductive toxicology. In few other disciplines are the results of experiments with laboratory animals so often inappropriately extrapolated to humans

KEY POINT

Experimental data from animal models are often inappropriately extrapolated to humans.

than in reproductive toxicology. Most of what is known relating to the mechanisms of action of well-defined reproductive toxicants is the result of experiments with laboratory rodents. In terms of human female reproductive toxicology, this presents an additional problem in both identifying hazards and establishing safe exposure standards.

Physiologically, male reproductive function is tonic in expression and relatively simple in its regulation. Female reproductive function, in contrast, is cyclic and complex in its regulation. It is easier to study the effects of environmental toxicants on male reproductive function because there is less risk of complicating factors confounding research design or obscuring interpretation of results. While the male model may be preferred in general for biomedical research, in some instances, attributes of the female reproductive system are required for specific kinds of studies. In such cases, more planning is required because of the cyclical dynamics of female reproductive processes. Single point-in-time sampling may not accurately reflect the interaction of these processes with exposures. Instead, serial sampling may be required to encompass time intervals of sufficient length to capture temporal changes. And, in the final analysis, a woman's fertility cannot be completely evaluated in the absence of a male partner or viable semen.

Humans, and animals selected as models for human reproduction, have basically the same organs, hormone structures, and processes. The anatomic and behavioral traits that vary between females of different species are the shape and location of the uterus, the development, size, and location of the mammary glands, and the behavioral responses to sex steroids. In contrast, the hypothalamic-pituitary-gonadal axis is represented by similar structures in different species. Even the chemical structures of the hormones that regulate reproductive processes are similar between species. Steroid hormones are identical in all mammals, fish, and birds, and protein hormones have highly conserved regions that maintain their biological activities. The main difference between species is the way in which similar hormones accomplish the same or comparable reproductive events through species-specific regulatory processes. The pituitary hormone, prolactin, for example, serves a variety of roles in different mammalian species and the various actions of this hormone are one reason that reproductive processes of rodents and primates are not comparable at the level of hormone action.

Much of our understanding of toxicology is a result of laboratory experiments using inbred stains of rodents. Such experimental data usually support and substantiate the adverse effects of reproductive toxicants in population-based epidemiologic studies or experiments using nonhuman primates. Examples of general, cross-species reproductive toxicants are those having targets of toxicity for the steroid hormone or arylhydrocarbon receptors, such as diethylstilbestrol, methoxychlor, bisphenol, several phenolic compounds, and the dioxins. A number of parallel rodent[6-9] and nonhuman primate[10-12] studies demonstrate ovarian, endometrial, central, and placental targets of toxicity and confirm the less convincing evidence from human exposures. These observations should not be surprising as these groups of toxicants are extremely potent, often slowly metabolized or cleared from the body, and act through highly conserved receptors. This is a combination of attributes that almost ensures cross-species consistencies. Far less consistency can be expected for putative reproductive toxicants that have the potential for species-specific differences in metabolism and targets of action. Certainly, a large percent of *polycyclic compounds* with phenolic or phenol-like moieties have the ability to target the Ah or steroid hormone nuclear receptor superfamily and to block steroid hormone and/or induce catabolic enzymes. Whether these compounds have similar adverse effects with similar exposure regimens in different species is still unknown.

KEY POINT

Species-specific differences in physiology confound the development of an effective nonhuman animal model for infertility.

Despite the relative uniformity of developmental processes across phylogeny, female reproductive processes, and, to a lesser extent, male reproductive processes, are species-specific in expression. It is important, therefore, to be cautious when nonprimate experimental data are the primary source of public concern. Species-specific differences in physiology confound the development of an effective nonhuman animal model for infertility. It is not known why there are so many diverse reproductive patterns, but most of the variation is expressed in female reproductive function, particularly in endocrine processes of ovulation, tubal transport, implantation, and gestation. When the unique qualities of reproduction in each possible model species are identified in the context of their adaptive significance, it is possible to identify unique physiologic traits that have evolved within each species and to understand why toxicants are likely to have different targets and different actions in different species. A quick review of basic comparative reproductive physiology provides the conceptual foundation necessary to understand how subtle differences between species can lead to major differences in the response to toxicants.

Comparative Reproductive Biology

Much of what we understand about environmental hazards to reproduction comes from reports of exposures to wildlife or laboratory experiments using rodent models. The positive results from such investigations often increase public concern particularly when infertility or pregnancy loss is indicated. Few reports deal with well-documented human exposures, and even fewer indicate mechanisms of action by which environmental hazards may act. This lack of information and limited understanding of mechanistic detail creates a major problem to regulators, scientists, and physicians. It is important, therefore, that there is comprehension of differences in reproductive physiology in order to understand similarities and differences in sites of toxic action. It is also important that there be an understanding of why adverse effects in one species may, or may not, translate directly to another.

There are a few broad generalizations that can be made regarding reproductive processes in mammalian species. These are internal fertilization, viviparity, and maternal care of the neonate. These few common traits are important to toxicologists because some of the physiologic mechanisms that control these processes are universal; hence, certain principals of toxic effects can be broadly applied. For example, it is a requirement of successful reproduction that a dam produce a fertilizable ovum (ovulate) within an appropriate environment (tubal transport) and that she provide adequate support for pregnancy (implantation and gestation). Meeting these requirements is dependent on the presence of healthy oocytes that are stimulated by gonadotropins to recruit undifferentiated stromal cells. The maturing oocyte and surrounding follicle complex produce sex steroids (estrogen and progesterone) that act to coordinate most of the other essential events in the reproductive tract. *Gametotoxins* are often non-species-specific and damage to oocytes is usually irreparable. Thus, environmental hazards that destroy oocytes, disrupt gonadotropin secretion or action, and that block sex steroid secretion or action, will likely be universal reproductive toxicants.

Circulating estrogen acts to prepare the reproductive tract for all reproductive processes and is produced by the vestments of the ovum or ova and can be produced only from intracellular androgen precursors. Toxicants such as dioxin, which block steroidogenic pathways, result in decreased circulating progesterone and/or estrogen. Progesterone creates and maintains an internal environment required for pregnancy and is produced by the remnants of the vestments of the ovum, the corpus luteum (CL). Progesterone production depends on gonadotropic support from the pituitary as well as the products of conception. There are species-specific mechanisms involved in forming and maintaining the CL, but its luteal function, progesterone production to support early pregnancy, is universal. The source of pregnancy-supporting progesterone varies greatly among different species, thereby making the CL a noncritical component of late pregnancy in some mammalian species. Early pregnancy loss is often associated with environmental hazards that prevent adequate progesterone production. With these simple, unifying concepts, the reproductive physiology of the more familiar mammalian species can be compared and contrasted.

KEY POINT

Interference with steroid hormone function has the greatest potential to adversely affect reproduction.

While peptide and protein hormones are essential for reproduction, it is the *steroid hormones* that are responsible for somatic development, support of the reproductive tract, and the coordination of most reproductive events. Steroid hormones are required for all steps in reproduction, and, like all efficient biological signals, must exist for only the interval of time they are biologically useful. Compounds with *steroid hormone-like* physical qualities, greater or lesser biological activities, and longer biological half-lives have the widest range of potential adverse effects and are likely to be least species-specific.

To facilitate comparisons between species, it is useful to categorize them into four groups. These groups are rodents, ungulates, carnivores (social and nonsocial), and the higher primates. For the purposes of brevity, detailed discussion will be limited to the two groups (rodents and nonhuman primates) most commonly used as models in biomedical and toxicologic research.

The first category to be considered is the Order Rodentia, which includes rats, mice, hamsters, guinea pigs, as well as squirrels, beavers, and porcupines. In terms of reproductive traits, rats, mice, hamsters, and guinea pigs are basically R-selected species that spend their energy producing many offspring and investing very little energy on parental care. In the wild, theirs is a "time and numbers" strategy: produce as many offspring as possible during a lifetime and a few will survive to reproduce themselves. These rodent species are short-lived. Nonpregnant female mice and rats ovulate every 4 or 5 days and mate "reflexively" with any male they encounter during their fertile period. The act of mating (which occurs exclusively during the fertile period) triggers a hormone response that is unique to rodents and that ensures that each mating has the highest likelihood of resulting in pregnancy. Fetuses are born small and altricial, but mature rapidly. For most rodents, litters are weaned within weeks of their birth and females are capable of fertile matings soon after. Male and female offspring reach adulthood within a few weeks, and, like their parents, they begin production of as many offspring as possible while investing as little as possible in their survival. Simply stated, since each surviving offspring also has the capacity to produce large numbers of offspring themselves, the species survival curve is maintained and "fitness," in evolutionary terms, is maintained. In some mouse species, the female's capacities to ovulate and to abort a pregnancy can be triggered by encountering a new potential mate or by the scent of a novel male. In the natural setting, the mother's immediate environment is the context of normal fertility and the success of individual pregnancies. In the laboratory, inbred strains have specific genetic attributes that permit investigators to preselect response characteristics. Different strains of mice may respond differently to the same toxicant.

Ovarian cycles in the absence of pregnancies are probably rare events in the life of noncaptive female rats and mice. In captive rats and mice, it is possible that nonconceptive ovarian cycles are an artifact of captivity or inbreeding since their natural physiologic adaptations are to save time and produce offspring.

The second group to be discussed includes the higher primates of the Order Primates, which includes Old and New World monkeys, the great apes, and humans. Primate species have evolved their own unique reproductive strategies and represent the

KEY POINT

In general, reproductive processes in rodents are extremely robust and very different from human and nonhuman primates, rendering them poor models for the study of several important human reproductive mechanisms.

smallest group in this arbitrary categorization of species groups. It is likely that primate reproductive strategies are the most recently evolved mammalian combination of physiology and behaviors. With the exception of the orangutan, all primate species are social, living in some social configuration, and exhibit complex and species-specific social-sexual patterns. The most common mating system is the single or age-graded male group in which one male actively breeds; however, in terrestrial Old World monkeys, some multimale groups have several breeding males.[13] True harems are characteristic of gorillas and hamadryas baboons, while monogamy is a specialized pattern that is characteristic of territorial species exhibiting little size dimorphism between males and females who share defense and care of the young.[13] The organization of the primate female reproductive cycle has evolved in concert with the development of these diverse social-sexual patterns. Higher primate females have an extended duration of sexual behavior compared to other species and this sexual behavior is associated with copulation outside of the fertile period. This trait, together with concealed ovulation, permits higher primate females to have some choice in terms of the paternity of offspring. This choice requires time between the previous nonconceptive cycle and the next ovulation and this increase in time increases the risk of adverse effects on oocyte maturation and ovulation resulting from an acute or episodic exposure to an environmental hazard. Once conception has occurred, however, neither the mother nor her immediate environment have a great deal of control on the progression of the pregnancy.

Humans and other higher primate females are more similar to female ungulates than they are to female rodents in terms of their mechanisms of ovulation, luteal function, and early pregnancy. Thus, hazards that reduce fecundity in ungulates are more likely to have a similar effect in humans compared to rodents. Both higher primate and ungulate females are spontaneous ovulators and do not require copulation to trigger normal luteal function. But unlike ungulates in which the uterus controls luteal function following ovulation, the products of conception take control of maternal ovarian function immediately following implantation in higher primates. This kind of control of luteal function and mechanism for supporting early pregnancy is not found outside of the higher primates and is one source of problems in modeling the menstrual cycle and early pregnancy in humans. The fact that these higher primate reproductive traits are markedly different from comparable traits in nonprimate species makes modeling for reproductive health extremely challenging. How can we interpret hormonal perturbations in one species when the function of that hormone is different in another? This question remains unanswered.

Animal Models in Reproductive Toxicology

Studies of animal models involve experimentation to confirm targets of toxicity or to verify that putative environmental toxins cause the types of reproductive failure commonly observed in human populations.[3] Only a few animal species are used routinely as animal models for human biomedical issues in experimental studies. The mouse, rat, sheep, pig, hamster, rabbit, guinea pig, and laboratory monkey contribute to most experimental studies in the broader biomedical sciences. Mice are used in over 90% of all scientific experiments and either mice or rats are used in approximately 66% of the experiments relating to reproduction. Production animals, e.g., cows, sheep, pigs, are also involved in scientific studies related to their own reproduction and not necessarily as models for human reproduction. When they are removed from the estimates of animal models used for human reproduction, it is likely that 70–80% of all experimental studies related to reproduction use mice or rats. Hamsters and guinea pigs also are used as animal models for gamete studies, increasing the percentage of rodent species used as models for studies directed toward reproduction and, more specifically, directed toward human reproductive health, to more than 90%. With respect to animal models used in toxicologic studies, over 80% use mice or rats, with rats predominating. In addition, when the gender of the mice or rats is given in the title of scientific reports, males are used almost 10 times more frequently than females. This is largely due to the intrinsic qualities of female reproductive biology that bring unwanted complexity to studies not specifically directed toward females. Thus, in experimental studies, the scales are balanced against learning a great deal about primate female reproductive toxicology.

As indicated above, the mouse is the animal model of choice in the majority of biomedical studies. It has limitations, however, in experiments requiring measurement of reproductive hormones. The combination of small size and short reproductive cycles limit the use of the mouse in the study of the endocrinology of ovulation, fertilization, tubal transport, and implantation. It is challenging to obtain adequate serial blood samples to permit the measurement of key hormones to characterize these events in routine experiments. Mice are very useful, however, in studies in which ovulation, conception, implantation, and the completion of pregnancy are endpoints because tissue samples can document these events by morphologic or histologic examination in the absence of hormonal measurements. When the hormone dynamics associated with these events must be documented, however, the mouse is of limited value and the rat becomes the superior model of choice.

The animal model most relevant to reproductive toxicology is the rat model, and, as such, will be the focus of the following discussion. The analytical levels for comparison of data generated by the rat model to the human are three: the anatomic, the organizational, and the mechanistic. Several processes may be examined as separate events (e.g., ovulation, preparation of the implantation site, implantation, and pregnancy), but it should be remembered that these processes occur in a tightly coupled sequence of interrelated events. There are a few common traits that apply to all species in terms of reproduction in general, that are useful in reproductive toxicology. These are as follows:

1. All reproductive events are mediated or controlled by steroid hormones and steroid hormone synthesis, secretion, action, and molecular structure are similar.
2. All steroid production related to reproduction is regulated by protein hormones derived from either the pituitary or placenta (i.e., trophoblast), and protein hormones secreted by the pituitary can be produced in slightly altered forms by the placenta.
3. Ovulation is associated with estrogen production that is essential for preparing the female reproductive tract for mating, fertilization, and the effects of progesterone for implantation.
4. Ovulation is triggered by a surge in pituitary luteinizing hormone (LH).

5. Each ovulating follicle produces a potentially fertilizable germ cell and then is converted into a discrete structure, the CL, which produces progesterone.
6. Progesterone is essential to all stages of pregnancy. The site or source of progesterone production and its regulation varies between species.

KEY POINT

Steroid hormones and their actions are similar between species.

These shared traits imply that although steroid hormones and their actions are similar, the protein hormones that regulate them, the mechanisms of regulation, and their source of production, however, can be different in different species. Thus, the targets of toxicity can be dissimilar despite the apparent similarity of the reproductive event and the hormones involved.

THE ANATOMIC LEVEL

Description of the anatomic level of comparison is relatively easy and straightforward. Rodents are anatomically designed to produce litters and not singleton offspring as are humans, with guinea pigs being an exception. Rodents have 8–12 small ovarian follicles that mature per cycle, a bicornuate tubular uterus, multiple mammary glands, and embryos that implant superficially with multiple cell layers separating them from their mother. Higher primates, including humans, by contrast, are designed to have one, sometimes two, offspring. They have large ovarian follicles, a simplex round uterus, two mammary glands, and embryos that invade to implant and have only one cell layer between them and their mother. Since each ovulation gives rise to discrete CL, rats have 8–12 corpora lutea per cycle compared to one in the primate. Corpora lutea formed in the absence of fertile mating in rodents are structurally and functionally different than those formed in a conceptive cycle. This is not the case in the primate and this difference is the basis of an important caveat in comparing the effects of environmental toxins in rodents and primates.

Neonatal rats are born before full neurologic processes are completed and this provides the opportunity for some processes to be altered following birth such as characteristics endowed by the sex steroids. Rodents have a short maturation period and an equally short life span. Male and female rodents maintain their fertility until death or shortly before. Primates, on the other hand, have evolved in the opposite direction and provide substantially different opportunities for toxicants to have adverse effects.

THE ORGANIZATIONAL LEVEL

The organizational level is more complex than the anatomic level and can be addressed here only superficially. This level is critical, however, in understanding targets of toxic action when exposure is episodic.

Although rats mature 8–12 follicles per cycle, the final selection occurs over 2–3 days. The final maturation of the single dominant follicle in the human takes 2–3 weeks. Similarly, the postovulatory/preimplantational period is much shorter in the rat than in the human. The rat even has mechanisms to truncate this time period further when mating does not occur or when a mating does not result in fertilized germ cells. Gestation in the rat, when compared to humans, is proportionately compressed, even more than follicular development and the postovulatory/preimplantational periods. Despite this truncation of reproductive events in the rat, the rat is as complex, if not more so, as the human in terms of the processes involved. Its very complexity makes the rat as vulnerable to insult from toxic environmental exposures as humans.

KEY POINT

Simply from a time-of-opportunity standpoint, then, the preovulatory period in humans is much longer and more vulnerable to environmental toxin exposure than is the same event in the rat.

THE MECHANISTIC LEVEL

Since even a superficial discussion of the mechanistic level cannot be contained in a few words, selected topics pertinent to the issue of environmental hazards to human reproductive health will be addressed.

In all mammals, ovulation is the result of resting primordial follicles being activated by the stimulation of pituitary hormones. The ovary is fully capable of normal function at birth and awaits gonadotropin stimulation. Puberty is the result of the maturation of the central nervous system in rats as well as in primates. The mechanism by which rodents regularly develop and ovulate many follicles, and by which primates generally develop and ovulate only one or two, is not known, but this difference implies different mechanisms. Generally, ovulation is under similar control in all mammals, with the exception of those that ovulate in response to mating (i.e., reflex ovulators such as cats, rabbits, squirrels, camels, and so on). In all species, follicular development and ovulation are under the control of the hypothalamus and pituitary, and are modulated by ovarian feedback. In most mammals, follicles are stimulated to develop by pituitary follicle-stimulating hormone (FSH), and assisted by LH. Hence, the effects of environmental exposures, at this level, generally are well correlated between species.

Luteal function and ovarian steroid production are the areas where the rat and the human are most dissimilar. The mechanism by which the rat creates and maintains luteal function involves a series of events requiring cervical stimulation as well as hypothalamic and pituitary responses to the products of conception, and, eventually, support from the placentae. In contrast, the primate CL forms spontaneously and is maintained by pituitary LH. In the rat, a true CL is not formed unless mating has taken place, which ensures the release of prolactin that is essential for luteal function. In short, formation of the CL in rodents requires copulation, so the demise of the CL is not an issue unless a sterile mating occurs. In the case of a sterile mating, the CL is formed but regresses in a few days if the products of conception are not present to contribute luteotropic factors. The primate CL is self-limiting in the absence of conception: 14 days following ovulation and spontaneous formation of the CL, the primate CL spontaneously regresses and permits the recruitment of the next cohort of ovarian follicles.

KEY POINT

Focusing on data generated from either the rodent or primate model, the questions to be addressed are how relevant are experimental data derived from studies on female rats to human female reproduction, and how should data from animal studies be viewed in terms of extrapolating findings and applying them to human reproductive health?

In both rodents and primates, early pregnancy requires the maintenance of the CL although the mechanism by which this is achieved is different. The CL is maintained in the rat by a series of events that involve both the products of conception and the pituitary and their combined effects extend into pregnancy. The primate also requires an LH-like luteotropic support from the products of conception, but only for a few days. Unlike the rodent, the higher primate ovary can be removed after the third or fourth week of pregnancy without interrupting it because the placenta produces sufficient progesterone and estrogen.

Gestation in both rodents and primates requires progesterone support, but the source of the progesterone is different between them. In rodents, the maternal ovaries continue to be the primary source of progesterone during gestation, and, in turn, gestation requires the support of secretions from both the products of conception and the ovary. In primates, the products of conception (i.e., the fetus and the placenta) are capable of secreting all of the progesterone necessary to maintain pregnancy following the fourth to fifth week of gestation (i.e., postimplantation). All mammalian species require estrogen support during pregnancy, and, like progesterone, estrogen is produced from different sources in different species. The rodent CL is the source of estrogen production using substrates produced by the products of conception. The primate placenta, however, is the primary source of estrogen production, using the substrates provided by the fetal adrenal.

What's the Evidence?

INTEGRATION OF EPIDEMIOLOGY, ANIMAL EXPERIMENTATION, AND CLINICAL STUDIES

Comprehensive investigation of environmental hazards to human fertility requires investigations at several levels. While much of the public concern relating to human fertility comes from observations of wildlife exposures, information regarding real and potential adverse effects to human populations is necessary to support or negate these concerns. In many species, the processes relating to reproductive function are more susceptible to environmental influences than they are in humans, and, as we mentioned before, spontaneous infertility may be inherently higher in humans than in other species. In addition, many wildlife species will experience exposures unlikely to ever occur in humans. Some environmental toxin exposures have similar adverse effects across species and these can generally be predicted based on the chemical structure and target of toxicity. Compounds that target conserved elements such as the endocrine disruptors that mimic or block hormone action, alter target cell function and differentiation, and alter the natural timing of cell death, will likely have similar adverse effects in laboratory animals and humans. Because investigations of humans will always be observational and retrospective, the *rodent models* have been, and will continue to be, the avenue by which progress will be made at the mechanistic level. For environmental exposures that are likely to be species-specific in their action, the correct classification as environmental toxins will most likely result from *population-based studies* in communities that have reason to suspect adverse reproductive outcomes. Such studies are now made possible by the advent of new tools for monitoring ovarian function and early pregnancy through self-collected urine samples.

Once identified, putative toxicants should be tested in both rodent and nonhuman primate animal models to confirm toxicity and to identify targets of toxicity in both models. This information should be used to design and execute *in vitro* studies to confirm the target and understand the mechanism(s) of action (see chap. 3 for details). Recent reports on the study of the toxic effects of bromodichloromethane (BDCM) are an example of this hierarchal progression of experimentation and provide an illustration of the importance of each level of investigation. Compounds such as diethylstilbestrol, DDT, DDE, dioxin, and methoxychlor also are examples of compounds that have been substantiated as hazards to human reproductive health in this manner.

Bromodichloromethane: A Model Compound

The current issues relating to the potential risk of chlorination by-products in drinking water provide a real-world example of the complexities involved. BDCM is a putative human reproductive toxicant and may cause late-term abortions in humans.

POPULATION-BASED STUDIES

While neither the specific toxicant(s) nor target(s) of toxic action of BDCM are known, epidemiologic data from several studies suggest that some form(s) of chlorinated hydrocarbons are responsible of an increase in human abortions observed in the communities studied to date.[14–17]

A population-based study by Waller et al.[14] prospectively investigated human pregnancies using a prepaid health plan as the vehicle for recruitment. Spontaneous abortions (defined as a loss of pregnancy at or before 20 weeks of gestation and confirmed by medical records) were identified and tabulated. The municipal utility company provided samples of drinking water that were analyzed for trihalomethane concentrations. Exposures were calculated based on the concentration of total trihalomethane during a woman's first trimester. An increased risk was found for spontaneous abortions in women who drank more than five glasses of tap water containing more than 75 µg/L total trihalomethanes, with the only individual trihalomethane to have a positive association with spontaneous abortions being BDCM at a concentration greater than 18 µg/L.[5]

In a separate population-based study by King et al.,[15] the risk of stillbirth in a human population was assessed through a retrospective cohort study also of trihalomethane exposure through drinking water. Approximately 50,000 singleton deliveries between 1988 and 1995 were evaluated by linking residence at the time of delivery to concentrations of trihalomethanes in local drinking water. The cause of death was also recorded when known, and this information provided some of the most interesting results. Both the total trihalomethane and specific trihalomethane were associated with increased incidence of stillbirths, with the strongest association found for BDCM. The risk of stillbirth was twice as high for exposures to BDCM at concentrations of 20 µg/L compared to concentrations of 5 µg/L or less.[15] Additionally, a stronger association was found between trihalomethane exposures and asphyxia-related deaths than was seen in unexplained caused of deaths or stillbirths overall,[14] and, although not indicated, suggests a placental target of toxicity.

Both of these studies were designed with reasonable cohorts, good recruitment procedures and screening protocols, adequate subject numbers, and relied on credible information regarding fetal losses. Thus, the association found in both studies between increased fetal loss in humans and exposure to trihalomethanes is a convincing and compelling reason for controlled laboratory experiments.

EXPERIMENTAL STUDIES

IN VIVO STUDIES   The results obtained from population-based studies stimulated experimental studies to investigate the adverse effects of candidate compounds such as BDCM on the maintenance of pregnancy. Narotsky et al.[18] tested the developmental toxicity of BDCM in different vehicles and established that it induced fetal loss in rats. A second report by Bielmeier et al.[19] extended the Narotsky et al.[18] study using a different rat strain to test the toxic effects of BDCM on pregnancy loss. Different time periods of exposure were compared and the endocrine mechanism was explored in this later study. The experimental design compared the F344 rat [as used in Narotsky et al.] to the Sprague Dawley (SD) rat and focused on aqueous gavage as the only vehicle delivered on gestational days 6–10 (GD6–10) or 11–15 (GD11–15). The F344 rats treated on GD6-10 were observed to have a 62% occurrence of full litter resorption compared to no losses in the SD strain. When the treatment period was shifted to GD11–15, the effect of exposure on pregnancy loss disappeared. Measurements of serum progesterone showed a decrease in progesterone secretion but not in LH 24 h following exposure.

The Bielmeier et al.[19] report reveals clear evidence of *strain differences* in toxicity and provides additional evidence that catabolic by-products may be involved. Again, there is no question regarding the specific exposure since the doses were delivered by gavage. This study also shows that a direct embryo-lethal action is not the complete story on the mechanism of action of BDMC since a change in *progesterone levels* is detected during the progesterone-dependent period of gestation (gestational days 6–10). The failure of BDMC to exert adverse effects after the progesterone-sensitive interval, the reduction of serum progesterone, and the unchanged serum LH levels suggests that the target of toxicity in the rat is the ovary and that the mechanism of action is a reduced sensitivity of the CL to LH.

IN VITRO STUDIES *In vitro* studies are designed to confirm the target cell and assess the mechanisms of toxicity at the biochemical and molecular levels. Chen et al. performed two *in vitro* studies[20,21] to address the mechanisms of BDCM action in inducing spontaneous abortion in humans. In the first report, primary cultures of human term trophoblast cells were used to test the hypothesis that BDCM targets the placenta. Multinucleated syncytiotrophoblast-like cells were derived from trophoblasts and incubated with different doses of BDCM. While trophoblast viability and morphology were similar between control and exposed cultures, exposed cultures exhibited a dose-dependent decrease in immunoreactive chorionic gonadotropin (CG) and bioactive CG secretion. This observation resulted in the conclusion that BDCM disturbs secretion of CG by differentiated trophoblasts *in vitro*, and supported the hypothesis that the placenta is a likely target of BDCM toxicity.[20]

A second study by Chen et al.[21] evaluated the effects of BDCM on morphologic differentiation of human mononucleated cytotrophoblast cells to multinucleated syncytiotrophoblast-like colonies. Formation of multinucleated colonies was inhibited in cytotrophoblast cultures exposed to BDCM in a dose-dependent manner as determined by immunocytochemical staining of desmosomes and nuclei. CG secretion was significantly inhibited, once again, in a dose-dependent manner and cellular levels of CG were also reduced. Trophoblast viability was not affected by BDCM exposure. The authors concluded that BDCM disrupted differentiation and inhibited CG secretion *in vitro*, which lends further support to the hypothesis that BDCM targets the placenta in primates. *In vivo* studies using the nonhuman primate animal model have not been done but are the logical "next step" in completing the investigation to correctly classify BDCM as a human reproductive toxicant.

Conclusion

The entry of large numbers of women in the workplace, the presence of potential hazardous chemicals in the home, and the recognition that women have gender-specific risks to toxicant exposure are the basis for real public concern regarding environmental exposure to toxicants and women's reproductive health. Solvents, metals, cigarette smoke, pesticides, wetting agents, and plasticizers are part of a growing list of the real and potential risks to human fertility. The classification of a large number of these compounds as environmental hazards to reproduction confirms the public's growing concern for reproductive health safety. But what portion of human infertility is a result of environmental hazards? Do adverse effects in wildlife predict similar effects in humans? How do we identify true hazards and establish appropriate guidelines? All these questions remain to be answered. A large national effort is currently underway to develop informative, high throughput screening assays that can keep abreast of the emergence of new compounds.

There is a paucity of mechanistic details, even with well-defined toxicants. Cigarette smoke, for example, leads to early menopause presumably through a depletion of primordial follicles. Despite numerous studies, the mechanism of this action is not known. Similarly, dioxin results in decreased estrogen production, decreased estrogen action, and early pregnancy loss. But the exact mechanisms are not well-defined and investigations to uncover them are likely to lead to previously unknown aspects of reproductive physiology.

The example of BDCM demonstrates three of the many challenges in female reproductive toxicology. First, how do we detect an increased incidence of reproductive failure with the unusually high degree of spontaneous reproductive failure in human populations? Second, when animal models with nonprimate reproductive traits are used to test a putative toxicant, how are those differences in physiology considered? Third, even when experiments in closely related primate species confirm the rodent studies, how do we set standards for safety that will safeguard women's health?

KEY POINT

The greatest limitation in identifying environmental hazards affecting reproduction is the lack of biomarkers that will accurately identify infertility or pregnancy losses attributable to exposure to environmental toxins in contradistinction to those losses that occur spontaneously.

While the potential of environmental hazards causing infertility and pregnancy loss is of great public concern, there are serious limitations to our ability to detect or identify agents that may be responsible for such events in women. Perhaps the greatest limitation in identifying environmental hazards that increase these adverse effects is the unavailability of biomarkers that will accurately identify infertility or pregnancy losses attributable to exposure to environmental toxins in contradistinction to those losses that occur spontaneously. As much as two-thirds of women's infertility and one-third of all failed human conceptions are thought to be the result of natural processes. This large percentage of disease and spontaneous losses can overshadow small increases of abortions that occur as a result of environmental exposures. New methods must be developed to deal with this problem. Great strides have been made in validating and applying such new methods. Several laboratories have focused on subtle differences in hormone secretion patterns that occur in the menstrual cycle and early in surviving and spontaneously failing pregnancies. Initial studies suggest that differences exist in the bioactivity of human chorionic gonadotropin in serum samples from surviving versus spontaneously failing pregnancies and that this difference could be used to predict pregnancy outcome in unexposed pregnancies.[22]

Many chemicals that are known to be reproductive toxicants are poorly metabolized, lipophilic, and often found in large quantities in the environment. Many will have documented adverse effects on wildlife, and many may have similar adverse effects in humans. Additional chemicals of a similar nature are developed each year and there are inadequate methods for adjudicating their safety. Public concern will continue to grow and women will become increasingly suspicious until methods are developed that give clinicians the ability to detect adverse effects on women's reproductive health caused by environmental hazards.

REFERENCES

1 National Research Council: Reproductive and developmental toxicants, regulatory actions provide uncertain protection. United States General Accounting Office, Report to the Chairman, Committee on Governmental Affairs, US Senate, GAO/PEMD-92-3, 1989.

2 Lawson CC, Schnorr TM, Daston GP, et al. An occupational reproductive research agenda for the third millennium. *Environ Health Perspect* 111(4):584, 2003.

3 Lasley BL, Overstreet JW. Biomarkers for human reproductive health, an interdisciplinary approach. *Environ Health Perspect* 106:955, 1998.

4 Enan E, Overstreet JW, Matsumura F, et al. Gender differences in the mechanism of dioxin toxicity in rodents and nonhuman primates. *Reprod Toxicol* 10(5):410–411, 1996.

5 Silbergeld EK, Flaws JA. Environmental exposures and women's health. *Clin Obstet Gynecol* 45:1119–1128, 2002.

6 Heimler I, Trewin AL, Chaffin CL, et al. Modulation of ovarian follicle maturation and effects on apoptotic cell death in Holtzman rats exposed to 2,3,7,8-tetrachlorodibenzo-p-dioxin in utero and lactationally. *Reprod Toxicol* 12(1):69–73, 1998.

7 Petroff BK, Gao X, Ohshima KI, et al. Effects of 2,3,7,8-tetrachlorodibenzo-p-dioxin (TCDD) on serum inhibin concentrations and inhibin immunostaining during follicular development in female Sprague-Dawley rats. *Reprod Toxicol* 16(2):97–105, 2002.

8 Ushinohama K, Son DS, Roby KF, et al. Impaired ovulation by 2,3,7,8 tetrachlorodibenzo-p-dioxin (TCDD) in immature rats treated with equine chorionic gonadotropin. *Reprod Toxicol* 15(3):275–280, 2001.

9 Gao X, Mizuyachi K, Terranova PF, et al. 2,3,7,8-Tetrachlorodibenzo-p-dioxin decreases responsiveness of the hypothalamus to estradiol as a feedback inducer of preovulatory gonadotropin secretion in the immature gonadotropin-primed rat. *Toxicol Appl Pharmacol* 170(3):181–190, 2001.

10 Moran FM, VandeVoort CA, Overstreet JW, et al. 2,3,7,8-Tetrachlorodibenzo-p-dioxin (TCDD) decreases estradiol production by altering the enzyme expression and activity of cytochrome P450c17, 20 lyase of human granulosa cells *in vitro*. *Endocrinology* 144(2):467–473, 2003.

11 Moran FM, Tarara R, Chen J, et al. Effects of dioxin on ovarian function in the cynomolgus monkey (*Macaca fascicularis*). *Reprod Toxicol* 14(4):377–383, 2001.

12 Golub MS, Hogrefe CE, Germann SL, et al. Effects of exogenous estrogenic agents on pubertal growth and reproductive system malnutrition in female rhesus monkeys. *Toxicol Sci* 74(1):103–113, 2003.

13 Jolly A. *The Evolution of Primate Behavior*, 2nd ed. New York, NY: Macmillan, 1985.

14 Waller K, Swan SH, DeLorenze G, et al. Trihalomethanes in drinking water and spontaneous abortion. *Epidemiology* 9:134, 1998.

15 King WD, Marrett LD. Case-control study of bladder cancer and chlorination by-products in treated water (Ontario, Canada). *Cancer Causes Control* 7:596, 2000.

16 Savitz DA, Andrews KW, Pastore LM. Drinking water and pregnancy outcome in central North Carolina: source, amount and trihalomethane levels. *Environ Health Perspect* 103:592–596, 1995.

17 Hertz-Picciotto I, San SH, Neutra RR, et al. Spontaneous abortion in relation to consumption of tap water: an application of methods from survival analysis to a pregnancy follow-up study. *Am J Epidemiol* 3:98–103, 1992.

18 Narotsky MG, Pegram RA, Kavlock RJ. Effect of dosing vehicle on the developmental toxicity of bromodichloromethane and carbon tetrachloride in rats. *Fundam Appl Toxicol* 40:30, 1997.

19 Bielmeier SR, Best DS, Guidici DL, et al. Pregnancy loss in the rat caused by bromodichloromethane. *Toxicol Sci* 59:309, 2001.

20 Chen J, Douglas GC, Thirkill TL, et al. Effect of bromodichloromethane on chorionic gonadotropin secretion by human placental trophoblast cultures. *Toxicol Sci* 76(1):75–82, 2003.

21 Chen J, Thirkill TL, Lohstroh PN, et al. Bromodichloromethane inhibits human placental trophoblast differentiation. *Toxicol Sci* 78(1):166–174, 2003.

22 Ho HH, O'Connor JF, Teiu J, et al. Characterization of hCG in normal and failing pregnancies. J Early Pregnancy: *Biol Med* 3(3):213–224, 1997.

7 The Psychologic Aspects of Infertility

Linda D. Applegarth

Introduction

KEY POINT

For most people, the inability to have a child leads to a crisis and creates many emotional pitfalls.

For most people, infertility can be a very disruptive and painful emotional experience. It brings on an array of powerful feelings that are sometimes difficult to manage. These feelings seem to stem from the fact that the desire and drive to have children is deeply rooted in our human culture as well as in our biology. When efforts to conceive and bear children are unsuccessful many people are left with not only feelings of anxiety and depression but also sadness and shame. The psychologic aspects of infertility can spread throughout the lives of a couple. Infertility affects career and financial decisions, relationships with partners, family, and friends, and it may ultimately affect one's basic sense of self-esteem and well-being. The purpose of this chapter is to describe the many psychologic and emotional responses to infertility, to discuss coping strategies that may be helpful during this difficult period, and to review a variety of family-building options which can lead to resolution. Within this context, there will also be a discussion of other conditions or circumstances which can contribute to or compound the experience of infertility. These can include age, pregnancy loss, secondary infertility, third-party reproduction, and psychosocial issues for single women and lesbian couples wanting to have children.

Guiding Questions

APPROACHING THE PATIENT

PSYCHOLOGIC CONSIDERATIONS

- How long has the patient/couple been trying to conceive? How willing are they to accept the diagnosis of infertility? What is their level of stress at this point in the process?

175

- What are some key components of the patient's emotional response to the infertility? What are some signs of significant anxiety or depression?
- To what extent is the patient depressed or anxious? Should he/she be referred to a mental health professional for counseling or psychotherapy?
- Does the couple appear to have a stable, supportive relationship? Are they allied with respect to treatment decisions or other parenting possibilities?
- How knowledgeable and well-informed is the patient regarding drug therapies, treatment possibilities, and options? Is the couple open to considering the treatment plan and recommendations?
- What is the individual's or couple's source of social support? Would a referral to a consumer support organization (such as *Resolve*) or to a mental health professional be a critical resource during this life crisis?
- Is the couple open to considering a range of parenting alternatives?
- What are some special circumstances which can occur during the infertility experience that require a unique understanding on the part of medical professionals?

The Emotional Crisis of Infertility

For many individuals and couples, the ability to conceive and give birth to a child is key to lifelong ideas about the meaning of life. Bearing children and parenting are often the foundations around which couples have built a loving, committed relationship. It is not only frustrating but also devastating for many who want to have children but cannot. Gay Becker notes in her book, *Healing the Infertile Family*, that parenting is the bond that seals the generations together, and the opportunity to pass along life experiences to the next generation is what, for many of us, gives life its meaning.[1]

The condition of infertility usually leads to a life crisis. The inability to conceive or give birth to a healthy child can threaten one's sense of identity as a woman or man, places one's values and motivations for parenthood in question, and often forces people to reevaluate the meaning of their relationship as a couple. It can also lead to financial hardship and uncertainty. As a result, many who experience infertility are thrust into a state of crisis or emotional disequilibrium.

A crisis generally requires significant coping abilities. However, it is not uncommon to find that infertility is the first major life crisis that many have confronted as individuals and as a partnership. Some writers, in fact, have described infertility as akin to the death of a loved one or a divorce. As a result, many people may find that their usual coping mechanisms are insufficient to manage the devastating impact of infertility. Self-esteem and self-confidence often plummet, and the relationship can suffer from blame, guilt, frustration, and disappointment.

The crisis of infertility is especially painful because it tends to be chronic. As a couple, individuals must often face setbacks and failure month after month, year after year. This condition can take a significant emotional toll. The infertility crisis is usually precipitated by *loss* or the *anticipation of loss*. As the menstrual cycle begins each month, this loss is experienced anew. This process can take on a life of its own, and it is not uncommon for couples to fear profoundly that they will never have a child. They fear that they will never be able to enter the world of parenthood that is, in so many ways, a rite of passage into adulthood. Many people, especially women, find it almost impossible to compartmentalize their infertility and not have it take over a major part of their lives.

As might be expected, most couples have tried to conceive on their own for a period of months or even years, and the ultimate diagnosis of infertility usually leads to a wide range of emotional responses. Barbara Eck Menning,[2] the founder of *Resolve*, the National Infertility Association, has described these responses as being similar to those defined by Elizabeth Kubler-Ross (*Death and Dying*) following the death of a loved one.[3] Initially, one may be in a state of *denial or shock*. He or she may ask, "How could I be infertile? I'm healthy, and I've spent so many years trying to be responsible and avoid an unwanted pregnancy. This just cannot be happening!" These feelings of surprise and shock are often followed by feelings of *anger and depression*. It is not uncommon for individuals to feel angry at their partners, at friends and family

KEY POINT

Infertility may represent a significant point of contention and crisis for a couple. The sense of loss may be intense, like a death in the family, and may be chronic.

members who seem to conceive so easily, at God, or at the medical profession for not caring enough or finding an immediate solution to the problem. There is no definite chronology to these feelings and they tend to ebb and flow as the infertile ride a precipitous emotional roller coaster.

If, on the final road to parenthood, a couple learns that they will not be able to have a child that is genetically related to them, they may then experience great feelings of *sadness*. As this loss is acknowledged, processed, and understood, a couple can ultimately move on to *acceptance* and *resolution*. This final stage allows people to go forward and make decisions about other parenting options or about childfree living.[2]

Common Emotional Responses to Infertility

When discussing the emotional responses to infertility, it may be helpful to emphasize that there are often differences between the ways in which men and women experience infertility. Despite advances in the feminist movement, there are still many cultural and social factors that influence women's and men's views of themselves as parents. In general, women are raised with expectations that they will be caregivers—mothers. Notwithstanding other life goals and expectations, the message has always been clear: motherhood is the primary job in a woman's life. For men, the expectations regarding fatherhood have been more vague. They may, in fact, not contemplate having a family, except in very general terms, until it becomes an issue or problem in a relationship. Women tend to accept primary responsibility for continuing the family lifecycle and a number of studies have supported the idea that women are more often adversely emotionally affected by infertility than men (Table 7-1).

In general, infertility patients most often describe the psychologic symptoms of infertility as depression and anger, guilt, and isolation.[4] These emotional responses are often a significant component of the infertility experience (see Table 7-2). The inability to do what many others do so easily and naturally is particularly painful. Some patients may openly describe themselves as feeling defective and worthless. They begin to question their adequacy as a person. The blow to self-esteem is often felt most acutely by those who are achievement oriented and who usually

Table 7-1. SOME GENDER DIFFERENCES AND
THE INFERTILITY EXPERIENCE

MEN	WOMEN
Expectations regarding fatherhood and family may be ambiguous	See motherhood as primary goal of adulthood
Men often initially assume that they are not the cause of the infertility	Women often initially assume that they are the cause of their infertility
In male factor infertility, men may experience strong guilt feelings but are reluctant to express these feelings. They may undergo treatments or move forward with parenting alternatives prematurely	In female factor infertility, women search endlessly for a cause and may reproach themselves for past "misdeeds"
Men often perceive their role as the optimist during the infertility crisis	Women become pessimistic regarding outcomes in an effort to protect themselves from disappointment
Workplace is seen by men as a distraction from the infertility crisis	Infertility often distracts women from efforts to be productive in the workplace
Express anger and irritation toward medical personnel	Feel depressed and helpless

Table 7-2. COMMON EMOTIONAL RESPONSES TO INFERTILITY

Guilt
One or both partners assume blame for the infertility. Self-reproach increases and self-esteem decreases.

Depression
One or both partners develop a sense of helplessness, loss or despair, tearfulness, fatigue, anxiety, sleep or eating disturbances, or an inability to concentrate. The onset of menstruation can often trigger a depression in many infertile couples.

Anger
The infertile couple often feels that life has treated them unfairly. They may feel out of control, resentful, and angry with others, including friends, family, and medical personnel.

Isolation
A sense of social separateness or feeling "left out" of the mainstream of life. Emotional and social isolation negatively impact self-confidence and self-esteem.

know how to go about reaching their goals. Many infertility patients have, in many cases, grown up with the belief that if they work hard enough and are "good" or competent, they will be justly rewarded. Infertility seldom seems to follow such a neat line of reasoning. It is unfair. The resulting sense of powerlessness is unfamiliar, frustrating, and very painful.

For those patients whose self-esteem is significantly dependent on the ability to do or to accomplish goals, the failure to conceive or bear a child becomes easily reinterpreted as *failure as a person*. Thus, it is understandable that individuals and couples may then tend to focus on what they do not have or have not accomplished, and to lose sight of the many positive, productive facets of their lives. Depression can ultimately result from this distorted style of thinking.

KEY POINT

Men and women may experience infertility quite differently. They should be encouraged to discuss these issues.

GUILT

Closely associated with the sense of personal failure is guilt. Some people describe themselves as feeling personally responsible for their infertility. Specifically, women tend to assume, before a thorough infertility work-up, that they are the cause of the infertility. If these assumptions prove true, they may suffer from guilt feelings and diminished self-confidence. All too often, they begin (often fruitlessly) searching for a cause. They may reproach themselves for a past legal abortion, for having had several partners before marriage, for using intrauterine devices (IUDs) or oral contraceptives, and so on. Some women may even go so far as to offer to divorce their husbands so as to free him for the opportunity to have children with someone else. (Not surprisingly, most husbands are aghast and hurt by such a suggestion.)

The attempt to determine how and why the infertility happened can take on an obsessional quality. As the condition persists, many patients feel increasingly out of control or powerless. These feelings lead to anxiety and ruminations that prevent individuals from thinking of little else but the infertility. Frequently, women describe their efforts to conceive as a "second job or career" and they may envy their partners' abilities to be more successful at compartmentalizing and disengaging emotionally from the day-to-day hurts and insults that accompany the infertility experience.

Guilt can also become translated into a belief that God is punishing a person or couple for past misdeeds, and fear that He is withholding the one thing that they value most—a child. This is a powerful aspect of infertility that can lead to a spiritual or religious crisis. Family, friends, or the clergy may also ask the couple to accept their childlessness as "God's will"—a request that for some may be comforting, but for others can lead further to feelings of powerlessness or shame.

Men may also experience guilt feelings, particularly if they have a significant male infertility factor. They may be reluctant, however, to express these feelings, as well as, those of disappointment or grief to their partners. Often the reasoning behind this restraint is the idea that the man will only contribute to the distress that both partners experience as a couple. If this is the case, it is imperative not to encourage treatments or other alternatives, such as donor insemination or adoption, prematurely so that couples don't make family-building decisions out of guilt or denial rather than as the result of an emotional resolution of the problem. This is often an appropriate time to refer couples to an infertility counselor to help them with this difficult and complex issue.

In general, men may perceive their role during the infertility crisis as being the "optimist" during difficult periods when their partners are distraught, discouraged, or depressed. Of interest is that this dynamic seems to happen regardless of which partner carries the diagnosis and it may be based on social and cultural factors which dictate male behavior. For most men, there appears to be a "code of silence" when it comes to expressing feelings. This can lead many men to feel emotionally distant from their partners and others, especially as couples go through the very private and personal aspects of infertility.

Feelings of guilt as well as a general sense of inferiority may be exacerbated by the overt and covert demands and expectations of family and friends. Women and men may experience overwhelming guilt and sorrow about disappointing or denying grandparents-to-be or potential aunts and uncles. Additionally, some couples may be consumed with guilt about failing to fulfill their duties and responsibilities related to "carrying on the family name" or providing an heir. Perceived family pressures placed on couples may or may not be real, but the powerful desire to join the world of parenthood can make some patients very sensitive to the slightest hurt or thoughtless comment.

DEPRESSION

People experiencing infertility seem to describe depression as their most universally experienced condition. Mild depression is expressed by feelings of sadness or despair, tearfulness, fatigue, a feeling of malaise, or a loss of interest in normal activities. The loss of a dreamed-of child with the arrival of each menstrual period, as well as the physical loss of reproductive capacity due to a known or unknown impairment, can be regarded as a significant trauma that may bring on a depressive state. Some infertility patients may experience long periods of profound depression, but most will commonly have short but recurrent episodes brought on by specific events such as family holidays and reunions, a failed *in vitro* fertilization (IVF) cycle, or the announcement of a friend's or family member's pregnancy.

Certainly, depression is a normal response to the emotional pain and loss brought about by infertility; however, severe, ongoing depression can develop resulting in feelings of hopelessness, an inability to function in daily living, severe anxiety or agitation, as well as suicidal thoughts or behavior. This condition requires immediate mental health intervention!

KEY POINT

Depression is the most commonly expressed condition among infertility patients.

Depression is frequently a response to loss, and there seem to be many losses, real or potential, that are an inherent part of infertility. These may include the loss of a dream, the loss of the opportunity to be a parent, the loss of self-confidence and self-esteem, the loss of the feeling of good health, the potential loss of status and prestige, and the potential loss of important relationships. Certainly, the loss of a sense of control over one's life and life plans is probably the one factor that significantly underscores the *life crisis* aspect of infertility. No matter how many doctors with whom they consult, no matter how many treatments they undertake, and no matter what they do, there are no certainties or guarantees that a couple will conceive or give birth to a child. This feeling of powerlessness and loss of control is probably very foreign to the majority of the infertile, and it can be very unsettling to them. Table 7-3 describes specific symptoms which can lead to minor or major depression.

ANGER

It is so common to feel anger as part of the infertility experience. This feeling again seems to stem from a sense of helplessness and a sense of the unfairness of it all. The individual's anger may be

***Table 7-3.* SIGNS OF DEPRESSION**[a]

Loss of interest in usual activities
Depression that doesn't lift
Agitation and anxiety
Marital discord
Strained interpersonal relationships
Obsession over the infertility
High levels of anxiety
Diminished ability to accomplish tasks
Difficulty concentrating
Change in sleep patterns
Change in appetite or weight
Increased use of drugs or alcohol
Thoughts about death or suicide
Social isolation
Persistent feelings of pessimism, guilt, or worthlessness
Persistent feelings of bitterness or anger

[a]Fewer than five symptoms: minor depression; more than five symptoms: major depression.
SOURCE: From *"Frequently Asked Questions—The Psychological Component of Infertility"* from The Mental Health Professional Group of the American Society for Reproductive Medicine (www.asrm.org).

directed at the partner, toward family members and friends, and frequently it is focused on the physician and medical staff, or adoption agency.

Couples often feel anger toward family and friends because they cannot understand the pain that infertility creates and seem insensitive to it. Ironically, these friends and family members usually provide an important source of emotional support under other circumstances. At the time the couple needs family or friends most, they find themselves withdrawing or distancing themselves so as to avoid uncomfortable moments. When anger is directed at one's partner, it can be especially destructive to the relationship. The need to assign blame for causing the infertility or to accuse one's partner of not caring enough or not understanding can have detrimental effects, and may require couples counseling.

Anger at physicians, nurses, and other medical personnel is also common. Some of this anger usually stems from the patient's anxiety, fear, and emotional anguish as well as there is a tendency to see the medical staff as exercising power or control over him or her. It is often helpful to educate physicians and staff about the many emotional aspects of infertility. The patient's frequent questions, demands, and overall neediness may require extra care and attention. Although these efforts can be quite time-consuming, it can often be very helpful to acknowledge the patient's anxiety and worry and to provide them with support and reassurance.

Some infertility patients may also develop more irrational targets for their angry and helpless feelings. They may feel enraged at every pregnant woman they see or at other couples who exhibit happiness and hopefulness about the future. Sometimes the anger will be expressed as belligerence and oppositionalism, and patients may be unaware that often this behavior stems from resentment at life and from sorrow and frustration about the infertility.

It should be stressed that anger is a very natural part of the infertility experience and it will need to be acknowledged and expressed on occasion. Problems can also arise if individuals are hesitant to acknowledge this powerful feeling. Many people are fearful of negative repercussions that might result from the expression of anger: a negative pregnancy outcome, or, rejection or abandonment by your spouse, family, friends, or medical personnel. Anger is a human feeling. It can be expressed appropriately and dealt with in such a way as to avoid offending or pushing away the people who care most. If the patient or couple is having difficulty in this area, it may be helpful to recommend an infertility counselor or suggest they contact *Resolve*, the National Infertility Association (www.resolve.org) at 617-623-0744 to locate a chapter or support resource nearby.

KEY POINT

Anger is quite common in infertility patients and caregivers must understand and accept this in the care of these patients. Taking time to explain and support couples with their questions may help.

ISOLATION

Infertility is inherently sexual and is often considered a "private" problem. As a result, many individuals and couples may find it exceedingly difficult to discuss this issue openly with others. They believe (often correctly) that no one else can understand the extent of the emotional pain, longing, and turmoil that it brings.

Perhaps feelings of isolation and social separateness began to develop as patients realize that others around them seem to conceive and bear children effortlessly. Unlike those experiencing infertility, they are able to plan for the future and "move on" with their lives. This sense of isolation may also develop if couples are continuously questioned or teased about their childlessness. The need to isolate themselves from the emotional pain brought on by curiosity or by social celebrations such as baby showers, christenings, and family religious and holiday events, is intense. These moments can leave infertility patients feeling left out of the mainstream of life.

Depending on the social and cultural environment, infertility can sometimes be experienced as shame and embarrassment. Emotional and social isolation can have a deleterious impact on one's self-confidence and self-esteem. The infertility can thus leave one feeling estranged from others, impaired, and prohibited from being a part of the larger social context. Having adequate social support is crucial as a way of coping more effectively with the isolation that can stem from the infertility crisis. Infertility support groups are often an invaluable source of mutual support and a productive means of connecting with others who share this experience.

Infertility and the Couple's Relationship

Perhaps one of the greatest stresses resulting from the infertility crisis is the strain that is placed on a marriage. Because many couples view having a child as a primary life goal, the inability to have a child may shake the very foundation of their relationship. Many may fear, in fact, that their marriage will be destroyed. This fear can seem very real to those who have placed parenthood as a central focus of a relationship. In addition, this focus is strongly supported not only by biological forces but also by most cultures and religions throughout the world. During this time of stress and vulnerability, feelings of guilt or blame may sabotage partners' interactions with one another (Table 7-4).

Within a couple's relationship, there seem to be many "gender-specific" or male versus female types of responses to infertility[6] (Table 7-1). These may at times undermine the intimacy and emotional bond that many partners experience with one another. Although couples have many, and often similar, feelings about infertility, they often tend to respond to them quite differently.

Table 7-4.   THE IMPACT OF INFERTILITY ON THE COUPLE'S RELATIONSHIP

1. When the lifelong goal of conceiving a child goes unmet, the couple may feel angry, anxious, and fearful.
2. Infertility may be the first life crisis that the couple has faced together, and they may be poorly prepared to cope effectively.
3. Partners may view their roles quite differently throughout the infertility experience yet each may feel misunderstood or uncared for.
4. Because of fear, anxiety, and emotional neediness, the infertile couple may have difficulty communicating with one another.

Frequently, there are expectations on the part of one person as to how his/her partner should react to the infertility crisis. For example, if her husband does not appear openly distressed or refuses to talk about the problem, the wife may believe that he doesn't really want a child or that he doesn't care about her fears and concerns. Men, on the other hand, often feel overwhelmed with their wives' desire to talk constantly about the infertility, and may feel helpless to change the situation. As a result, as partners, the couple may withdraw from one another, feeling angry, hurt, and alone.

KEY POINT

Men and women often respond differently to the infertility experience. This can lead to breakdown in communication between partners. The stress of infertility can also result in sexual dissatisfaction or dysfunction.

Furthermore, society has supported, and even encouraged, emotional expression on the part of women. Societal expectations for men, however, have focused on the suppression of emotions. It is not surprising therefore the woman may tend to react to the infertility with significant emotional upset whereas her partner may respond with calm, reason, and optimism. In fact, men sometimes consciously suppress their own concerns and anxieties in an effort to console and comfort their partners. Although these diverse responses to the infertility crisis may provide some balance in a relationship, there may be periods in which the couple is unable to work through differences with respect to treatment decisions, parenting options, and so forth. In these cases, couples often benefit from brief counseling aimed at helping them develop more effective communication skills that ultimately enable them to feel closer on this issue.

The sexual relationship may also suffer during the long months or years of infertility. Infertile couples have reported problems ranging from lack of desire, pleasure, or spontaneity to overt sexual dysfunction. With the inability to conceive, there may be a tendency for sexual intercourse to become either mechanical or contrived, and perceived as "sex on demand." Many couples feel either required or obligated to be sexually active so as not to miss the optimally fertile days of the menstrual cycle. The pleasure and enjoyment that were once intrinsic to lovemaking now become illusive. As infertility testing and treatment continue, couples often feel a greater pressure to perform sexually.

Because fertility is so intimately tied in most people's minds to sexuality and identity as a sexual being, some may find themselves feeling inadequate as well as sexually undesirable. With the disappointments that come with months of trying to conceive, partners may feel more and more isolated from one another in the one place they have felt closest and most intimate—the bedroom. Sexuality then takes on a new definition: failure and despair. It is certainly not surprising that infertile couples have difficulty feeling positive about themselves as healthy and "normal." Although they are not able to protect themselves from all the threats that infertility presents to a satisfying, fulfilling sexual relationship, there are things that couples can do to help come to terms with their "bedroom demons." Health and mental health professionals can offer the following suggestions:

1. Try to bring sexual issues into the open by talking about them. It is important to understand that you are not sexually maladjusted but responding normally to the strains that infertility puts on the sexual relationship.
2. Try to be innovative about sexual practices so as to counteract the sexual monotony and routine that arises from such purposeful lovemaking. Consider having sexual intercourse on days that you know that it is unlikely you can conceive.
3. If you are depressed or feeling helpless, consider meeting with a mental health professional. Depression and anxiety can often interfere with sexual desire.

Marriage, or a long-term, committed partnership, is a complex relationship, and there is no single test that can predict with accuracy how it will weather the long, often unabating storm of infertility. Given the nature of the infertility experience, many couples are frequently not prepared to cope with the uncertainties, fears, and potential losses involved. Ultimately, only the couple can truly know the sacrifices and rewards of their relationship, and only they can decide its future. It is important to encourage them to keep lines of communication open during this most difficult and stressful time.

Although this section has focused on the potentially negative impact of infertility on a couple's relationship, it should be emphasized that most healthy relationships can withstand the infertility crisis. Many couples, in fact, find that their relationship has been strengthened by this powerful life event and that they have been able to cope together as a supportive, unified partnership.

Emotional Factors as a Cause of Infertility

As recently as 30 years ago, it was believed that there was a direct psychologic basis underlying many cases of infertility. This condition was thought to be the direct result of emotional conflicts around femininity or masculinity or a conflicted or ambivalent relationship with one's mother. Men and women were both seen as experiencing psychosexual maladjustments that resulted in the inability to conceive. It is certainly not surprising that infertile couples hid their condition as best they could and seldom discussed it with even their closest family members and friends. With the refinement of diagnostic techniques and treatments for infertility as well as increased research into the psychologic bases of infertility, it was later concluded that there are numerous organic or physiologic reasons for infertility. In fact, infertility is more likely to *cause* distress rather than being the result of it.

KEY POINT

There is little hard evidence to support the notion that stress causes infertility. However, learning stress management techniques can be very useful in coping with this emotionally difficult life event.

Despite this current view regarding the psychologic component of infertility, both patients and clinical investigators have recently questioned the roles that stress may play in reproduction.[7] Researchers have now begun to consider the hormonal changes that occur in the human body during stressful periods, and many infertility patients have expressed concerns about the effects of tension, anxiety, and/or worry and their impact on pregnancy outcomes.

Although scientific research in this area is still in its infancy, there are studies which point to a circular aspect of stress and infertility. As the infertility investigation and treatment become more prolonged and difficult, the resulting stress may have an adverse effect on fertility. One recent study[8] suggests that psychologic interventions in the form of support groups or cognitive-behavioral (mind/body) groups may lead to increased pregnancy rates in women. However, a word of caution: this type of research is very preliminary, and it could be easy for patients to blame themselves or see themselves as a failure if they joined a group and did not conceive. Clearly, there are many reasons that people are infertile and it is especially important to encourage couples not to fall into the trap of believing that "if I take a vacation or join a support group, I will get pregnant." Psychologic support groups are important and helpful in many ways that go beyond the possibility of getting pregnant: they help infertile people feel better and cope more effectively with their condition.

Helping Patients Cope with the Medical Evaluation and Treatment

KEY POINT

Developing more effective strategies for coping with anxiety and depression during infertility can create a greater sense of control, improved social relationships, and improved decision-making abilities. Dependence on the medical team can also be mitigated.

The ability to develop useful coping strategies during the infertility crisis seems to make it more manageable and less anxiety-producing for most patients. To gain and maintain a more balanced sense of control, patients should be encouraged to communicate as openly, honestly, and directly as possible with their physician. This communication can include establishing a long-term treatment plan and responding to specific questions about that plan. The communication might also include providing information about the physical and emotional implications of various diagnostic tests and drug therapies as well as about the medical treatment alternatives and costs that couples should consider.

A useful way of addressing feelings of helplessness is to provide patients with as much information as possible. In general, the more informed and educated patients are, the more positive their medical treatment-experience as a whole, and, more specifically, the better the physician-patient relationship. Whenever it is possible, encourage patients to attend medical consultations together as a couple. Because these meetings are sometimes stressful, patients often miss or forget important pieces of information. With both partners present at medical consultations, it is less likely that there will be confusion or misunderstanding. In addition, *Resolve*, the National Infertility Association (www.resolve.org), and the American Society for Reproductive Medicine (www.asrm.org) make informational fact sheets and patient education booklets available to patients who require information about all aspects of infertility treatments and options.

Treatment Decisions and Other Family-Building Options

For many individuals and couples, the path to parenthood is a slow and arduous process. It usually begins with the least invasive medical tests and procedures, and may slowly expand toward high technology treatments that can lead to tough decisions. These involve medical, emotional, and financial considerations. Other patients may have received a clear diagnosis early during the infertility evaluation, leaving them shocked and devastated. In either case, many infertile couples are faced with treatment choices and family-building alternatives which are ultimately an emotional and financial gamble.

THE ASSISTED REPRODUCTIVE TECHNOLOGIES

The advancement in medical and scientific technology in reproductive medicine has been meteoric. The assisted reproductive technologies (ARTs) have brought new hope to many patients whose parenting options only a decade ago were considerably more limited. Despite the hope and potential success of these medical advances [IVF, micromanipulation of eggs and sperm, including intracytoplasmic sperm injection (ICSI), sperm and egg donation, preimplantation genetic diagnosis, and so on], they are accompanied by additional emotional factors and other stressors that may be unique to each procedure. These include significant financial expense, less than optimal statistical success rates, medical risks, removal of sexual intercourse as part of conception, and potential legal, moral, and ethical conflicts.

Most couples enter IVF and its related treatments seeing it as a last, best option for having a child that is biologically related to them. The emotional stakes are quite high in light of the potential for great disappointment and loss. At the same time, there is new hope that these treatments will finally result in a healthy child. This is a crucial time for individuals and couples to take care of themselves emotionally because, in all likelihood, they have already experienced long months, perhaps years, of infertility treatment. Thus, patients often enter these high technology treatments already feeling fatigued, depressed, or anxious. If they have limited financial resources and/or are relying heavily on insurance coverage for assistance, they may have only one or two attempts at these procedures. The emotional strain and anxiety can therefore be especially fierce.

Each stage of treatment can create new fears and tensions for couples, and the failure to achieve pregnancy will understandably cause a significant grief reaction. Being adequately prepared emotionally for these ARTs procedures can be very helpful. This can include getting accurate and adequate information about success rates as well as medical, financial, emotional, and logistical aspects of the procedure. Psychologic support groups or telephone support from peers as well as access to a mental health professional can also make coping with the procedure much easier. Open communication between partners as well as with medical personnel is also imperative. Ultimately, the vast majority of infertility patients who enter treatment in the ARTs—despite the outcome—will feel that trying these procedures is worth the effort. Of interest is the fact that many couples lose sight of their ultimate goal—to become parents. They get caught up in the singular aspect of conception. It is important to assist couples who need to leave treatment or move to other parenting alternatives feeling that they have done the best they could.

GAMETE (EGG AND SPERM) DONATION

Although the use of donated eggs or sperm appears to be a quick and "reasonable" solution to some couples' infertility problems, it is a decision fraught with long-term psychosocial and emotional implications. The use of donor gametes is not, in fact, another "treatment" or "cure" for infertility. When recommending gamete donation to a couple as a potential means of having a child, there are a number of important issues to be considered.[9]

First, this recommendation in all likelihood follows a statement that there are no medical treatments available that will enable you to have a child that is fully genetically related to both partners. The finality of the individual or couple's infertility must then be accepted. It is common at this point that patients may need some time to grieve this loss before moving to another alternative. Frequently, in the midst of their grief, couples may suddenly be confronted with an option that feels either completely untenable or is seen as a "quick fix" to a seemingly unbearable pain. It is for this reason that it is important for patients to be given time to adequately resolve the finality of their infertility, and they may also need time to consider other options that lead to parenthood. Referral to an infertility counselor at this point may be a healthy and productive way for individuals or couples to obtain information about gamete donation as well as adoption and discuss which of these alternatives feel most comfortable and why.

It is also important to acknowledge that sperm or egg donation is dramatically different than having a child using one's own gametes. Most couples initially set out to have a genetic child, and when this goal cannot be reached, every effort must be made to come to terms with the long-term ramifications of donor conception. These include issues of secrecy and disclosure, the use of a known or anonymous donor, and social and religious attitudes. The decision to use donor gametes can also have an impact on the marriage, and it most assuredly has an impact on the potential child.[10]

ADOPTION

Adoption is a wonderful resolution for many people. After long months and years of infertility treatment, many couples may come to the conclusion that becoming a parent is more important than experiencing pregnancy and childbirth. As the authors of *Resolving Infertility* (HarperCollins Publishers, 1999) point out, there are many worries that people have when considering adoption. However, most are myths and stereotypes.[5] The vast majority of adoptions are tremendously satisfying for both parents and couples as well as other family members. There are also ways to make adoption affordable, and the best way to ensure a legally safe adoption is advise patients to work with a reputable agency or adoption attorney. Again, it is crucial that, if patients are considering adoption, they be encouraged to allow themselves time to grieve the loss of their fertility and obtain as much information as possible before moving forward. Infertility counselors or consumer organizations such as *Resolve* can often be helpful to individuals or couples wishing to adopt, and usually have many available resources and referrals.

CHILDFREE LIVING
KEY POINT

Depending on their emotional stamina and social support, financial resources, medical diagnosis, and degree of need to have a genetic offspring, couples may turn to a wide variety of family-building options or decide to remain "childfree."

At the end of the infertility crisis, some couples decide that they would like to consider a life that does not include parenthood. The term "childfree" suggests that they have made this a choice rather than being "childless" as the result of treatment failure.[11] In choosing this option, some partners may also choose to reverse this decision at a later time. Others may find themselves surprisingly comfortable with this choice, and they may also seek out friends who are also childfree or who have older children who do not require as much focused attention. Some couples may still want to have children in their lives in a variety of ways (such as spending time with nephews and nieces, or doing volunteer work with children). The pleasure that they take in them will no doubt be very different than the painful feelings they experienced during the infertility crisis.

Special Infertility Conditions and Considerations

PREGNANCY LOSS

The loss of a pregnancy can have complex psychologic ramifications for a couple. Although a woman may be able to conceive without difficulty, she may view herself as a failure because of the inability of her body to carry a healthy child to term. Often those who have suffered a pregnancy loss feel personally responsible for the loss and thus experience overwhelming guilt and fear. A pregnancy loss is mourned regardless of whether the loss was early in the pregnancy or after birth, and the expression of grief may be as great with a miscarriage as with a stillbirth. The intensity and duration of the grief, however, tend to be less in a miscarriage.

Nonetheless, professionals as well as the general community still tend to regard miscarriage as a relative insignificant event from which a woman can quickly recover with few, if any, lasting psychologic effects on either the woman or her partner. With pregnancy loss in general, there has been cultural denial with respect to its impact on the couple and a tendency not to define miscarriage or stillbirth as a legitimate source of grief.[12]

Some women, who have experienced a pregnancy loss, have noted that they were not encouraged to cry, grieve, or talk about the loss. As a result, they may sense that their feelings are unjustified, and they have tried to deny them—to themselves as well as to others. Interestingly, medical personnel can also perpetuate these feelings of isolation by tending to minimize the emotional and psychologic effects of the loss.

Those patients who have been able to conceive after infertility treatment and subsequently suffer a pregnancy loss, in all likelihood, will experience this differently than those who have no difficulty with conception. Their grief may be especially profound, as they fear, sometimes realistically, that this was their only chance at bearing a child.

There are several factors that are important in coping with a pregnancy loss and these can influence couples' adjustment to this loss. Physicians, for example, can play an invaluable role in alleviating feelings of guilt, grief, and frustration. It is also very helpful for patients to have emotional support from family and friends as well as from others who have experienced a similar loss. For those patients who are severely depressed or are having difficulty recovering from their grief, it is recommended that they seek help from a mental health professional.

INFERTILITY AND MIDLIFE

Many women in their late 30s and early 40s have postponed childbearing to obtain their educations, establish themselves in careers, or become financially secure. These aspirations frequently work against the decision to have children. Other midlife women may have only recently found a suitable partner. The importance of the "biological clock" cannot be overlooked, and for women over 35, some may discover that it is more difficult to conceive than expected. If this is the case, physicians and other health professionals may encourage a woman to be more aggressive in her efforts to conceive. As women age and the opportunity to conceive and bear children becomes closed to them, it seems that the loss of the ability to choose to have a child can also result in painful disappointment.[13] The realization of this "missed opportunity" can also lead to self-recrimination and depression. As with younger couples, these patients may have to come to terms with this loss and consider other family-building alternatives. Occasionally, this difficult emotional circumstance can lead to the need for mental health intervention.

SECONDARY INFERTILITY

The emotional impact of secondary infertility can, for some couples, be no less severe than for those who never conceived or bore a child. Couples with secondary infertility experience great sadness, longing, anxiety, and pain. They describe the joy of parenthood and feel profoundly deprived because it now eludes them.

The couple who already has a child(ren), often finds themselves in the paradoxical position of being a biological parent and being infertile. For many, it is an emotionally confusing state. The couple is grateful for the child they have, but also yearn for another. Patients who are experiencing primary infertility are seldom a source of support for this population. Some patients with secondary infertility may feel resentful of those who are easily able to have a second or third child, or feel guilty that they can't give their child a sibling. Although they maintain an active parenting role, they tend to feel different and apart from the "normal" family. Bound to all of these emotional dynamics is also the societal pressure to produce more than one child.

Like other infertile couples, it is important to encourage them to develop and use coping strategies to deal with their pain and frustration.[14] Support from *Resolve* or help from a trained mental health professional can be useful in helping patients sort through the many complex issues and feelings that arise during the difficult struggle with secondary infertility.

SINGLE WOMEN AND LESBIAN COUPLES

In some parts of the modern world, there appears to be less social stigma toward people who wish to become single parents or same-sex parents. For both groups, however, the idea of motherhood by choice has only recently been more widely acknowledged by physicians and other health professionals. Those who present to infertility clinics are not necessarily infertile or known to be infertile. Rather, they have chosen to have the assistance of medical professionals rather than choosing to conceive via intercourse or self-insemination. It has been pointed out that the motivations for parenting given by single women and lesbian couples do not differ from those of married women.[15] Many of these women state that they have always wanted to have children or hope to fulfill the expectations of family. To that extent, single women and lesbians should not be asked to convince medical practitioners of their desire for children more clearly than married women do. Of interest is the fact that there are little or no data that indicate that children of single mothers by choice or lesbian couples are less well-adjusted or mentally healthy than children born of heterosexual couples.[15]

Although most of these women tend to be thoughtful and deliberate in their decisions to conceive, there are those who may make this decision impulsively and without discussing the issue with family or friends. Many who move forward with this decision have a sound financial situation, have solid social support, and have dealt with their own uncertainties and fears about this life-changing event. In addition, it is important that these women have considered how they will tell the child about his/her conception through the use of donor insemination. While there are definite benefits, the decision to use a known donor will also have potential social and legal ramifications that must be considered. This is usually not the case with the use of an anonymous sperm donor. If the lesbian couple has not come out to family members, work mates, and so on, it is crucial that they give careful thought to what it might be like for a child to carry the burden of this secret. Lesbian couples wishing to have a child together should complete the process of coming out as part of their preparation for parenthood. Meeting with a mental health professional to discuss these and other potential parenting issues can be immensely helpful to single women and lesbian couples if they have not fully processed their decision.

Conclusion

For most individuals and couples, the desire to have children has roots deeply imbedded in our social, cultural, and biological histories. The meanings of infertility for a man and woman may differ, but ultimately most of those who experience prolonged infertility confront a variety of feelings and thoughts, such as anger, guilt, isolation, and depression. As a couple, partners are often forced to undertake an in-depth examination of their relationship as well as their personal beliefs, values, and goals concerning parenthood.

This chapter has touched broadly on a number of important areas and issues that many people, as individuals and couples, will confront during the infertility experience. Other psychosocial topics not discussed here but of equal importance include infertility and stepfamilies, other medical conditions, such as cancer, which impact fertility, the issue of multiple gestations following infertility treatment, and the emotional aspects of pregnancy after infertility.

As medical professionals come to understand the psychologic aspects of infertility, it can be useful to know that patients' feelings and reactions are frequently a normal part of a difficult and unanticipated life crisis. Infertility resolution is a process. Many people feel enormous relief when they are able to make decisions about treatment and parenting so that they are able to move forward. Some may, in fact, welcome the physician's recommendation that they end treatment and consider other parenting options. Keep in mind that it should not be the goal of the medical professional to "fix" everyone's fertility problem; rather, some patients will need to be encouraged to deal with their loss and pain, and leave treatment feeling that they have done the best they could. Infertility changes couples, but hopefully they will come to know that there is life after this experience. Infertile people are likely to cope better with adequate support from others as they make their way through the infertility maze. It is important for them to know that they will survive this ordeal. As with most life crises, individuals and couples can learn to cope more effectively with their infertility. In doing so, they will ultimately develop new strengths and self-understanding that will serve them well throughout a lifetime.

Discussion of Cases

CASE 1

A 36-year-old woman presents to an infertility specialist. She and her husband have attempted to achieve a pregnancy for the past 18 months. She has been seeing her gynecologist who has subsequently referred her to the specialist. Her husband has a normal sperm analysis. The woman is well-nourished and appropriately dressed in business attire. She is an attorney working in a large law firm. On the second visit, the woman becomes tearful and describes herself as facing the infertility alone. She finds herself unable to concentrate at work despite many pressures. She tends to think only about her infertility. Although her husband is sympathetic and supportive, she resists depending on him for emotional support. She states several times that no one understands how she feels, and that she is helpless to manage. She avoids seeing family and friends, and resists going out of the house on weekends. She is having trouble sleeping, and worries that her stress and fatigue are contributing to her infertility. She loves her husband but has offered to divorce him so that he can marry someone who can give him children. She describes herself as being "damaged goods." She tends to be extremely private about her infertility and most of her friends and family members are unaware of the couple's efforts to conceive.

What is your general impression of this patient?

This patient appears to be suffering from a major depression. It is important to ask her whether she has had suicidal ideation. She should be referred to a mental health professional as soon as possible. It may also be a good idea to reassure her that there are a number of antidepressant medications that are safe to take before and during pregnancy.

Is there something that can be done to assist this patient in gaining more social support?

This patient could benefit greatly from talking with others who have experienced infertility. She appears ashamed of her condition and unwilling to seek out her usual sources of support. She should be encouraged to contact *Resolve* or other patient support organizations that can provide confidential support and care. If this type of organization is unavailable, the patient could again benefit from working with an infertility counselor. One goal would be to assist the patient in managing her stress and anxiety more effectively. Another goal would be to build self-esteem and help the patient to find ways that she can reach out to others, including her husband. A counselor experienced in working with infertility patients can be especially helpful with this type of individual.

Is there anything more that can be done to provide relief to this patient?

It is likely that this patient would benefit from having a clear treatment plan. This would allow her to anticipate the treatment steps and regain some sense of control. She should also be encouraged to include her husband at medical consultations as often as possible. This should relieve some of the feeling of carrying the burden of infertility alone.

CASE 2

A 39-year-old woman and her 43-year-old husband present to the infertility specialist. They report that they have been trying to conceive "on and off" for the past 6 years. They have been married for 10 years. They both reported that they had not been interested in having children for the first 4 years of marriage. During the past 6 years, the husband has become more desirous of having children. His wife is still ambivalent, but is willing to look into beginning an infertility work-up. The husband states at the outset that he will not consider adoption under any circumstance. He adds that he wants his wife to begin IVF as soon as possible, and that she'll get "used" to the idea of motherhood eventually. The wife is generally silent throughout the consultation and displays little or no affect. She asks no questions. The husband comments that he wants a "blood heir" and would prefer to have male offspring. The wife notes, toward the end of the interview, that she and her husband's family are estranged. The partners are of different religions, and her in-laws refused to attend their wedding or develop a relationship with her. She is aware, however, that they also want grandchildren and are pressuring her husband on this issue. She also comments offhandedly that perhaps IVF is a good treatment option because she can avoid having sexual relations with her husband.

In addition to doing some basic medical testing with this couple, what other issues should be addressed?

This couple has provided important information about their relationship. Clearly, the marriage is troubled and a referral to a couple's counselor is recommended. The wife's ambivalence about parenthood may be indicative of a desire to leave the marriage. The husband's aggressive stance toward treatment may also be stemming from anxiety and is his way of attempting to hold the marriage together. The couple's delay in seeking medical treatment and problematic sexual relationship are also indicators of marital problems.

What other issues or concerns might there be with these individuals?

Each of these people may have psychologic or personality issues which are specific. The wife appears depressed and intimidated: it is possible that she is being abused emotionally and/or physically by her husband. The husband, who acted against his parents' wishes when he married, appears caught in the middle of this triangle. He may be making an effort to control both sides of this difficult situation. These individuals could benefit from individual psychotherapy to help sort out what emotional "baggage" each is bringing into the relationship.

Should this couple be required to get counseling before proceeding with treatment?

Although this is a tough call for most medical professionals, it would be very difficult to move forward with treatment knowing that there are significant problems in this marriage. This could be seen as a situation in which the physician must act in the "best interest of the potential child." In establishing a requirement for mental health intervention prior to undergoing treatment, the couple may choose to seek out another physician or clinic. More likely, however, is the possibility that the wife will sabotage the treatment as long as she is ambivalent. Her age also compounds the issue and hopefully these psychologic and marital problems can be resolved as quickly as possible.

REFERENCES

1 Becker G. *Healing the Infertile Family: Strengthening Your Relationship in the Search for Parenthood.* New York, NY: Bantam Books, 1990.

2 Menning B. Emotional needs of infertile couples. *Fertil Steril* 34:313–319, 1980.

3 Kubler-Ross E. *On Death and Dying.* New York, NY: Scribner, 1969.

4 Lalos A, Lalos O, Jacobson L. Depression, guilt and isolation among infertile women and their partners. *J Psychosom Obstet Gynecol* 15:197–206, 1986.

5 Aronson D, Clapp D, Hollister M, Resolve staff. *Resolving Infertility: Understanding the Options and Choosing Solutions When You Want to have a Baby.* New York, NY: HarperCollins, 1999.

6 Abbey A, Andrews FM, Halman LJ. Gender's role in responses to infertility. *Psychol Women Q* 15:295–316, 1991.

7 Stanton AL, Dunkel-Schetter C (eds.). *Infertility: Perspectives from Stress and Coping Research.* New York, NY: Plenum Press, 1991.

8 Domar AD, Clapp D, Slawsby EA. Impact of group psychological interventions on pregnancy rates in infertile women. *Fertil Steril* 73:805–811, 2000.

9 Zolbrod AP, Covington SN. Recipient counseling for donor insemination. In: Burns LH, Covington SN (eds.), *Infertility Counseling: A Comprehensive Handbook for Clinicians.* New York, NY: Parthenon Publishing, 1999, p. 325.

10 Greenfeld DA. Recipient counseling for oocyte donation. In: Burns LH, Covington SN (eds.), *Infertility Counseling: A Comprehensive Handbook for Clinicians.* New York, NY: Parthenon Publishing, 1999, p. 345.

11 Carter J, Carter M. *Sweet Grapes: How to Stop Being Infertile and Start Living Again.* Indianapolis, IN: Perspectives Press, 1989.

12 Covington SN. Pregnancy loss. In: Burns LH, Covington SN (eds.), *Infertility Counseling: A Comprehensive Handbook for Clinicians.* New York, NY: Parthenon Publishing, 1999, p. 227.

13 Applegarth LD. Psychosocial effects of infertility and age on women. In: Jansen R, Mortimer D (eds.), *Towards Reproductive Certainty: Fertility & Genetics Beyond 1999.* New York, NY: Parthenon Publishing, 1999, p. 21.

14 Simons HF. *Wanting Another Child. Coping with Secondary Infertility.* New York, NY: Lexington Books, 1995.

15 Jacob MC. Lesbian couples and single women. In: Burns LH, Covington SN (eds.), *Infertility Counseling: A Comprehensive Handbook for Clinicians.* New York, NY: Parthenon Publishing, 1999, p. 267.

Medical Management of the Anovulatory Infertile Female

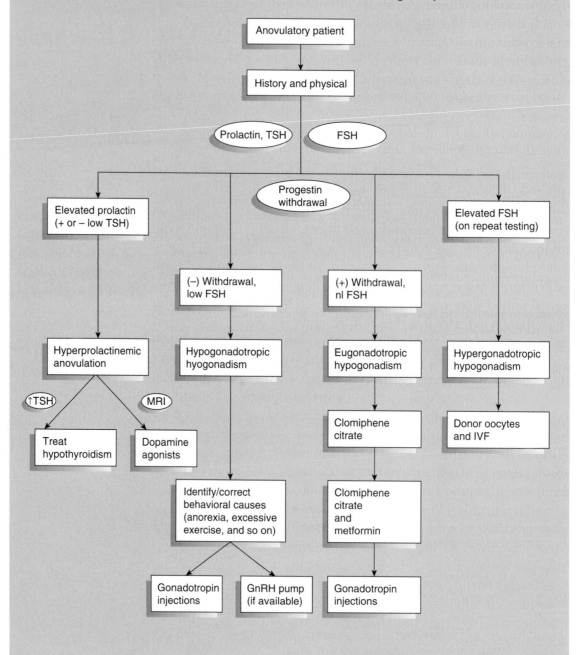

8

Medical Management of the Anovulatory Infertile Female

Kenneth K. Moghadam
Michael Thomas

Introduction

Among the many advances in reproductive medicine during the past 50 years, the successful medical induction of ovulation remains a significant achievement. Beginning with the Food and Drug Administration (FDA) approval of clomiphene citrate (CC) in 1967,[1] clinicians have been able to induce menstrual cycle regularity and ovulation in 75% or more of previously anovulatory patients.[2] The emergence of gonadotropins and gonatropin-releasing hormone (GnRH) analogs provided further treatment alternatives, and now forms the cornerstone of assisted reproductive technologies.

As is often the case, however, success has its limitations. Multiple stimulation cycles are frequently required to attain pregnancy rates comparable to fertile norms, escalating costs, and potential complications. Women also continue to postpone childbearing until their later reproductive years, which can heighten the desire for immediate results in the face of declining treatment efficacy. With a broad range of diagnostic and therapeutic modalities available to the patient, the physician must possess a complete knowledge of ovulation induction to individualize treatment.

KEY POINT

Ovulatory dysfunction represents the most frequent cause of female infertility.

Chronic ovulatory dysfunction is present in 20–25% of infertile females,[3] and is the manifestation of a heterogeneous group of disorders. In this chapter, we will review the causes of anovulation and their medical management, with an emphasis on treatment of anovulation in the polycystic ovarian syndrome (PCOS).

Guiding Questions

- Does the patient have evidence of endogenous estrogen?
- Are there lifestyle modifications that should be made (weight loss or gain, change in exercise, and so on)?
- What would be the most physiologic approach?
- Are there medical illnesses which need correction?
- What are the risks of my treatment recommendations?

Background and Etiology

DIAGNOSIS

The initial interview should focus on the menstrual history. In general, patients with secondary amenorrhea or oligomenorrhea (cycles longer than 35 days) are likely to have ovulatory dysfunction. Alternatively, regular, predictable menses at 25–35-day intervals with moliminal signs (breast discomfort, bloating, and mood changes) are suggestive of normal ovulation. Cycles with an interval of <25 days, while they can be ovulatory, should be suspect for subtle defects of ovulation and particularly a sign of ovarian aging in the woman who has noticed a shortening in her intermenstrual interval. Other elements of the history that relate to ovulatory function include change in weight, temperature intolerance, change in bowel habits, change in hair growth or texture of the hair, vaginal dryness, vasomotor symptoms, or a family history of endocrine disorders. Relevant physical findings would include acne, hirsutism, thyromegaly, acanthosis nigricans (velvety hyperpigmentation of the neck and hair-bearing areas), virilization (clitoral enlargement, voice deepening, male-pattern hair loss), and galactorrhea. Attention should be paid to the vital signs checked routinely by the nursing staff. An elevated blood pressure, in the face of anovulation and hirsutism, may indicate need to evaluate for adrenal abnormalities. While the pulse is a very good bioassay of thyroid status, an additional piece of information that is often mentioned but overlooked in practice is the body mass index (BMI):

$$\text{BMI} = \frac{\text{Weight (kg)}}{\text{Height}^2 \ (\text{m}^2)}$$

The patient's BMI is easily calculated and can help guide therapy. Both obese (BMI greater than 30 kg/m^2) and underweight (BMI less than 18 kg/m^2) women are at increased risk for ovulatory disorders and infertility.[4] Huber-Buchholz and associates demonstrated in a small group of obese PCOS patients that a modest reduction (2–5%) in body weight can reestablish ovulation.[5] Furthermore, sustained weight loss can enhance fertility treatment. In a study of 67 anovulatory, obese subjects who lost an average of 10.3 kg over 6 months in a directed weight loss program; 90% of these women resumed spontaneous ovulation, with significant increases in pregnancy and live birth rates and substantially lower treatment costs.[6] Similarly, Bates et al. noted high (73%) pregnancy rates in a study of previously anovulatory underweight women after weight gain.[7] These results notwithstanding, clinicians should remember that circumstances (including the stress of infertility) may render patients hesitant or even unable to readily make these changes. Nonetheless, recommendations for dietary and lifestyle modification in selected patients should be considered initially and discussed in conjunction with other modes of treatment.

In patients with suspected ovulatory dysfunction, basal body temperature (BBT) testing has been advocated as a cost-effective means of documenting the presence or absence of ovulation. When charting demonstrates a biphasic pattern with sustained temperature rise for greater than 10 days, the couple can be instructed to have intercourse, alternating days during the 5 days before and 1 day following ovulation.[8] However, the BBT is limited in the management of ovulation induction because it is laborious and the progesterone-induced temperature rise is noted only *after* ovulation has already occurred. Patients need to be instructed that ovulation occurs approximately 2 days *prior* to temperature elevation and delaying intercourse until the rise is noted will accomplish effective contraception! The use of BBT charting has decreased significantly since a careful history of *regular, cyclic, predictable* menses is as, or more, predictive of ovulation as is testing with BBT. Given the importance of time for the infertility evaluation and the desire to not contribute the patient's stress level, the usefulness of BBT charting should be questioned in modern fertility care. (See Chap. 1 for a full discussion of ovulation detection.)

Serum progesterone concentrations are elevated following ovulation. Values over 3 ng/mL correlate well with the development of secretory endometrium, but midluteal values above 8.8 ng/mL are typically observed in conception cycles.[9] These levels may also be higher in ovulation induction cycles if the development of multiple corpus luteum cysts is demonstrated.

Luteinizing hormone (LH) prediction kits are frequently employed in clinical settings for ovulation detection. Physicians will typically identify one or two commercially available kits that patients can use and interpret with reliability. The urinary LH surge trails the rise in serum LH by about 5–12 h. It is also important to remember that ovulation can occur in the absence of urinary LH surge detection.[10] In these situations, transvaginal sonography can be used as a back-up technique in monitoring follicular growth and rupture.

The routine use of endometrial biopsy to detect ovulatory response by noting secretory endometrium should be limited. Although this test is the gold standard in assessment of adequacy of the endometrial response to ovarian stimulation, it is frequently a source of patient discomfort and it adds little to the basic infertility evaluation. In current practice, the use of endometrial biopsy is best restricted to women in whom endometrial pathology (hyperplasia or cancer) or a luteal phase defect is suspected. Additionally, it has been shown that women with proven fertility exhibited the same incidence of asynchronous biopsies as those with infertility problems.[11]

WHO CLASSIFICATION In 1993, the World Health Organization (WHO) devised a classification scheme[12] for women who do not ovulate, dividing them into three major categories (Table 8-1). Patients who have hypothalamic amenorrhea as the cause of ovulatory dysfunction comprise *WHO group I*. Such individuals generally have low to low-normal gonadotropin secretion with estradiol concentrations in the postmenopausal range. As a result, affected women do not commonly exhibit withdrawal bleeding when administered

Table 8-1. **WORLD HEALTH ORGANIZATION CLASSIFICATION OF OVARIAN DYSFUNCTION**

CLASS	EXAMPLES
I. Hypothalamic hypogonadism	Kallman's syndrome Anorexia nervosa Exercise-induced amenorrhea Isolated gonadotropin deficiency
II. Euestrogenic chronic anovulation	Polycystic ovarian syndrome Hyperthecosis
III. Hypergonadotropic hypogonadism	Premature ovarian failure

exogenous progestins; these women should also have normal thyroid-stimulating hormone (TSH) and prolactin levels. Disorders in this category include Kallman's syndrome, isolated gonadotropin dysfunction, and some secondary causes of amenorrhea (anorexia nervosa, psychogenic or exercise-induced amenorrhea). *WHO group II* individuals are euestrogenic, often exhibiting an abnormally elevated LH:FSH ratio, though gonadotropins are typically in the normal range. These women represent the majority of anovulatory patients clinicians will encounter, and include women with PCOS. Elevated levels of gonadotropins and hypoestrogenism are characteristic of *WHO group III* patients. Premature ovarian failure and gonadal dysgenesis are examples of conditions in this group. Women with hyperprolactinemia comprise a separate group of patients and we will first consider their management.

Treatment of Hyperprolactinemia

Hyperprolactinemia causes a decrease in GnRH pulsatility through a direct effect of prolactin on the hypothalamus. The three most common etiologies of hyperprolactinemia include pituitary prolactin-secreting adenomas, intake of psychotropic and other medications, and primary hypothyroidism. Basic evaluation ideally includes measurement of fasting serum prolactin and TSH levels,[13] and a review of the patient's current medications. In women with subclinical hypothyroidism and hyperprolactinemia, it is controversial whether thyroxine administration will result in improvement of infertility,[14] although most physicians will treat this clinical entity. If a prolactinoma is the suspected diagnosis, a magnetic resonance image (MRI) study of the head should be obtained to identify the presence of a macroadenoma (tumor greater than or equal to 10 mm in diameter) or microadenoma (tumor less than 10 mm). In the absence of severe visual field and central nervous system disturbances, macroadenomas are approached medically as an initial treatment, as with microadenomas, with reduction of tumor size and resumption of cycle regularity.[15]

BROMOCRIPTINE

Though surgery and radiation can be used for treatment of prolactinomas, medical therapy is the more common approach. Bromocriptine mesylate (Fig. 8-1) is an ergot derivative that stimulates dopaminergic receptors in the brain and anterior pituitary.[16] It is rapidly absorbed and primarily metabolized in the liver, with peak serum levels noted after 3 h. As mentioned, a reduction in tumor diameter can be accomplished with bromocriptine, attributable to a decrease in overall DNA synthesis and cellular proliferation; the response time is variable, from several weeks to several months.[16]

Bromocriptine is usually started at a dose of 1.25 mg each evening for the first 7–14 days to decrease possible side effects. It can then be increased in 1.25 mg increments every 2–3 weeks until normoprolactinemia is achieved. Treatment response rates are high with 80–90% of patients establishing ovulatory menstrual cycles and 70–80% conceiving.[17] When pregnancy occurs in a woman with a known prolactinoma, we advise that the dopamine

Figure 8-1: Chemical structure of bromocriptine.

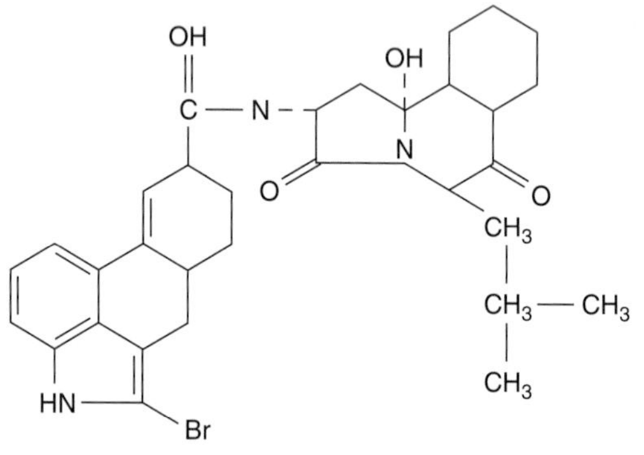

Bromocriptine

agonist be discontinued. With macroadenomas, however, many clinicians will continue therapy throughout pregnancy to reduce the risk of tumor enlargement.[16] Although this approach is a subject of debate, studies of bromocriptine during pregnancy have failed to demonstrate a significant change in pregnancy outcomes.[16]

It is important to note that bromocriptine therapy can be associated with side effects in up to 60% of patients. Gastrointestinal disturbances, such as nausea and vomiting, are the most common reactions, but will lead to discontinuation in only 3–5% of these women.[16] Three other frequent complaints are orthostatic hypotension, nasal congestion, and headache. Many of these symptoms will resolve when the therapeutic dose is established, but an alternative method to minimize these effects is vaginal administration. When given intravaginally, bromocriptine has been shown to be equally efficacious with a longer duration of action.[18] In addition, this approach has not been shown to negatively impact sperm activity or viability.[15] A long-acting depot injectable preparation is also available. In the 10% of patients who are unable to tolerate bromocriptine, pergolide or cabergoline can be substituted. Clinical data with pergolide at doses of 50–100 µg/day have shown comparable results to bromocriptine in efficacy, though it lacks FDA approval for ovulation induction.[19]

CABERGOLINE

During the last several years, the dopamine agonist cabergoline (Fig. 8-2) has been increasingly used in the treatment of hyperprolactinemia. It possesses several advantages over bromocriptine, including a longer half-life that allows for semiweekly dosing and a higher binding capacity for pituitary dopamine (D_2) receptors.[16] Administration is begun at 0.25 mg twice weekly and can be increased in 0.25 mg increments to a maximum of 1 mg twice weekly. In a study of 27 patients who were resistant to bromocriptine or a nonergot dopamine agonist (quinagolide), Colao et al. demonstrated normalization of prolactin levels in 22 of these subjects using cabergoline, with symptomatic improvement in 25 subjects. Side effects were similar to those reported for bromocriptine, but were not as frequent and did not result in discontinuation.[20] It can also be given vaginally to improve tolerance. Cabergoline is a relatively new medication, but continues to show promising results.

For the infrequent patient that fails to show an ovulatory response to dopamine agonists, once the hyperprolactinemia is

KEY POINT

Dopamine agonists are the mainstay of treatment in hyperprolactinemic, anovulatory patients.

Figure 8-2: Chemical structure of cabergoline.

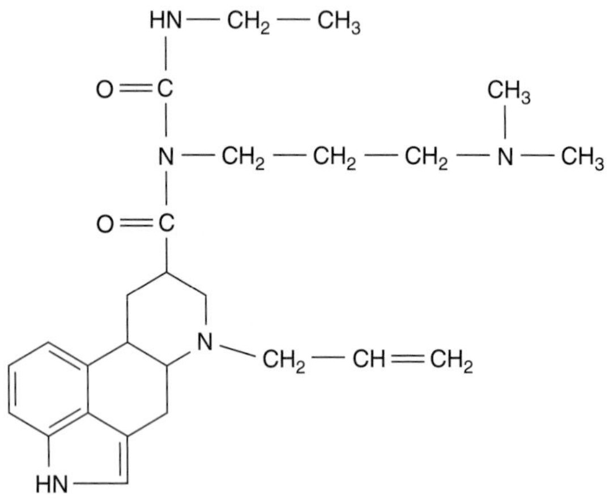

Cabergoline

corrected, the addition of clomiphene citrate or exogenous gonadotropins may be necessary.

Standard Therapy in Ovulation Induction—Estrogenized Anovulation

CLOMIPHENE CITRATE   Owing to its ease of administration, affordability, and successful clinical record, clomiphene citrate (Fig. 8-3) is extensively used in the management of anovulatory infertility. A nonsteroidal compound with weak estrogenic effects, clomiphene is produced as a combination of the isomers enclomiphene (*trans*) and zuclomiphene (*cis*); the more potent *cis*-isomer comprises over one-third of this mixture.[1] Clomiphene is readily absorbed with a half-life of approximately 5 days, and primarily excreted

Figure 8-3: Chemical structure of clomiphene citrate.

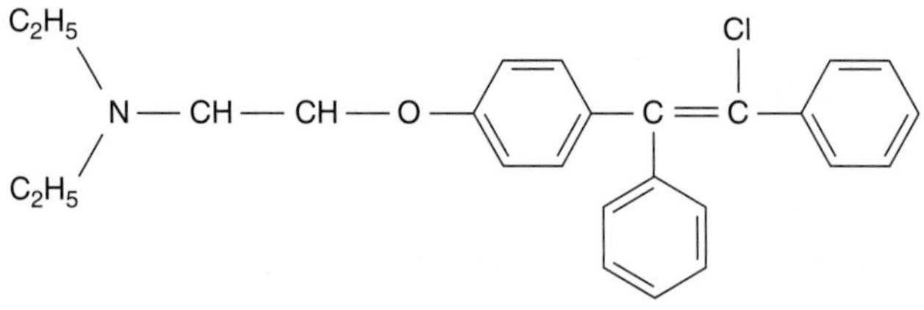

Clomiphene citrate

in the feces. Of note, studies using ^{14}C-labeling demonstrated that clomiphene can be identified in the feces up to 6 weeks following administration.[1] This extended presence allows clomiphene to compete for estrogen-receptor binding sites.

When clomiphene binds to estrogen receptors in the hypothalamus, central perception of circulating estrogen levels is prevented, dampening or abolishing the usual negative feedback response. As a consequence, GnRH pulsatility and gonadotropin secretion are enhanced, which further results in the stimulation of follicular growth and development. Moreover, clomiphene may also affect the pituitary and the ovary directly, enhancing gonadotropin secretion and synergistically augmenting FSH-induced aromatase activity in these sites, respectively.[1] Clomiphene may also exhibit antiestrogenic properties in other areas of the female reproductive tract; particularly the endometrium and cervix (thickened cervical mucus). These antiestrogenic effects may adversely affect likelihood for conception. Some investigators have observed significantly decreased sonographic endometrial thickness[21] and altered morphometric endometrial histology (decreased gland number and increased vacuolated cells)[22] in clomiphene cycles, but others dispute whether these effects exist or have an adverse effect on pregnancy rates.[23] No stimulation of cortisol, androgen, or progestin receptors is noted with clomiphene administration.[24]

As we will discuss, clomiphene is primarily indicated for ovulation induction in the euestrogenic, anovulatory patient (*WHO group II*), most of whom will have PCOS. Treatment is usually begun following spontaneous menses or a progestin withdrawal bleed. Clomiphene is prescribed for 5 days, beginning with cycle days 2–5; variation of the initiation day has not been shown to have an effect on ovulation rates, pregnancy rates, or the endometrium.[25] Nevertheless, it is essential to begin early in the follicular phase to ensure adequate follicular recruitment. The starting dosage of clomiphene is typically 50 mg, but a dose of 25 mg can be considered for lower weight patients, while a dosage of 100 mg may be more appropriate for obese patients. If no ovulatory response is noted using one of the methods mentioned previously, the dose should be increased in future cycles by 50 mg until ovulation is noted, or a maximal dose of 150 mg is reached. While the FDA recommends a prescribed daily maximum of 250 mg, the aforementioned amounts are in concert with common clinical usage. Physicians should also strive to use the lowest dose that induces ovulation, since higher doses have not been shown to improve pregnancy outcomes, and may theoretically have a negative influence on endometrial thickness and implantation. If ultrasound monitoring of follicular maturation is employed, the leading follicle is considered to be mature when it reaches a mean diameter of 18–20 mm. For patients who exhibit sonographic follicular enlargement but fail to ovulate, urinary human chorionic gonadotropin (u-hCG) or recombinant hCG can be used to facilitate mature ovum release and precisely time coitus or insemination. Again, this approach is frequently incorporated in medical practice, but it is unclear if hCG administration improves pregnancy outcomes with clomiphene.[26] When ultrasound is not used, scheduled intercourse should commence every other day starting 3 days after the last clomiphene dose, or it can be timed using a urinary LH surge detection kit.

Women with chronic anovulation as their only source of infertility can expect excellent results—half of these patients will ovulate at the 50 mg dose and an additional 25% will ovulate at the 100 mg dose. Clinicians should keep in mind, however, that these results are cumulative over three to six cycles, and 18% or more of patients will remain anovulatory at the 250 mg clomiphene dosage.[27] In pharmaceutical clinical trials, pregnancy followed in 34.8% (2635/7578) of women given CC, with comparable pregnancy continuation and live birth rates to the general population. An equivalent number of congenital anomalies were also noted. The incidence of multiple gestations was elevated at 8%; the majority of these (86.5%) being twins.[28] Patients should be counseled on the possibility of multiple pregnancies prior to starting medication. Though the risk of ovarian, breast, or cervical cancers has not proved to increase with ovulation induction agents, limitation of use is warranted. Since 95% of those women who conceive on clomiphene will do so in the first 6 months of therapy, it would seem reasonable to limit patients to six consecutive cycles, with no more than a dozen lifetime cycles.[29]

Two of the most significant side effects of clomiphene citrate administration include mild ovarian enlargement (13.6%) and multiple gestations, reviewed in the Chap. 9. Other notable adverse reactions include vasomotor flushing (10.4%), abdominal bloating (5.5%), and rarely visual disturbances (1.5%).[28] While visual symptoms such as night blindness, scotomata, and blurring are usually seen with higher doses and are reversible with clomiphene cessation, many authorities recommend immediate discontinuation and ophthalmologic assessment with these abnormalities due to a few reported instances of optic nerve injury.[30]

Patients who fail to ovulate, or ovulate but fail to conceive after three to four clomiphene cycles should undergo reassessment. For patients who ovulate but do not conceive after four cycles, the "infertility" evaluation should be completed, including a semen analysis and hysterosalpingogram. While some clinicians perform this on all couples at the beginning of the infertility evaluation, in young women with obvious ovulatory defects, this part of the initial workup may be deferred until after ovulation is established without evidence of pregnancy.

KEY POINT

Clomiphene citrate is an effective and inexpensive initial treatment in euestrogenic, anovulatory patients.

For patients who fail to ovulate after increasing the clomiphene dosage, with or without hCG, there are three adjuvant therapies that merit mention. First, for women with hyperandrogenism and elevated dehydroepiandrosterone (DHEAS) levels (above 2 µg/mL), *dexamethasone* can be administered at a dose of 0.5 mg at bedtime to diminish adrenal androgen exposure, with resumption of clomiphene at the 50 mg dose and incremental increase until ovulation is achieved. Dexamethasone is continued until pregnancy is confirmed. Two different investigators provide evidence that anovulatory, clomiphene-resistant patients with hyperandrogenism and DHEAS levels below the 2 µg threshold may benefit from a combined clomiphene and dexamethasone protocol as well.[31,32] A second approach involves pretreatment with *oral contraceptives* for ovarian suppression. Branigan and colleagues demonstrated in a cohort of clomiphene-resistant patients that a 2-month course of oral contraceptives followed by treatment with clomiphene at the 150 mg dose led to ovulation in 69 of 95 cycles (72.6%) and 22 pregnancies in 35 patients (58%).[27] Finally, the use of *insulin-sensitizing agents* such as metformin (either alone or with ovulation induction agents) has had a profound impact on treatment of the anovulatory PCOS patient, and will be discussed later in this chapter. If the patient does not respond or is not a candidate for clomiphene, we proceed to administration of exogenous gonadotropins. A sequential regimen of clomiphene and gonadotropins (clomiphene cycle days 3–7 with low-dose—1 ampule—gonadotropin beginning cycle day 8) may also be used to decrease the risk for over-response and the overall amount of gonadotropin required for ovulation induction.

GONADOTROPINS The first exogenous gonadotropins used for ovarian stimulation were produced from animal pituitary extracts. Despite significant homology, patients rapidly formed antibodies to these immunogenic peptides that neutralized their clinical effect.[33] Investigators then turned to the preparation of cadaveric human pituitary gonadotropins (hPG), but difficulty in harvesting adequate amounts of pituitary tissue and the development of Creutzfeldt-Jakob's disease in recipients resulted in removal of hPG from clinical use.[34] It was later discovered that gonadotropins (in a 1:1 ratio of LH:FSH) could be isolated from the urine of menopausal women. Interestingly, one pituitary gland contains as much FSH as 2–5 L of menopausal urine, but manufacturers were able to perfect urinary extraction techniques. The urinary human menopausal gonadotropins (hMG) were the only available gonadotropin regimen for three decades. As the purification process advanced, researchers focused their efforts on increasing the percentage of FSH in these compounds. This ultimately led to the development of urinary FSH (uFSH) and highly purified urinary FSH (u-hpFSH) derivatives. Both of these forms have negligible or absent biological LH activity,[33] and u-hpFSH has the added feature of more than 95% purity after removal of urinary protein contaminants.[35] Additionally, recombinant FSH (rFSH) preparations were synthesized by transfection of an ovarian cell line from the Chinese hamster with the complete FSH-beta coding sequence together with the alpha subunit minigene; rFSH possesses nearly 100% FSH receptor stimulation without added LH.[36]

What's the Evidence?

Existence of multiple formulations presents a complex choice for the clinician and patient. While much of the existing information comes from *in vitro* fertilization (IVF) studies, some broader observations can still be made. A prospective, randomized trial showed that addition of recombinant LH (rLH) to u-hpFSH did not improve pregnancy rates compared to cycles with u-hpFSH alone, providing support for the concept that only a minimal amount of baseline LH (0.5 IU/L) is required in most instances for successful ovarian stimulation.[37] Superiority of individual FSH preparations, on the other hand, remains controversial. Frydman and colleagues demonstrated in a randomized, double-blinded trial that IVF cycles using u-hpFSH produced significantly fewer oocytes and embryos, and required more ampules and treatment days with similar pregnancy results to IVF cycles using rFSH.[38] These results directly contrast with a recent multicenter trial that showed no significant difference in follicular or embryonic development, treatment course, medication requirement, ongoing pregnancy rates, or tolerability in IVF subjects given u-hpFSH versus rFSH.[39] An ongoing metaanalysis of 18 randomized trials offers a large body of evidence to suggest that pregnancy rates in IVF are 3.7% higher (statistically significant) with rFSH than urinary FSH.[40] Unfortunately, this analysis considers u-FSH and u-hpFSH collectively, preventing individual comparison to rFSH. More research is required to determine if rFSH indeed has an advantage over urine-derived gonadotropins, particularly u-hpFSH.

Since gonadotropins have water-soluble structures that are easily denatured by gastrointestinal enzymes, all gonadotropin preparations must be given through an intramuscular or subcutaneous route.[33] The newer recombinant and purified urinary forms allow for subcutaneous dosing. When administered in the early follicular phase, exogenous gonadotropins directly stimulate the ovaries to rescue some of the 20–40 follicles which possess sufficient granulosa cell receptors. Dosing is tailored to each patient but in general, 1–2 weeks of daily gonadotropin administration will result in adequate follicular recruitment. A baseline cycle day 2–3 ultrasound and estradiol level are obtained to exclude the presence of functional ovarian cysts (mean diameter greater than 10 mm), as these have a potential negative impact on controlled ovarian hyperstimulation with or without IVF.[41,42] We will also typically document an antral follicle count at this time. The patient and her partner undergo injection teaching and start gonadotropin administration that evening, usually at a dosage of 75–150 IU/day (one to two ampules).

Following 4–5 days of medication, the patient returns for repeat sonography and estradiol measurement. Endometrial thickness measurement is frequently added to this and future sonographic assessments. An increase in estradiol levels above 100 pg/mL and the presence of early follicular growth is consistent with a response; the patient is maintained at the current dose and reevaluated in 2 days. Alternatively, some patients will require an increase in medication and return for blood work and sonography in 3 days. The patient is then followed closely at 1–2-day interval until at least one mature lead follicle is seen. Physicians should note that the peak follicular diameter with gonadotropin treatment is 16–18 mm, which is less than that observed with clomiphene. When follicular maturity is attained, hCG is given at a dose between 5000 and 10,000 units to mimic the LH surge and prompt final maturation and oocyte release. Insemination is performed 36 h after injection, or the couple is instructed to have intercourse on two occasions at 12 and 36 h after the injection time.

KEY POINT

The usage of exogenous gonadotropins requires monitoring by a skilled clinician and incurs additional risk.

The approach detailed above is far from absolute and, as we will see, there are significant variations to the theme among patient groups. In certain women, ovulation and pregnancy rates approach 90% over six cycles,[43] though this can differ considerably depending on the patient's age and diagnosis.[43,44] Ovarian hyperstimulation syndrome is a concern with gonadotropin therapy; therefore, estrogen levels merit close surveillance when they approach the 2000–3000 pg/mL range. We strongly recommend that physicians thoroughly advise their patients on all these points before *initiation* of gonadotropin therapy. For patients with three or more mature follicles, it is imperative to address the issue of a high-order multiple pregnancy and the option of therapeutic fetal selective reduction prior to hCG administration.

Treatment of Hypogonadotropic Hypogonadism

Women with hypothalamic anovulation have diminished GnRH secretion, with resultant low gonadotropin and estrogen levels. Hypoestrogenism is verified by low serum estradiol levels or the absence of a progestin withdrawal bleed.[12] In *WHO group I* patients with modifiable causes of anovulation such as high-intensity exercise, eating disorders, and excessive stress, behavior modification is a valuable preliminary intervention. Kallman's syndrome, affecting 1 out of 50,000 females, is characterized by anosmia and hypogonadism, and results from aberrant development and migration of GnRH neurons from the olfactory placode *in utero*.[45] Rare pituitary causes include craniopharyngiomas (tumors of Rathke's pouch arising from the pituitary stalk) and Sheehan's syndrome (pituitary ischemic insult from obstetric hemorrhagic shock), in which gonadotropin secretion is compromised or absent. Since these patients have a blunted endogenous signaling system for folliculogenesis, clomiphene will not provide sufficient stimulation to induce ovulation. Hypogonadotropic anovulation is best approached with either pulsatile GnRH (in nonpituitary causes) or exogenous gonadotropin therapy.

The GnRH pump devices used for ovulation induction are essentially modified insulin pumps that allow a pulse frequency of 60–120 min with GnRH doses of 1–200 µg/pulse. Dose delivery can be accomplished either intravenously or subcutaneously, at optimal dosages of 1–5 µg/pulse or 10–25 µg/pulse, respectively. When the proper dose is achieved, 80–100% of patients will ovulate with a conception rate of 25% per cycle. Monofollicular development occurs most commonly with the use of the GnRH pump, but increasing the amount of GnRH infused can produce multiple follicles.[46] Prior to administration of GnRH, patients may be given exogenous estrogen for 2 months to increase GnRH receptor expression. The GnRH pump is perhaps the best means of ovulation induction in *WHO group I* patients with an intact pituitary response, but the apparatus can be cumbersome and difficult to obtain commercially. If the pump is employed, however, luteal phase support, using either hCG or progesterone, is imperative as these patients will otherwise have a high spontaneous abortion rate of 24–32%.[47]

KEY POINT

The use of pulsatile GnRH is the most physiologic treatment for WHO category I anovulation. The recent difficulty in obtaining this product has increased the usage of exogenous gonadotropins with the inherent increase of multiple gestations.

Given that women with hypogonadotropic hypogonadism have inadequate LH production, most authorities agree that, when using exogenous gonadotropins, a combination of LH and FSH should be administered. With use of FSH alone, follicular growth takes place, but inadequate estradiol production correlates with poor oocyte and endometrial development. As only small amounts of LH are required, several authors have found that adequate LH may be delivered through injection of a single ampule of rLH daily, in addition to the daily dose of the selected FSH preparation.[34] For dosing simplicity, we will routinely use hMG in these patients. Ovulation and pregnancy rates with gonadotropins are high, similar to those mentioned with GnRH administration, but the latter is much more likely to produce a singleton gestation.[48] Luteal support is again the standard.

Treatment of Hypergonadotropic Hypogonadism

Defined as exhaustion of ovarian function before age 40, premature ovarian failure affects approximately 1% of all females.[49] The majority of these women have completed their childbearing, but the remainder desiring fertility pose a difficult dilemma for the physician. A progestin-induced withdrawal bleed may or may not be present, but the diagnosis is confirmed through documentation of two serum FSH levels above 40 mIU/mL in separate cycles.[49] Once the finding is established, few treatment options are available. Patients will intermittently ovulate with a 5% chance of spontaneous pregnancy, but predicting the likelihood and timing of remission individually is not currently feasible. There are case reports of pregnancies following high-dose gonadotropin therapy, but due to the financial cost and the lack of a proven benefit we cannot recommend ovulation induction with gonadotropins. In fact, following review of 52 case reports, 9 uncontrolled studies, 8 observational studies, and 7 controlled trials, van Kasteren and Schoemaker concluded that none of the described treatments demonstrated a significant improvement over nonintervention.[50] The only approach that has been beneficial in women with premature ovarian failure is IVF with donor oocytes. Some data also suggest that egg donation from siblings of these patients results in decreased pregnancy rates.[49]

KEY POINT

Oocyte donation is the most appropriate option for women with premature ovarian failure.

The diminished ovarian reserve, in advanced reproductive age, does not represent ovarian failure, but does have a profound impact on success of ovulation induction techniques. As the potential pool of follicles ages, early follicular phase FSH levels rise due to decreased secretion of inhibin B from these follicles. Buyalos and associates observed that in patients over 35 with cycle day 3 FSH values greater than 13, no live births resulted from the use of clomiphene and/or hMG protocols in conjunction with insemination.[51] The importance here is not the above FSH cutoff value; this will be assay-dependent and physicians should familiarize themselves with the FSH assay of their chosen laboratories. Rather, FSH testing furnishes an additional tool in counseling the patient and planning treatment. Another screen of ovarian reserve is the clomiphene citrate challenge test. Following measurement of cycle day 3 FSH, patients are administered clomiphene citrate, 100 mg, from days 5–9, with repeat cycle day 10 FSH testing. Elevation of either FSH value predicts a markedly decreased response to ovulation induction.[52] Patient expectations should be gauged accordingly, and the option of oocyte donation should be offered when appropriate.

Treatment of Eugonadotropic Hypogonadism

Stein and Leventhal were the first to describe the association of polycystic ovaries with hirsutism and amenorrhea over 65 years ago. Today, PCOS is the most frequently encountered cause of female infertility in the United States and a common endocrinopathy found in 6–10% of reproductive age women.[53] In a 1990 National Institute of Child Health and Human Development (NICHD) conference on PCOS, authorities agreed that the two main diagnostic features of the syndrome are menstrual/ovulatory irregularity and hyperandrogenism in the absence of other endocrine disorders.[54] Two additional pertinent hallmarks of PCOS include obesity (60–70%) and hyperinsulinemia (50–70%). The health-related implications of this disorder extend well beyond fertility issues, but infertility will be the primary complaint in 40% of these patients.[55] As detailed at the beginning of this chapter, a thorough history and physical will readily identify most PCOS patients. Laboratory evaluation of TSH and prolactin levels is then performed, as well as testosterone and DHEAS levels. Obese PCOS patients should be offered consultation with a dietician and provided information on weight loss programs.

PCOS-related insulin resistance is a frequent obstacle to ovulation induction. Most reproductive endocrinologists concur that elevated serum insulin levels stimulate ovarian theca cell production of androgens and alter normal follicular growth. Multiple methods to diagnose insulin resistance in patients have been presented with no prevailing opinion as to which approach is best. A decreased fasting glucose:insulin ratio (less than 4.5) may be employed as a specific indicator of insulin resistance,[56] but limiting intervention to patients who test positive excludes others that might benefit from insulin-sensitizing agents. Lack of a consensus in this area has led many practitioners to proceed with the assumption that all women with PCOS may ovulate with insulin-sensitizing medications. Particularly in obese PCOS patients, empiric treatment with an insulin sensitizer is not an unreasonable starting point. Though lacking FDA approval for ovulation induction, the three most widely studied insulin-sensitizing agents in ovulation induction include D-*chiro*-inositol, troglitazone, and metformin. Several studies of troglitazone showed improvement of insulin sensitivity and ovulation, but reports of liver toxicity ultimately led to its removal from the market; the newer thiazolidinediones, pioglitazone and rosiglitazone, may have similar effects on insulin resistance but have not been extensively studied.[56] D-*chiro*-inositol enhanced ovulation over placebo in a study of obese PCOS patients, but is only available for research purposes at this time.[53]

A wealth of information has permeated fertility literature regarding metformin during the past decade. Metformin is an orally administered biguanide that acts at the cellular level to reduce hepatic gluconeogenesis and augment insulin receptor sensitivity.[57] As it does not directly effect insulin secretion, hypoglycemia is an extremely rare occurrence with metformin therapy, and glucose levels do not need to be monitored. Furthermore, since metformin is a pregnancy category B drug, it has a good safety profile in early pregnancy. Prior to giving metformin, clinicians should confirm normal kidney function (serum creatinine less than 1.5 mg/dL) and normal liver function in each patient. Women undergoing surgery or intravenous contrast administration should also discontinue metformin before and until 48 h after these procedures. We begin dosing at 500 mg daily for the first week and increase the daily dosage by 500 mg each week to a maximum of 1500–2000 mg/day. In responders, ovulation will occur within 6–8 weeks.[56] Gastrointestinal side effects such as bloating, flatulence, and diarrhea are fairly common, leading to intolerance and discontinuation in 5% of patients. Symptoms are related to dosage and may be circumvented through a stepwise dose increase as above.[57]

What's The Data?

A randomized, double-blinded, placebo-controlled trial revealed that women with PCOS who took metformin over at least 6 months had significant improvement in plasma insulin levels, insulin resistance, and menstrual regularity (50% experienced complete cycle normalization).[58] Nestler and colleagues also demonstrated in obese PCOS patients that an ovulatory cycle pattern could be established more readily with the use of clomiphene and metformin (19 of 21 subjects) than clomiphene and placebo (2 of 25 subjects).[59] Regarding pregnancy, a recent study showed that previously anovulatory, clomiphene-resistant PCOS patients given metformin and clomiphene ovulated, and then conceived significantly more often (6 of 11 women) than patients taking placebo and clomiphene (1 of 14 women).[60] Larger numbers of patients are needed to further reinforce these outcomes, but these and other studies provide evidence that metformin is an important therapy in anovulatory PCOS patients. Studies directly comparing metformin and clomiphene monotherapy, as starting treatments, are currently ongoing and may provide new guidance for clinicians in the near future. Even so, authors have begun to advocate metformin as a first-line medication in euestrogenic, normogonadotrophic women for ovulation induction.[56]

Clinicians should be advised that women who were previously clomiphene-resistant at higher doses should be restarted at lower doses of clomiphene when used in conjunction with insulin-sensitizing agents. If patients do not ovulate with clomiphene and/or metformin therapy (or one of the previously described adjuvant clomiphene treatments is not applicable) gonadotropins may be necessary. PCOS patients generally have increased pituitary LH pulsatility, and many exhibit elevated baseline LH levels; they are also at greater risk for ovarian hyperstimulation syndrome. Therefore, a low-dose, step-up FSH-only regimen is often used.[61] Patients are given a 2-week course of 1 ampule/day, with small dose adjustments as needed. Ovulation rates and pregnancy rates approach 70 and 30%, respectively, although insulin resistance can have a negative impact in this area as well.[61,62] To date, there is insufficient evidence to support combined metformin/gonadotropin therapy in clomiphene-resistant patients.

Future Directions

Primarily used in metastatic breast cancer, aromatase inhibitors may prove to be a useful treatment in clomiphene-resistant, anovulatory women. The postulated antiestrogenic effect of clomiphene on the endometrium coupled with its long half-life may contribute to poor cycle implantation and pregnancy rates in some patients. Letrozole is a relatively short-acting (45-h half-life) nonsteroidal aromatase inhibitor that prevents estrogen synthesis from andro-gen precursors.[63] Hence, administration of letrozole in the early follicular phase can release the hypothalamus from negative feed-back, increasing GnRH release. This is accomplished without lin-gering antiestrogenic effects in the reproductive tract. In 12 women with PCOS that failed to ovulate or exhibited a thin (5 mm or less) endometrium with clomiphene, letrozole significantly improved endometrial thickness, with ovulation occurring in 9 of 12 subjects (75%), resulting in three pregnancies (25%).[63] Aromatase inhibitors may indeed prove to be a safe and effective alternative to gonadotropin therapy in these patients.

Discussion of Cases

CASE 1

History A 26-year-old woman presents to your office complaining of irregular cycles and the inability to achieve pregnancy over the past 2 years. She states that her menses have been unpredictable since puberty, and now occur at a 50–70-day interval. On further discussion, the patient admits to significant problems with acne for which her dermatologist prescribed isotretinoin several years ago with some improvement. Her family history is significant for adult-onset diabetes in her father and pater-nal grandmother, and hypothyroidism in her sister. She denies galactorrhea or hirsutism. Her last menstrual period was 6 weeks ago.

Physical Examination On physical assess-ment, the patient's height is 5 ft 5 in. and her weight is 188 lb (BMI 31.3). Inspection of her neck reveals acanthosis nigricans. Her thy-roid is not enlarged and has no palpable nod-ules. Breast examination is negative for expressible discharge or any other abnormali-ties. Her pelvic examination is also unremark-able, with evidence of normal vaginal rugae and secretions.

What testing would you recommend at this point?

- **TSH and prolactin levels are obtained and found to be normal.**
- **As the patient has not had a recent men-strual period, a progestin challenge is administered and the patient has a with-drawal bleed.**

What is your diagnosis and initial manage-ment for this patient?

- **The patient has PCOS.**
- **Since she has evidence of adequate estrogenization, an appropriate initial treatment is clomiphene citrate. The patient is also offered referral to a dieti-cian, and counseled that concurrent exercise and weight loss may improve her chances of ovulation and pregnancy.**
- **She undergoes a hysterosalpingogram which is normal. Her husband's semen parameters are within normal limits.**

The patient fails to ovulate despite three clomiphene cycles with successive dosing increases. What are the next steps in her management?

Following review of her history and stimulation cycles, the best intervention would be initiation of metformin over the next several weeks to a maximal dose of 1500–2000 mg. If the patient does not ovulate on this regimen over one to two cycles, clomiphene is restarted at the 50 mg dose and increased to 100 mg as necessary. If ovulation does not occur in two to three cycles of combined therapy, the patient should be treated with gonadotropins.

CASE 2

History A 33-year-old female presents to your office following 6 months of amenorrhea and desires fertility. The patient discontinued her oral contraceptives after 12 years of continuous use, and has not yet resumed spontaneous cycles. Multiple home pregnancy tests have been negative. The patient has not had any previous difficulties with irregular cycles and denies galactorrhea, weight changes, vasomotor symptoms, hirsutism, or acne. Her past medical history is negative for illnesses other than frequent headaches in the past year; she has also had some associated blurring of her vision recently and plans to see her ophthalmologist next week to update her eyewear prescription.

Physical Examination On physical examination, the patient's height is 5 ft 8 in. and her weight is 145 lb (BMI 22.1). Extraocular movements are normal with no evidence of exophthalmos. Her thyroid is normal in size with no palpable nodules. Breast examination reveals a small amount of milky discharge that is easily expressed bilaterally. She has no palpable masses or lymphadenopathy. Her pelvic examination in unremarkable. The breast is inspected more closely under the microscope and fat lobules are noted.

What testing is warranted to further evaluate this patient?

- **A prolactin level is obtained and found to be elevated at 176 ng/mL. The patient's TSH level is within normal limits, and her pregnancy test is negative.**
- **MRI of the head was performed revealing a 12 mm macroadenoma.**
- **Visual field testing was undertaken and showed no deficits.**

How would you manage this patient's hyperprolactinemia?

- **The most appropriate treatment is a dopamine agonist. In this case, the patient was begun on cabergoline 0.25 mg orally two times weekly. Prolactin levels are followed every 3–4 weeks for improvement and doses are adjusted accordingly.**
- **The patient responded to 0.5 mg twice weekly and resumed ovulatory cycles after 3 months of treatment.**

REFERENCES

1 Dickey RP, Holtkamp DE. Development, pharmacology, and clinical experience with clomiphene citrate. *Hum Reprod Update* 2:483, 1996.

2 Imani B, Eijkemans MJ, te Velde ER, et al. Predictors of patients remaining anovulatory during clomiphene citrate induction of ovulation in normogonadotrophic oligomenorrheic infertility. *J Clin Endocrinol Metab* 83:2361, 1998.

3 van Santbrink EJ, Hop WC, Fauser BC. Classification of normogonadotrophic infertility: polycystic ovaries diagnoses by ultrasound versus endocrine characteristics of polycystic ovarian syndrome. *Fertil Steril* 67:452–458, 1997.

4 Grodstein F, Goldman MB, Cramer DW. Body mass index and ovulatory infertility. *Epidemiology* 5:247–250, 1994.

5 Huber-Buchholz MM, Carey DG, Norman RJ. Restoration of reproductive potential by lifestyle modification in obese polycystic ovary syndrome: role of insulin sensitivity and luteinizing hormone. *J Clin Endocrinol Metab* 84:1470–1474, 1999.

6 Clark AM, Thornley B, Tomlinson L. Weight loss in obese infertile women results in improvement in reproductive outcome for all forms of fertility treatment. *Hum Reprod* 13:1502–1505, 1998.

7 Bates GW, Bates SR, Whitworth NS. Reproductive failure in women who practice weight control. *Fertil Steril* 37:373–378, 1982.

8 Wilcox AJ, Weinburg CR, Baird DD. Timing of sexual intercourse in relation to ovulation. *N Engl J Med* 333:1517–1521, 1995.

9 Hull MGR, Savage PE, Bromham DR, et al. The value of a single serum progesterone measurement in the midluteal phase as a criterion of a potentially fertile cycle ("ovulation") derived from treated and untreated conception cycles. *Fertil Steril* 37:355, 1982.

10 Ponto KL, Barnes RB, Holt JA. Quantitative and qualitative tests for urinary luteinizing hormone: comparison in spontaneous and clomiphene citrate-treated cycles. *J Reprod Med* 35:1051, 1990.

11 Davis OK, Berkeley AS, Naus GF, et al. The incidence of luteal phase defect in normal fertile women, determined by endometrial biopsies. *Fertil Steril* 51:582, 1989.

12 Rowe PJ, Comhaire FH, Hargreave TB, et al. *WHO Manual for the Standardized Investigation and Diagnosis of the Infertile Couple.* Cambridge, MA: Cambridge University Press, 1993.

13 Reichlin S. Neuroendocrinology. In: Wilson JD, Foster DW, Kronenberg HM, Larsen PR (eds.), *Williams Textbook of Endocrinology.* Philadelphia, PA: WB Saunders, 1998, pp. 165–248.

14 Bals-Pratsch M, Geyter CD, Muller T, et al. Episodic variations of prolactin, thyroid-stimulating hormone, luteinizing hormone, melatonin and cortisol in infertile women with subclinical hypothyroidism. *Hum Reprod* 12:896–904, 1997.

15 Blackwell RE. Hyperprolactinemia: evaluation and management. *Endocrinol Metab Clin North Am* 21:105–124, 1992.

16 Molitch ME. Medical treatment of prolactinomas. *Endocrinol Metab Clin North Am* 28:143–169, 1999.

17 Molitch ME. Prolactinomas. In: Melmed S (ed.), *The Pituitary.* Cambridge, MA: Blackwell Science, 1995, pp. 443–477.

18 Katz E, Weiss BE, Hassell A, et al. Increased circulating levels of bromocriptine after vaginal compared with oral administration. *Fertil Steril* 55:882, 1991.

19 Conner P, Fried G. Hyperprolactinemia: etiology, diagnosis and treatment alternatives. *Acta Obstet Gynecol Scand* 77:249–262, 1998.

20 Colao A, Di Sarno A, Sarnacchiaro F, et al. Prolactinomas resistant to standard dopamine agonists respond to chronic cabergoline treatment. *J Clin Endocrinol Metab* 82:876–883, 1997.

21 Nakamura Y, Ono M, Yoshida Y, et al. Effects of clomiphene citrate on the endometrial thickness and echogenic pattern of the endometrium. *Fertil Steril* 67:256–260, 1997.

22 Sereepapong W, Suwajanakorn S, Triratanachat S, et al. Effects of clomiphene citrate on the endometrium of regularly cycling women. *Fertil Steril* 73:287–291, 2000.

23 Check J, Dietterich C, Lurie D. The effect of consecutive cycles of clomiphene citrate therapy on endometrial thickness and echo pattern. *Obstet Gynecol* 86:341–345, 1995.

24 Mikkelson TJ, Kroboth PD, Cameron WJ, et al. Single-dose pharmacokinetics of clomiphene citrate in normal volunteers. *Fertil Steril* 46:392–396, 1986.

25 Triwitayakorn A, Suwajanakorn S, Triratanachat S, et al. Effects of initiation day of clomiphene citrate on the endometrium of women with regular menstrual cycles. *Fertil Steril* 78:102–107, 2002.

26 Agarwal SK, Buyalos RP. Corpus luteum function and pregnancy rates with clomiphene citrate therapy: comparison of human chorionic gonadotropin-induced versus spontaneous ovulation. *Hum Reprod* 10:328, 1995.

27 Branigan E, Estes MA, et al. Treatment of chronic anovulation resistant to clomiphene citrate (CC) by using oral contraceptive ovarian suppression followed by repeat CC treatment. *Fertil Steril* 71:544–546, 1999.

28 Merrill Dow Pharmaceutical Company. Product Information Bulletin. Cincinnati, OH: National Laboratories, 1972.

29 Hammond MG, Halme JK, Talbert LM. Factors affecting the pregnancy rate in clomiphene citrate induction of ovulation. *Obstet Gynecol* 62:196, 1983.

30 Lawton AW. Optic neuropathy associated with clomiphene citrate. *Fertil Steril* 61:390–391, 1994.

31 Trott EA, Plouffe L, Hansen K, et al. Ovulation induction in clomiphene-resistant anovulatory women with normal dehydroepiandrosterone sulfate levels: beneficial effects of the addition of dexamethasone during the follicular phase. *Fertil Steril* 66:484, 1996.

32 Parsanezhad ME, Alborzi S, Motazedian S, et al. Use of dexamethasone and clomiphene citrate in the treatment of clomiphene citrate-resistant patients with polycystic ovary syndrome and normal dehydroepiandrosterone sulfate levels: a prospective, double-blind, placebo-controlled trial. *Fertil Steril* 78:1001–1004, 2002.

33 Dumble LD, Klein RD. Creutzfeldt-Jakob disease legacy for Australian women treated with human menopausal gonadotropins. *Lancet* 340:848, 1992.

34 Howles CM. Role of LH and FSH in ovarian function. *Mol Cell Endocrinol* 161:25–30, 2000.

35 Zwart-van Rijkom JE, Broekmans FJ, Leufkens HG. From HMG through purified urinary FSH preparations to recombinant FSH: a substitution study. *Hum Reprod* 17:857–865, 2002.

36 Germond M, Dessole S, Senn A, et al. Successful in vitro fertilization and embryo transfer after treatment with recombinant FSH. *Lancet* 339:1170, 1992.

37 Sills ES, Levy DP, Moomjy M, et al. A prospective randomized comparison of ovulation induction using highly purified follicle-stimulating hormone alone and with recombinant human luteinizing hormone in in-vitro fertilization. *Hum Reprod* 14:2230–2235, 1999.

38 Frydman R, Howles CF, Truong R. A double-blind, randomized study to compare recombinant human follicle-stimulating hormone (FSH; Gonal-F) with highly-purified urinary FSH (Metrodin-HP) in women undergoing assisted reproductive techniques including intracytoplasmic sperm injection. *Hum Reprod* 15:520–525, 2000.

39 The European and Israeli Study Group on Highly Purified Menotropin versus Recombinant Follicle-Stimulating Hormone. Efficacy and safety of highly-purified menotropin versus recombinant follicle-stimulating hormone in in vitro fertilization/intracytoplasmic sperm injection cycles: a randomized, comparative trial. *Fertil Steril* 78:520–528, 2002.

40 Daya S. Updated meta-analysis of recombinant follicle-stimulating hormone (FSH) versus urinary FSH for ovarian stimulation in assisted reproduction. *Fertil Steril* 77:711–714, 2002.

41 Akin JW, Shepard MK. The effects of baseline ovarian cysts on cycle fecundity in controlled ovarian hyperstimulation. *Fertil Steril* 59:453–455, 1993.

42 Segal S, Shifren JL, Isaacson KB, et al. Effect of a baseline ovarian cyst on the outcome of in vitro fertilization-embryo transfer. *Fertil Steril* 71:274–277, 1999.

43 Fluker MR, Urman B, Mackinnon M, et al. Exogenous gonadotropin therapy in World Health Organization groups I and II disorders. *Obstet Gynecol* 83:189–196, 1994.

44 Sahakyan M, Harlow B, Hornstein M. Influence of age, diagnosis, and cycle number on pregnancy rates with gonadotropin-induced controlled ovarian hyperstimulation and intrauterine insemination. *Fertil Steril* 72:500–504, 1999.

45 Battaglia C, Salvatori M, Regnani G, et al. Successful induction of ovulation using highly purified follicle-stimulating hormone in a woman with Kallman's syndrome. *Fertil Steril* 73:284–286, 2000.

46 Liu JH, Durfee R, Muse K, et al. Induction of multiple ovulation by pulsatile administration of gonadotropin-releasing hormone. *Fertil Steril* 40:18, 1983.

47 Santoro N. Efficacy and safety of intravenous pulsatile gonadotropin-releasing hormone: Lutrepulse for injection. *Am J Obstet Gynecol* 163:1959, 1990.

48 Martin KA, Hall JE, Adams JM, et al. Comparison of exogenous gonadotropins and pulsatile gonadotropin releasing hormone for induction of ovulation in hypogonadotropic hypogonadism. *J Clin Endocrinol Metab* 77:125–129, 1993.

49 Anasti JN. Premature ovarian failure: an update. *Fertil Steril* 70:1–15, 1998.

50 van Kasteren YM, Schoemaker J. Premature ovarian failure: a systematic review on therapeutic interventions to restore ovarian function and achieve pregnancy. *Hum Reprod Update* 5:483–492, 1999.

51 Buyalos RP, Daneshmand S, Brzechffa PR. Basal estradiol and follicle-stimulating hormone predict fecundity in women of advance reproductive age undergoing ovulation induction therapy. *Fertil Steril* 68:272–277, 1997.

52 Csemiczky G, Harlin J, Fried G. Predictive power of clomiphene citrate challenge test for failure of in vitro fertilization treatment. *Acta Obstet Gynecol Scand* 81:954–961, 2002.

53 Nestler JE, Stovall D, Akhter N, et al. Strategies for the use of insulin-sensitizing agents to treat infertility in women with polycystic ovary syndrome. *Fertil Steril* 77:209–215, 2002.

54 Dunaif A. Insulin resistance and the polycystic ovary syndrome: mechanism and implications for pathogenesis. *Endocr Rev* 18:774–800, 1997.

55 Guzick D. Polycystic ovary syndrome: symptomatology, pathophysiology, and epidemiology. *Am J Obstet Gynecol* 179(Suppl):89–93, 1998.

56 Barbieri RL. Induction of ovulation in infertile women with hyperandrogenism and insulin resistance. *Am J Obstet Gynecol* 183:1412–1418, 2000.

57 Kirpichnikow D, McFarlane SI, Sowers JR. Metformin: an update. *Ann Intern Med* 137:25–33, 2002.

58 Moghetti P, Castello R, Negri C, et al. Metformin effects on clinical features endocrine and metabolic profiles and insulin sensitivity in polycystic ovary syndrome: a randomized, double-blind, placebo-controlled 6-month trial followed by open, long-term clinical evaluation. *J Clin Endocrinol Metab* 85:139–146, 2000.

59 Nestler JE, Jakubowicz DJ, Evans WS, et al. Effects of metformin on spontaneous and clomiphene-induced ovulation in the polycystic ovary syndrome. *N Engl J Med* 338:1876–1880, 1998.

60 Vandermolen DT, Ratts VS, Evans WS, et al. Metformin increases the ovulatory rate and pregnancy rate from clomiphene citrate in patients with polycystic ovary syndrome who are resistant to clomiphene citrate alone. *Fertil Steril* 75:310–315, 2001.

61 Homburg R, Howles CM. Low-dose FSH therapy for anovulatory infertility associated with polycystic ovary syndrome: rationale, results, reflections and refinements. *Hum Reprod Update* 5:493–499, 1999.

62 Dale PO, Tanbo T, Haug E, et al. The impact of insulin resistance on the outcome of ovulation induction with low-dose follicle-stimulating hormone in women with polycystic ovary syndrome. *Hum Reprod* 13:567–570, 1998.

63 Mitwally MF, Casper RF. Use of an aromatase inhibitor for ovulation induction in patients with an inadequate response to clomiphene citrate. *Fertil Steril* 77:776–780, 2002.

9

Complications of Ovulation Induction

Tracey L. Telles

Introduction

Ovulation induction agents have been used with increasing frequency since the 1960s. Since then, a multitude of agents have been derived, all with the single purpose of restoring or increasing the chance for conception. These can be used in different clinical scenarios, including ovulation induction, superovulation, and superovulation in conjunction with assisted reproductive technologies. With ovulation induction, the intention is to induce unifollicular development to restore normal cycle fecundity. In contrast, in patients with regular menstrual cycles who are unable to achieve pregnancy spontaneously, the induction of multiple follicles with fertility medications can improve fecundity rates. Unfortunately, the release of several mature oocytes, available for fertilization, presents a risk for multiple pregnancies. This risk can be controlled with assisted reproductive technologies, by limiting the number of embryos transferred into the uterus, and compelling arguments have been made that this is a safer route to achieve pregnancy. However, many couples cannot afford the costs associated with assisted reproductive technologies and elect to accept the risks associated with superovulation.

While these medications offer specific benefits, more and more attention has been focused on the potential risks associated with the use of these medications. Some of these risks are shared,

KEY POINT

*As with all
treatment
strategies, both
benefits and risks
of ovarian
stimulation must be
discussed with
patients.*

such as the risk for multiple pregnancy, ovarian hyperstimulation syndrome (OHSS), and extrauterine pregnancy. Some of the newer agents, such as insulin sensitizers, have unique risks, including significant metabolic disturbances. In addition, there is increasing awareness of the possible linkage between the use of fertility medications and an increased risk for gynecologic cancers. The most recent literature does not support this link; thus, there does not appear to be any carcinogenic effects of ovulation induction agents. Whether infertile women constitute a high-risk population for developing a gynecologic cancer remains uncertain, and further epidemiologic studies are needed.

Multiple Pregnancy

A common strategy to improve cycle fecundity is to increase the number of oocytes released for fertilization in a single menstrual cycle, so-called "superovulation." This can be achieved by using antiestrogens, such as clomiphene citrate or tamoxifen, or exogenous gonadotropins, and is usually combined with intrauterine insemination (IUI). While multifollicular development imparts a greater chance for pregnancy, there can be substantial risk that a multiple gestation will result. There is a general consensus that attempts must be made to create guidelines for practioners, to enable physicians to reduce the incidence of multiple gestations, without diminishing the success rate of such treatment.

INCIDENCE

In 1999, the U.S. Department of Health and Human Services reported that infertility treatments accounted for more than 225,000 *excess* multiple births between 1980 and 1997.[1] Multiple pregnancies can be expected in up to 40% of superovulation cycles, including a 26% rate of twins, 6% rate of triplets, and up to 5% rate of quadruplets.[2] When clomiphene citrate is used, in those that achieve pregnancy, the risk of a twin gestation is approximately 10%, and triplets occur in up to 1% of patients.[2] In contrast, the use of injectable gonadotropins causes a greater risk for high-order multiple gestations, especially in patients less than 32 years of age, and in patients with polycystic ovarian syndrome.[3] Multiple pregnancy is seen in up to 30–40% of patients who conceive using exogenous gonadotropins.

COMPLICATIONS

Although many couples may desire a multiple pregnancy after having difficulty conceiving spontaneously, the perinatal morbidity and mortality, and maternal morbidity, seen with high-order gestations is alarming, and patients should be counseled appropriately prior to treatment. The maternal complications frequently associated with multiple gestations include preterm labor, preterm delivery, preeclampsia, and gestational diabetes mellitus (Table 9-1).[4] These complications, which occur three to seven times more often than with a singleton pregnancy, increase in frequency as the number of fetuses present increases.[2] Maternal complications at delivery are also more common with multiple gestations, including postpartum hemorrhage, uterine atony, and placental abruption.[2] In addition, the likelihood of requiring cesarean delivery is increased with multiple gestations, subjecting the patient to risks associated with surgery.

Perinatal mortality and morbidity is increased 4- to 10-fold in twins, and is even greater with high-order multiple gestations.[2] Among the most common fetal complications seen are those associated with prematurity. These include growth restriction, pulmonary immaturity, retinopathy of prematurity, and cerebral palsy, all of which may have debilitating long-term effects. Since the average gestational length for twins is 37 weeks and for triplets is 33.5 weeks, it is likely that many of these children will be delivered prematurely and therefore be at risk for such complications. It is incumbent on the physician to appropriately counsel patients regarding these risks, *prior* to the initiation of treatment.

While much attention has been focused on the medical aspects of multiple gestations, there are important social factors that must

Table 9-1. **RATES OF MAJOR MATERNAL COMPLICATIONS**

NUMBER OF FETUSES	PRETERM LABOR (%)	PRETERM DELIVERY[a] (%)	GESTATIONAL DIABETES MELLITUS (%)	PREECLAMPSIA (%)
1	15	10	3	6
2	40	50	5–8	10–12
3	75	92	7	25–60
4	>95	>95	>10	>60

[a]Delivery at <37 weeks' gestation.
SOURCE: With permission from Ref. 4.

be considered as well. Language development does seem to be delayed in twin siblings, largely due to shared parental attention.[2] In addition, individualization may be delayed due to interdependence, leading to behavior difficulties later in development. In addition, the financial burden that the parents may face, especially with high-order multiples, can be overwhelming, particularly when chronic medical complications exist.

PREVENTION

As the evidence mounts demonstrating increased risk, as well as the enormous costs, associated with multiple gestations, it becomes clear that our goal should be to minimize this risk by reducing the incidence of multiple gestations. Multiple studies have attempted to identify markers that would reliably predict those at greatest risk for such pregnancies, including the maximum estradiol concentration on day of human chorionic gonadotropin (hCG), the number of preovulatory follicles visualized on transvaginal ultrasound, and total number of motile sperm inseminated.[2,3,5–7] Although these studies have failed to consistently identify such markers, some trends can be seen. One study showed that in human menopausal gonadotropin/IUI (hMG/IUI) cycles, the incidence of high-order multiple gestations was 13.2% for women younger than 35 years of age, with six or more follicles measuring 12 mm or more, compared to 4% for those with one to five follicles.[5] In patients over 35 years of age, the incidence of high-order multiple gestations in cycles with more than six follicles was 5.3%, compared to 4.8% in cycles with one to five follicles.[5] Another study showed that, in women younger than 32 years of age, those with six or more follicles measuring 10 mm or greater, and an estradiol level greater than 862 pg/mL, the incidence of high-order multiple gestations was 18%.[3] For women 32 years of age or older, with the same clinical response, the risk of high-order multiple gestations was 3.3%.[3]

These studies highlight that patients should be followed closely during these treatments to minimize their risk for a multiple pregnancy, especially in those at greatest risk, such as younger patients and patients with polycystic ovarian syndrome. Although no specific guidelines have been established, one algorithm for management in patients less than 35 years of age, those at greatest risk, is shown in Fig. 9-1. The literature supports that, in patients less than 32 years of age with six of more follicles >10 mm, and an estradiol

KEY POINT

Multiple gestation represents the greatest risk of ovarian stimulation. This risk is highest in young women and presents significant risk for the resultant child(ren).

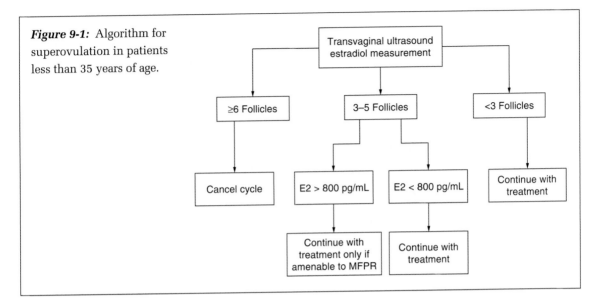

Figure 9-1: Algorithm for superovulation in patients less than 35 years of age.

greater than 862 pg/mL, the risk for high-order multiple gestations is substantial, and these cycles should be abandoned.[3] The risk for high-order multiple gestations in patients 35 years and older is reduced, but these patients still require careful monitoring. More prospective studies are needed to determine more detailed guidelines, with specifications for age, to minimize the risk of high-order multiple gestations, without unduly affecting overall fecundity rates.

MULTIFETAL PREGNANCY REDUCTION

Despite efforts to minimize the incidence of high-order multiple gestations, this risk will never be eliminated completely. For those patients facing the potential complications of a high-order multiple pregnancy, multifetal pregnancy reduction offers an opportunity to reduce those risks, by selectively reducing the number of gestations developing. Specifically, at 11–12 weeks of gestation, under ultrasound guidance, 1–2 mL of KCl is injected into the thoracic cavity of a developing fetus, inducing the cessation of cardiac activity.[2] Although there is some risk that the remaining pregnancy may be jeopardized, the risks associated with maintaining a high-order multiple pregnancy are greater. Of course, the emotional burden of having to consider such a procedure cannot be understated, and patients, even those who support abortion, often struggle to make this decision. Although efforts should be made, in all cases, to minimize the risk of multiple pregnancy, this is especially true in patients who are not amenable to multifetal pregnancy reduction.

Ovarian Hyperstimulation Syndrome

Ovarian hyperstimulation syndrome is potentially the most serious medical complication of ovulation induction. This syndrome consists of a spectrum of clinical findings, along with physical signs and laboratory abnormalities. Several classifications have been published to describe the intensity of this syndrome (Table 9-2).[8] Mild OHSS is characterized by abdominal distention, due to bilateral ovarian enlargement. This is the most commonly seen form of OHSS, is usually time-limited to a short duration, and requires minimal intervention. In contrast, moderate and severe OHSS is often complicated by more pronounced abdominal distention and discomfort due to increasing ascites. This can lead to several serious, potentially life threatening, complications including pleural effusion, pericardial effusion, hyperkalemia, hypovolemia, impaired renal function, thromboembolic episodes, and respiratory compromise.[9] Patients,

Table 9-2.   **CLINICAL CLASSIFICATION OF OHSS**

MILD **OHSS**		*SEVERE* **OHSS**	
Grade 1	Abdominal distention and discomfort	Grade 4	Features of moderate OHH Clinical evidence of ascites
Grade 2	Features of grade 1 plus nausea, vomiting, and/or diarrhea Variably enlarged ovaries	Grade 5	Hct > 45% (>30% increase over baseline) WBC > 15,000 Oliguria, creatinine 1.0–1.5 Creatinine clearance ≥50 mL/min
MODERATE **OHSS**		*CRITICAL* **OHSS**	
Grade 3	Features of mild OHSS Ultrasonic evidence of ascites	Grade 6	Tense ascites ± hydrothorax Hct > 55% WBC > 25,000 Creatinine > 1.6 Creatinine clearance 50 mL/min Thromboembolic phenomenon ARDS

SOURCE: With permission from reference 8.

with severe OHSS, require immediate hospitalization and very close surveillance to minimize the chance for untoward events.

Although rare case reports exist of this occurring in natural menstrual cycles, OHSS is nearly exclusively iatrogenic. While all patients should be considered at risk for developing OHSS, some patients are at greater risk given predisposing factors, such as polycystic ovarian syndrome. Therefore, diligent surveillance during a treatment cycle should be performed to minimize such risk.

INCIDENCE

The variable classifications make determining the exact incidence of OHSS difficult. Based on one report, consistent with other estimations, mild OHSS with ovulation induction is thought to occur in 5–10% of cycles, with severe OHSS seen less frequently in 0.2–0.5% of patients.[9] This incidence is higher when ovarian stimulation is performed in conjunction with assisted reproductive technologies. Those at greatest risk include patients with polycystic ovarian syndrome, due to the excessive follicular activity that is often seen as a result of stimulation. Other risk factors include young age (<35 years of age), pregnancy, high serum estradiol concentration, and multiple follicles, even if immature.[10] That is, there is a strong correlation between the total number of follicles and OHSS. Again, while all patients should have appropriate surveillance during treatment, those patients with specific risk factors for OHSS may require heightened surveillance.

PATHOPHYSIOLOGY

There has been considerable effort to elucidate the mechanisms that trigger OHSS. While there is a correlation between serum estradiol levels and the incidence of OHSS, estradiol alone does not seem to be causative.[9] That is, patients treated with high doses of estrogen do not develop OHSS. Rather, it is the stimulation of the ovary, with estradiol serving as a marker of the *extent* of that stimulation, that presents the risk for OHSS. It is likely that other factors, produced concurrently with estradiol, are causative. Attention has been directed at trying to identify those factors. One such factor is vascular endothelial growth factor (VEGF). VEGF seems to be responsible for the increased capillary permeability seen in OHSS.[9] It is this increased permeability that leads to the massive transudation of fluid from the hypervascular ovary, causing the accumulation of ascites in the peritoneal cavity, and possibly the pleural cavities and pericardial cavity as well.

The presence of hCG, either exogenous or endogenous, is also correlated with the occurrence of OHSS. Many patients receive exogenous hCG at the time of follicular maturation, and this can trigger symptoms of OHSS. Because this is metabolized fairly rapidly, the symptoms are likely to improve within several days. However, if *conception* occurs, hCG levels will begin rising by 10–14 days postconception, and it is at that time when the more severe symptoms may develop. hCG can also be used for luteal phase supplementation, but should be avoided in patients at risk for OHSS.

The renin-angiotensin system also seems to play a critical role is the development of OHSS. Navot et al.[11] evaluated plasma renin activity and aldosterone in patients with OHSS. He demonstrated that there is a direct correlation between the magnitude of plasma renin activity and severity of OHSS. The actions of the renin-angiotensin system explain several of the clinical consequences seen with OHSS.

Other factors thought to be critical in the development of OHSS include cytokines, such as interleukin 1 (IL-1), secreted by activated macrophages. IL-1 activity is correlated with hematocrit and plasma estradiol levels, and may be responsible for the increased capillary permeability, hemoconcentration, and other acute phase reactions.[9] Other factors thought to contribute to the increased vascular permeability include IL-8 and endothelin-1.[9]

COMPLICATIONS

The vast majority of clinical findings seen with OHSS are directly the result of intravascular volume depletion. Because of the increased vascular permeability, there is a massive fluid-shift that results in the accumulation of protein-rich fluid into the abdominal cavity. This can lead to serious consequences, including abdominal pain, pleural effusions, and pericardial effusion. Fatalities have been reported in the literature as a direct result of massive pulmonary edema.[12] In addition, the increased abdominal pressure can cause intraluminal compression of the inferior vena cava, thereby reducing blood flow to the renal arteries, resulting in renal impairment. This increased pressure can also reduce preload to the heart, diminishing cardiac output and compromising respiratory function.

Another consequence of the extreme intravascular depletion that can be seen with OHSS is hemoconcentration. There are several case reports in the literature documenting the occurrence of thromboembolic events as a result of OHSS, including bilateral internal jugular vein thrombosis,[13] multiple cerebral infarctions,[14] and ischemic stroke.[15] These reports demonstrate that patients can suffer permanent, debilitating consequences with OHSS. One recent study prospectively evaluated the prevalence of thrombophilia in women hospitalized for severe OHSS, and found that women with severe OHSS were more likely to be carriers of thrombophilia mutations than controls (85% versus 27%, respectively).[16] This study suggests that all women with severe OHSS should be screened for thrombophilias, and that patients with these mutations should be treated with anticoagulant prophylaxis.

TREATMENT

The vast majority of patients with OHSS will demonstrate mild symptoms and do not require hospitalization. These patients will often improve with supportive measures alone, such as limitation of activity and maintenance of hydration. Patients with moderate-to-severe OHSS require greater surveillance and often need to be hospitalized, especially when there is concern regarding respiratory status. Hospitalized patients should be placed on oxygen saturation monitoring, and strict input/output accounting should be employed. Intravenous hydration should be initiated to treat the intravascular depletion. In addition, laboratory testing should include serial electrolytes, complete blood counts, renal function tests, and liver function tests.[8] Patients may require pain medication, as well as antiemetics, due to the extreme abdominal distention and resultant gastrointestinal effects.

Those patients with significant ascites may require intravenous macromolecules to increase intravascular oncotic pressure, creating a gradient and inducing fluid back into the vascular space. This can be accomplished with either intravenous albumin or intravenous hydroxyethyl starch solution (Hetastarch). Since albumin is a human product, some concerns have been raised regarding both safety and side effects, including allergic reactions.[10] In contrast, Hetastarch is a nonbiological substitute and may be better tolerated. Since both are equally effective at treating OHSS, preference may be to use Hetastarch, as it is also less expensive.

In the face of extreme hemoconcentration, such as a hematocrit >50%, consideration should also be given to the administration of thromboembolism prophylaxis. This can be achieved with low molecular weight heparin, such as enoxaparin. In addition, patients should also be screened for thrombophilias, due to the correlation between severe OHSS and the presence of thrombophilia mutations.[16]

The accumulation of ascites can lead to severe consequences and may require intervention. Paracentesis may be needed to relieve the increased abdominal pressure seen with ascites, thereby improving venous return to the heart and improving renal blood flow. Patients also see a reduction in symptoms, such as abdominal pain, shortness of breath, and nausea. Although placement of indwelling catheters has been described,[17] which allows continuous drainage of peritoneal fluid, more commonly an ultrasound-guided abdominal paracentesis can be performed, removing up to 2 L of peritoneal fluid in a single session. It may be necessary to repeat this procedure every few days, until the patient's clinical course stabilizes.

Ectopic and Heterotopic Pregnancy

Release of several potential oocytes in one cycle also creates an increased risk for an ectopic gestation. Despite earlier detection, largely due to improved quality of transvaginal ultrasound imaging and increased sensitivity of serum β-human chorionic gonadotropin (β-hCG) immunoassay, ectopic pregnancy remains the most common cause of maternal mortality in the first trimester.[18] In addition, this may occur with a concurrent intrauterine pregnancy (heterotopic pregnancy) frequently delaying the diagnosis. While the incidence of heterotopic pregnancy in natural cycles is rare,[19] the risk is significantly increased with ovulation induction agents.[20–22] Heightened awareness for this clinical scenario should exist in patients taking fertility medications, as the presence of an intrauterine pregnancy does not exclude the existence of a concomitant extrauterine pregnancy.

INCIDENCE

The incidence of ectopic pregnancy is estimated to be 2.0% of all pregnancies in the United States.[23] However, this is increased with fertility medications, reportedly as high as 3.1% in patients

KEY POINT

A high index of suspicion for tubal pregnancy, is required when evaluating all pregnancies after ovulation induction with or without assisted reproductive technologies.

undergoing ovulation induction or superovulation, in the presence of apparently normal fallopian tubes,[24] and even higher with assisted reproductive technologies. The incidence of heterotopic pregnancy in natural cycles is rare (1 in 30,000 pregnancies), but this is markedly higher when fertility treatments are used to achieve pregnancy, as high as 1% of pregnancies conceived either through the induction of multiple ovulations or with *in vitro* fertilization (IVF).[25] Therefore, clinical suspicion should be raised when fertility treatments are used, even if an intrauterine pregnancy is documented by transvaginal ultrasonography.

COMPLICATIONS

The complications that can arise due to an ectopic pregnancy can be life threatening. Most patients will present with early symptoms that will raise suspicion of the diagnosis, such as abnormal vaginal bleeding and pelvic pain. Other gynecologic causes of these symptoms must be ruled out, including miscarriage, hemorrhagic ovarian cyst, pelvic infection, and ovarian torsion. In addition, in the presence of multiple follicles induced for ovulation, ovarian hyperstimulation syndrome may mask the diagnosis of ectopic pregnancy. Tubal rupture often presents more acutely, with evidence of hemorrhage, extreme abdominal pain, hypotension, and tachycardia. This constitutes a medical emergency and requires immediate surgical intervention. In this setting, patients often require transfusion of blood products and should be counseled regarding the risks of viral transmission via blood products prior to surgery.

TREATMENT

Options for treatment will depend on the clinical stability of the patient, as well as diagnostic findings. The most commonly used tools for diagnosis include serum quantitative β-hCG determination, transvaginal ultrasound, and clinical examination.[24] In the presence of a β-hCG level greater than 1500 IU/L, an intrauterine gestational sac should be seen with transvaginal ultrasonography, if present. This discriminatory zone has been shown to have a diagnostic sensitivity of 95–99% and specificity of 95–100% for ectopic pregnancy.[24] In general, options for treatment include conservative medical management, conservative surgical treatment, or more aggressive surgical treatment.

Table 9-3 shows the American College of Obstetrics and Gynecology criteria for medical management of ectopic gestations.[26]

Table 9-3. **CRITERIA FOR RECEIVING METHOTREXATE**

ABSOLUTE INDICATIONS	RELATIVE INDICATIONS
Hemodynamically stable without active bleeding or signs of hemoperitoneum	Unruptured mass ≤ 3.5 cm at greatest dimension
Nonlaparoscopic diagnosis	No fetal cardiac motion detected
Patient desires future fertility	Patients whose β-hCG level does not exceed a predetermined value (6000–15,000 mIU/mL)
General anesthesia poses a significant risk	
Patient is able to return for follow-up care	
Patient has no contraindications to methotrexate	

SOURCE: With permission from Ref. 26.

If a patient meets these criteria, this is the preferred method of treatment, as it likely eliminates the need for surgery, and is associated with a 90% success rate.[23] This is usually accomplished with intramuscular methotrexate, either in a single dose (50 mg/m^2 of body surface area) or in multiple doses (1.0 mg/kg every other day for 5–7 days) (Table 9-4).[23] Methotrexate is a folic acid antagonist

Table 9-4. **ADMINISTRATION OF DOSAGE OF METHOTREXATE TO TREAT AN ECTOPIC PREGNANCY**

	SINGLE DOSE	MULTIDOSE
Dose		
Methotrexate (MTX)	50 mg/m^2	1 mg/kg
Leucovorin (LEU)	None	0.1 mg/kg
Frequency of dose	One dose: repeat in 1 week if necessary	Up to four doses of each (MTX and LEU): alternate daily doses of MTX and LEU until serum hCG declines by 15%
Monitor hCG level	Baseline (day 0), day 4, and day 7	Baseline (day 0), day 1, day 3, day 5, and day 7 until hCG declines 15% from the previous value
When to administer additional dose(s)	Second dose on day 7 if hCG value did not decline 15% between days 4 and 7	Give second, third, or fourth dose if hCG value has not declined 15% from the prior value; maximum four doses
Surveillance hCG (after initial treatment response)	Weekly until hCG is not detectable	Weekly until hCG is not detectable

SOURCE: With permission from Ref. 23.

that inhibits DNA and RNA synthesis, thereby inhibiting the rapidly dividing trophoblastic cells of a developing pregnancy. A recent metaanalysis compared the efficacy of single versus multiple dose treatment, and found that, while the single dose regimen was associated with fewer side effects, it was also associated with a greater chance for failure of treatment.[23] Common side effects include nausea, diarrhea, mouth sores, and pelvic pain, as a result of the induced tubal abortion. The presence of pelvic pain may complicate the identification of treatment failure. However, up to 4% of patients will not respond to medical therapy and/or will suffer tubal rupture, necessitating surgical intervention.[24] Factors associated with treatment failure included increasing β-hCG levels and detectable embryonic cardiac activity on transvaginal ultrasonography.[23] Therefore, all patients receiving medical treatment for ectopic pregnancy require close monitoring, as tubal rupture requires immediate intervention.

In patients who are clinically ineligible for medical treatment (Table 9-5), surgery is indicated. Patients who are hemodynamically unstable should undergo emergent laparotomy with salpingectomy. These patients are likely to require blood transfusion

Table 9-5. **CONTRAINDICATIONS TO MEDICAL THERAPY**

ABSOLUTE CONTRAINDICATIONS	*RELATIVE CONTRAINDICATIONS*
Breastfeeding	Gestational sac $\geq$ 3.5 cm
Overt of laboratory evidence of immunodeficiency	Embryonic cardiac activity
Alcoholism, alcoholic liver disease, or other chronic liver disease	
Preexisting blood dyscrasias, such as bone marrow hyperplasia, leukopenia, thrombocytopenia, or significant anemia	
Known sensitivity to methotrexate	
Active pulmonary disease	
Peptic ulcer disease	
Hepatic, renal, or hematologic dysfunction	

SOURCE: With permission from Ref. 26.

and should be counseled appropriately prior to surgery. In most patients, the preferred surgery is laparoscopy, with either linear salpingostomy or salpingectomy. Linear salpingostomy does carry the risk of leaving residual trophoblastic tissue in the tube at the time of surgery, and may require additional medical treatment. This occurs in up to 20% of linear salpingostomy cases.[24] However, the intrauterine pregnancy rate in subsequent pregnancies following linear salpingostomy is 60%, therefore this should be performed if the pregnancy is unruptured. To minimize the chance for residual trophoblastic tissue, extensive irrigation should be performed at the time of surgery to remove all products of conception from the tube. Overall, the advantages of laparoscopy, compared to laparotomy, include shorter hospital stay, fewer postoperative pain medication needs, reduced cost, and lower risk of pelvic adhesions.

KEY POINT

Treatment for tubal pregnancy includes medical and surgical options based on specific patient characteristics.

If a heterotopic pregnancy is diagnosed, surgical treatment is the only viable option. The most common surgery performed is laparoscopic salpingectomy. In terms of the intrauterine pregnancy, one review found that approximately one-third of patients will subsequently have spontaneous abortion.[25] These authors could not identify any cause for this increased incidence of spontaneous loss, and they specifically noted that the presence of maternal hemoperitoneum did not increase this risk.

Cancer and Fertility Medications

Perhaps one of the most controversial areas regarding ovulation induction agents is their proposed association with hormone-related cancers, such as ovarian, breast, and endometrial cancer. There have been many reports either supporting or denying this suspected association. Most of the published data suggesting a causal relationship between fertility drugs and these cancers have been retrospective epidemiologic studies, and many have indicated their studies are limited by an insufficient number of patients, as well as other factors, such as recall bias. There is also the problem of identifying the appropriate control group. Because of the frequency with which these medications are prescribed, and the still unanswered question regarding their potential harm, more comprehensive studies are currently being completed to define the role of fertility drugs and hormone-related cancers with greater certainty.

BREAST CANCER

Breast cancer is the most common malignancy in women in developed countries, and in the United States, the lifetime risk for developing breast cancer is 12.5%.[27] Several metaanalyses have shown that recent oral contraceptive pill use and long-term use of hormone therapy may be associated with a slightly increased risk for breast cancer.[27] This has raised concern that fertility medications, which acutely increase estradiol levels, may also increase the risk breast cancer.

Many studies have been done to address this very issue. An Australian cohort study[28] found an increased risk in breast and uterine cancer within the first 12 months of treatment in patients undergoing *in vitro* fertilization, but the overall incidence was no greater than expected. Similarly, a case-control study conducted in Northern Italy did not find any association between fertility drug treatment and breast cancer risk.[29] Another recent metaanalysis showed that neither the presence of subfertility nor the use of medications to treat subfertility was associated with an increased risk of breast cancer.[30]

OVARIAN CANCER

In the United States, the lifetime risk for developing ovarian cancer is 1.75%.[27] There is evidence that oral contraceptive pills and parity impart a protective effect. Conversely, there has been a suggestion that subfertility may be due to a genetic defect, which may also predispose a woman to developing ovarian cancer.

Although multiple studies have tried to link the use fertility medications with an increased risk for developing an ovarian malignancy, there does not appear to be any causal relationship between ovulation induction agents and ovarian cancer. In 1994, Rossing et al.[31] performed a case-cohort study evaluating 3837 infertile women, and found that there was an increased risk for ovarian cancer in women who had been exposed to clomiphene citrate for more than 12 months. These findings have never been reproduced, despite many subsequent studies. In 2002, Ness et al.[32] performed a metaanalysis analyzing the risk of infertility, fertility drugs, and ovarian cancer, by pooling eight case-control studies. This revealed that among nulliparous, subfertile women, neither fertility drug use nor a duration of use greater than 12 months was associated with an increased risk of ovarian cancer.

The Rossing study had also found that prolonged use of clomiphene citrate may increase the incidence of borderline ovarian tumors,[31] and this was corroborated by Ness et al. (OR 2.43, CI 1.01–5.88).[32] One other study[33] did find a statistically increased incidence of borderline tumors, while others have shown trends toward an increased incidence, although not statistically significant.[34,35]

ENDOMETRIAL CANCER   Factors that predispose patients to the risk of endometrial cancer may also be associated with infertility, such as polycystic ovarian syndrome and estrogenized anovulation. In the United States, over 40,000 new cases of endometrial cancer can be expected in 2003, and the vast majority will be diagnosed in the postmenopausal state. There is a general consensus that it is the long-term state of unopposed estrogen that results in both infertility, as well as the potential risk for endometrial cancer.

Several studies have been published attempting to link fertility medications with the development of endometrial cancer. Modan et al.[36] found that there was no statistically significant increased incidence of endometrial cancer in patients who received treatment, as compared to those who did not receive treatment, and this has been confirmed by additional studies.[28]

KEY POINT

There is no strong evidence to support an increased risk of hormone-dependent malignancies in women taking fertility drugs.

Other Potential Complications

OVARIAN TORSION   There have been several reports in the literature describing adnexal torsion following fertility treatment. Child et al.[37] reported that their patient had received gonadotropins with insemination, and subsequently developed symptoms consistent with ovarian torsion at approximately 6 weeks of gestation. Laparoscopy, followed by minilaparotomy, was performed to remove the right ovary, which was nonviable. At the time of surgery, the patient's left ovary appeared enlarged, consistent with recent ovarian stimulation, but no evidence of torsion was noted. Unfortunately, 3 days later, she required repeated laparotomy for subsequent left ovarian torsion.

Other reports describe similar findings, that is, an increased incidence of ovarian torsion following ovarian stimulation.[38] According to reported cases, common factors that seem to increase risk for torsion include ovarian stimulation, OHSS, and pregnancy. As such, the majority of reported cases are in pregnant patients. One review found that, among 154 patients hospitalized for OHSS, 16% of the pregnant patients developed adnexal torsion, compared to 2.3% of the nonpregnant patients.[38] Therefore, in patients receiving fertility medications, and especially in those with symptoms of OHSS and/or in those who are pregnant, adnexal torsion should be considered in the differential diagnosis when patients present with pelvic pain.

INSULIN SENSITIZERS   Metformin has been used for the purpose of ovulation induction in women with polycystic ovarian syndrome, and, presumed, hyperinsulinemia. This oral biguanide decreases hepatic glucose production and hence decreases insulin levels. A resultant decrease in androgen levels occurs. Whether by this mechanism, or due directly to the fall in insulin levels, patients treated with metformin are more likely to either ovulate spontaneously, or become more responsive to ovulation induction agents, such as clomiphene citrate. One randomized-controlled trial demonstrated that, in clomiphene-resistant PCOS patients, metformin, coupled with clomiphene citrate, markedly improved ovulation and pregnancy rates.[39]

The side effects of metformin may cause early discontinuation of this medication. Those most commonly seen include diarrhea, nausea, abdominal discomfort, and anorexia, and these are encountered in approximately 30% of patients.[40]

There have been several reports of serious metabolic consequences suffered in patients unable to metabolize this drug. One report stated the incidence of lactic acidosis to be 5/100,000 in treated patients.[41] The mortality rate of lactic acidosis is 50% when associated with metformin therapy. Because of this, careful evaluation prior to dispensing this drug should be undertaken, including measurement of serum AST and creatinine. In addition, contraindications to this drug include liver disease, heart or respiratory failure, alcohol abuse, and kidney disease. Metformin should not be dispensed if serum creatinine is above 1.4 mg/dL in women, as mortality with lactic acidosis is more likely with impaired renal function.

Conclusion

Ovulation induction may be a necessary treatment in those patients unable to conceive spontaneously. While most patients will tolerate these treatments with no significant complications, some patients may be at higher risk for complications, and all efforts should be made to minimize this risk. Patients should be informed prior to the onset of treatment regarding such risks. The presence of risk factors may necessitate heightened surveillance during treatment.

Progress is being made in terms of understanding any linkage between fertility medications and gynecologic malignancies. Currently the only consistent finding is that there is an increased incidence of borderline ovarian tumors in women given fertility medications. No causal relationship has been established between fertility drugs and invasive ovarian cancer.

Further studies are needed to develop more formal guidelines to reduce the risk of complications, without reducing the cycle fecundity. Once these guidelines can be generated and enacted, we can help patients reach their goal of achieving and maintaining a healthy pregnancy, as safely as possible.

What's the Evidence?

- Multiple gestation risk is increased with six or more follicles measuring 12 mm or more.[5] However, evidence would suggest the patient's age is a strong, concurrent predictor.[3,5]
- OHSS can lead to serious, permanent, debilitating consequences, including thromboembolic events.[13-15] A recent study suggested women with OHSS were more likely to be carriers of a thrombophilic mutation and thus, women with OHSS should be screened for these mutations and treated prophylactically.[16]
- Surgery is the most appropriate treatment for heterotopic pregnancy, but puts the intrauterine pregnancy at risk with one-third of patients subsequently undergoing a first trimester loss.[25]
- A case-control study from Northern Italy did not find any association between fertility drug treatment and breast cancer risk.[29] A recent metaanalysis show that neither the

presence of subfertility nor the use of medications to treat subfertility was associated with an increased risk of breast cancer.[30]

- A 2002 metaanalysis by Ness et al.[32] showed no increased risk for ovarian cancer in women taking fertility drugs.

Discussion of Cases

CASE 1

You are a third-year OB/GYN resident on call, covering the emergency room (ER). You are paged to the ER, asking that you evaluate a patient who has presented with complaints of shortness of breath and abdominal pain. She also has a positive serum qualitative β-hCG. You proceed to the ER to find out the details. She is a 34-year-old G0 who reports she had noticed increasing abdominal distention over the past few days, but this has progressively worsened in the past 24 h. She states she is having moderate right-sided pelvic pain that has been steady for the past 3 h, and this is what prompted her to visit the ER. She denies any vaginal bleeding. Her history is remarkable for recent treatment at a fertility clinic. She states she has been trying to get pregnant for about 1.5 years. She has taken various medications, but recently was treated with injectable gonadotropins, along with insemination. She states their evaluation has revealed that her husband's sperm counts are fair, but the motility is low. They had tried several cycles of clomiphene citrate, but she did not get pregnant. She states she has some bloating around the time of the insemination, but this improved after a few days. She noticed a few days ago, about 11 days since the insemination, the bloating returned. She states she

started having increased right-sided pelvic pain about 3 h ago, and this has continued. As you are talking with her, you notice that her respirations are slightly labored. The ER has noted that her vitals signs are all stable.

What tests would you order?

- **Complete blood count**
- **Serum electrolytes**
- **Chest x-ray**
- **Pelvic ultrasound with Doppler studies**

Since hemoconcentration is common with ovarian hyperstimulation syndrome, a complete blood count should be drawn. In patients with a hematocrit greater than 50%, thromboembolic prophylaxis should be started. This can be achieved with enoxaparin, 30–40 mg subcutaneously bid. Serum electrolytes will demonstrate if hyperkalemia is present. If elevated, it may be warranted to obtain an electrocardiogram to ensure no cardiac abnormalities are present. A chest x-ray is necessary, to evaluate for the presence of pleural effusions. This patient has localized right-sided pelvic pain that is constant, therefore the possibility of ovarian torsion should be considered, and requires Doppler studies

with the study. However, in the absence of localized symptoms, pelvic ultrasound is not necessary.

You are called back to the ER once the lab results return. In the meantime, she has received some intravenous pain medications and reports that her pain is improving. The ER physician tells you all her labs have returned within normal limits. He shows you the chest x-ray which is normal. The pelvic ultrasound is significant for bilaterally enlarged ovaries. Both ovaries were noted to have appropriate blood flow. She was found to have a moderate amount of free-fluid, but no active bleeding was seen. Since she is feeling better and all her testing was normal, the ER physician is getting ready to discharge her home. The patient seems relieved.

What instructions would you give this patient at discharge?

- **She should weigh herself everyday**
- **She should stay well-hydrated, especially by drinking water and tomato juice**

- **She should limit her physical activity until her symptoms resolve**

If she gains more than 3–4 lb in 1 day, she is likely excessively retaining fluid and would need reevaluation. Because intravascular depletion is a main component of OHSS, she should drink fluids that are likely to improve this, including tomato juice. Even though the Doppler studies were normal, she is still at risk for developing ovarian torsion, and limitation of activity is warranted.

What type of follow-up does this patient need?

- **She should see her fertility physicians the following day.**
- **She should be followed closely by her physicians, as she is at risk for worsening of symptoms.**

CASE 2

A patient of your colleagues' left a message earlier in the day on the nursing phone message center that she is having mild pelvic pain and wants to come in for evaluation. Your nurse is able to get in touch with her at work. She tells you that she started having some left-sided pain yesterday, but it went away within 30 min. The patient is an attorney and has been catching up at work since completing her *in vitro* fertilization cycle about 4 weeks ago. Her pregnancy test was positive 2 weeks ago, and she is scheduled for an ultrasound soon. She describes the pain as mild but constant, at times radiating toward her back. She did notice

some vaginal spotting yesterday, but denies any further bleeding.

What should your next step be?

- **Physical examination**
- **Pelvic ultrasound**
- **Serum quantitative β-hCG**

This patient should be evaluated immediately to rule out an ectopic pregnancy. The pelvic ultrasound should detect an intrauterine pregnancy, if present, given that she is approximately 6 weeks in gestation. The presence of

a heterotopic pregnancy should also be considered. The β-hCG level will provide clinical information regarding the viability of the pregnancy, as well as determine if she is a candidate for medical treatment if an ectopic gestation is found.

She presents to your office for an examination. She has her β-hCG level drawn in your office, then is placed in an examination room. Clinically she looks stable. Her vital signs are all stable. She states the pain is still present, but seems to be getting better, just like the day prior. You perform an ultrasound in the office. You visualize the uterus, which appears empty. Her ovaries are still slightly enlarged. You find an adnexal mass measuring 2.2 cm in greatest diameter. A yolk sac is seen, but no fetal pole is seen. She tolerates the ultrasound well, without any discomfort. You discuss these findings with her and her husband. They are understandably disappointed, but seem focused on dealing with her current situation.

What are the treatment options?

- **Medical therapy with methotrexate**
- **Conservative surgical treatment**

This patient is a candidate for medical treatment, as long her β-hCG level is less than 10,000 mIU/mL. Specifically, she is hemodynamically stable, with no contraindications to medical management. If her β-hCG level is over 10,000 mIU/mL, then she is more likely to fail conservative therapy and needs appropriate counseling. She will need preliminary testing, including complete blood count, liver enzymes, and renal function tests. You confirm that she is Rh positive. Your office staff already obtained her height and weight.

The patient and her husband want to avoid surgery, if possible. You confirm her general health, and she has no identifiable contraindications to medical treatment of the ectopic pregnancy. The lab results return within a few hours, and she is in fact a candidate for medical treatment. You counsel her about side effects of the medication, and potential risks and benefits of treatment, including the risk of failed treatment. Your nurse administers the medication.

What follow-up will she need?

- **Serial blood testing**

She will need to repeat the β-hCG level on day 4 (day 0 is day of medication administration) and again on day 7. If the β-hCG level has not decreased by 15% from day 4 to day 7, then a second injection is required. In addition, the complete blood count, liver function tests, and renal function tests are also repeated on day 7, to ensure the patient can tolerate the second dose. Once the β-hCG level is shown to be decreasing appropriately, she will need weekly β-hCG levels to confirm complete resolution of the pregnancy.

REFERENCES

1 U.S. Department of Health and Human Services. *Trends in Twin and Triplet Births: 1980-97.* National Vital Statistics Report No. 24. Washington, DC: Centers of Disease Control and Prevention, 1999.

2 The ESHRE Capri Workshop Group. Multiple gestation pregnancy. *Hum Reprod* 15:1856, 2000.

3 Tur R, Barri PN, Coroleu B, et al. Risk factors for high-order multiple implantation after ovarian stimulation with gonadotropins: evidence from a large series of 1878 consecutive pregnancies in a single center. *Hum Reprod* 16:2124, 2001.

4 American Society of Reproductive Medicine. *Multiple Pregnancy Associated with Infertility Therapy*, 2000.

5 Dickey RP. A year of inaction on high-order multiple pregnancies due to ovulation induction. *Fertil Steril* 79:14, 2003.

6 Gleicher N, Oleske DM, Tur-Kaspa I, et al. Reducing the number of high order multiple pregnancy after ovarian stimulation with gonadotropins. *N Engl J Med* 343(1):2–7, 2000.

7 Pasqualotto EB, Falcone T, Goldberg JM, et al. Risk factors for multiple gestation in women undergoing intrauterine insemination with ovarian stimulation. *Fertil Steril* 72:613, 1999.

8 Dourron NE, Williams DB. Prevention and treatment of ovarian hyperstimulation syndrome. *Semin Reprod Endocrinol* 14:355, 1996.

9 Schenker JG. Clinical aspects of ovarian hyperstimulation syndrome. *Eur J Obstet Gynecol Reprod Biol* 85:13, 1999.

10 Delvigne A, Rozenberg S. Epidemiology and prevention of ovarian hyperstimulation syndrome (OHSS): a review. *Hum Reprod Update* 6:559, 2002.

11 Navot D, Margalioth EJ, Laufer N, et al. Direct correlation between plasma renin activity and severity of ovarian hyperstimulation syndrome. *Fertil Steril* 48:57, 1987.

12 Semba S, Moriya T, Youssef EM, et al. An autopsy case of ovarian hyperstimulation syndrome with massive pulmonary edema and pleural effusion. *Pathol Int* 50:549, 2000.

13 Ellis MH, Nun IB, Rathaus V, et al. Internal jugular vein thrombosis in patients with ovarian hyperstimulation syndrome. *Fertil Steril* 69:140, 1998.

14 Yoshii F, Ooki N, Shinohara Y, et al. Multiple cerebral infarctions associated with ovarian hyperstimulation syndrome. *Neurology* 53:225, 1999.

15 Hwang WJ, Lai ML, Hsu CC, et al. Ischemic stroke in a young women with ovarian hyperstimulation syndrome. *J Formos Med Assoc* 97:503, 1998.

16 Dulitzky M, Cohen SB, Inbal A, et al. Increased prevalence of thrombophilia among women with severe ovarian hyperstimulation syndrome. *Fertil Steril* 77:463, 2002.

17 Al-Ramahi M, Leader A, Claman P, et al. A novel approach to the treatment of ascites associated with ovarian hyperstimulation syndrome. *Hum Reprod* 12:2614, 1997.

18 Lemus JF. Ectopic pregnancy: an update. *Curr Opin Obstet Gynecol* 12:369, 2000.

19 Varras M, Akrivis C, Hadjopoulos G, et al. Heterotopic pregnancy in a natural conception cycle presenting with tubal rupture: a case report and review of the literature. *Eur J Obstet Gynecol Reprod Biol* 106:79, 2003.

20 Duce MN, Ozer C, Egilmez H, et al. Heterotopic pregnancy: a case report. *Abdom Imaging* 27:677, 2002.

21 Pan HS, Chuang J, Chiu SF, et al. Heterotopic triplet pregnancy: a report of a case with bilateral tubal pregnancy and an intrauterine pregnancy. *Hum Reprod* 17:1363, 2002.

22 Thakur R, El-Menabawey M. Combined intra-uterine and extra-uterine pregnancy associated with mild hyperstimulation syndrome after clomiphene citrate ovulation induction. *Hum Reprod* 11:1583, 1996.

23 Barnhart KT, Gosman G, Ashby R, et al. The medical management of ectopic pregnancy: a meta-analysis comparing "single dose" and "multidose" regimens. *Obstet Gynecol* 101:778, 2003.

24 Abusheikha N, Salha O, Brinsden P. Extra-uterine pregnancy following assisted conception cycles. *Hum Reprod Update* 6:80, 2000.

25 Tal J, Haddad S, Gordon N, et al. Heterotopic pregnancy after ovulation induction and assisted reproductive technologies: a literature review from 1971–1993. *Fertil Steril* 66:1, 1996.

26 American College of Obstetricians and Gynecologists. *Medical Management of Tubal Pregnancy*, 1998.

27 Klip H, Burger CW, Kenemans P, et al. Cancer risk associated with subfertility and ovulation induction: a review. *Cancer Causes Control* 11:319, 2000.

28 Venn A, Watson L, Bruinsma F, et al. Risk of cancer after use of fertility drugs with in-vitro fertilization. *Lancet* 354:1586, 1999.

29 Ricci E, Parazinni F, Negri E, et al. Fertility drugs and the risk of breast cancer. *Hum Reprod* 14:1653, 1999.

30 Venn A, Healy D, McLachlan R. Cancer risks associated with the diagnosis of infertility. *Best Pract Res Clin Obstet Gynaecol* 17:343, 2003.

31 Rossing MA, Daling JR, Weiss NS, et al. Ovarian tumors in a cohort of infertile women. *N Engl J Med* 331:771, 1994.

32 Ness RB, Cramer DW, Goodman MT, et al. Infertility, fertility drugs, and ovarian cancer: a pooled analysis of case-control studies. *Am J Epidemiol* 155:217, 2002.

33 Shushan A, Paltiel O, Iscovich J, et al. Human menopausal gonadotropin and the risk of epithelial ovarian cancer. *Fertil Steril* 65:13, 1996.

34 Harlow BL, Weiss NS, Lofton S. Epidemiology of borderline ovarian tumors. *J Natl Cancer Inst* 78:71, 1987.

35 Mosgaard BJ, Lidegaard O, Kjaer SK, et al. Ovarian stimulation and borderline ovarian tumors: a case-control study. *Fertil Steril* 70:1049, 1998.

36 Modan B, Ron E, Lerner-Geva L, et al. Cancer incidence in a cohort of infertile women. *Am J Epidemiol* 147:1038, 1998.

37 Child TJ, Watson NR, Ledger WL. Sequential bilateral adnexal torsion after a single cycle of gonadotropin ovulation induction with intrauterine insemination. *Fertil Steril* 67:573, 1997.

38 Mashiach S, Bider D, Moran O, et al. Adnexal torsion of hyperstimulated ovaries in pregnancies after gonadotropin therapy. *Fertil Steril* 53:76, 1990.

39 Vandermolen DT, Ratts VS, Evans WS, et al. Metformin increases the ovulatory rate and pregnancy rate from clomiphene citrate in patients with polycystic ovary syndrome who are resistant to clomiphene citrate alone. *Fertil Steril* 75:310, 2001.

40 De Leo V, la Marca A, Petraglia F. Insulin-lowering agents in the management of polycystic ovary syndrome. *Endocr Rev* 24:633, 2003.

41 Misbin R, Green L, Stadel B. Lactic acidosis in patients with diabetes treated with metformin. *N Engl J Med* 338:265, 1998.

Surgical Management of the Infertile Female

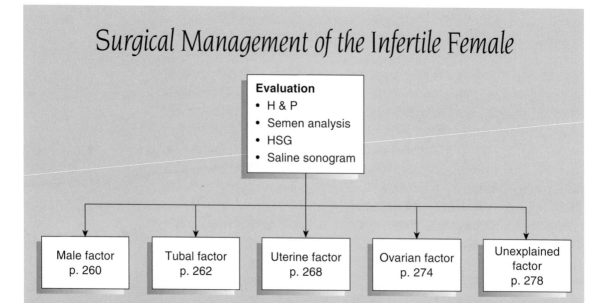

Evaluation
- H & P
- Semen analysis
- HSG
- Saline sonogram

| Male factor p. 260 | Tubal factor p. 262 | Uterine factor p. 268 | Ovarian factor p. 274 | Unexplained factor p. 278 |

Surgical Management of the Infertile Female

10

Sae H. Sohn
Danielle Lane

Introduction

In the 1970s it became apparent that surgical techniques could be applied to the realm of infertility with some success. Examples included reparation of obstructed fallopian tubes and congenital anomalies of the Müllerian ducts, and treatment of endometriosis, polycystic disease of the ovaries, and pelvic adhesive disease.[1] The 1970s also brought the development of microsurgical technology with the use of compound microscopes and surgical loupes. This concept was advanced and practiced throughout the 1980s. The development of the laparoscope, in the 1980s, lead to the replacement of open laparotomy with minimally invasive approaches to pelvic disease. Laser technology was also introduced in the 1980s and was applied to the treatment of pelvic disease through the laparoscope. As assisted reproductive techniques began to expand in the early 1980s, reparative surgery continued to play a large role.

Also during the late 1970s, there was great interest in the use of hysteroscopy.[2] While this technique was first developed in 1869, it was not until the concern regarding trans-tubal spread of intrauterine pathology had been alleviated that its use became accepted in the field of gynecology. And by the 1980s, hysteroscopy had replaced dilatation and curettage (D&C) as the standard procedure for diagnosis of intrauterine pathology.

KEY POINT

Indications for surgery in infertile women have changed as a result of wide availability and significant increase in success rates of in vitro fertilization.

As these surgical advancements were progressing, great strides were also being made in the realm of *in vitro* fertilization (IVF). Success rates for IVF have now risen from the single digits up to 50% per cycle in women under 35 years of age. This dramatic improvement in IVF, or as it is more broadly known, assisted reproductive technology (ART), has had a huge impact on reproductive medicine, especially reproductive surgery. It can be said that these two fields, reproductive surgery and assisted reproduction, have evolved together. This coincident evolution has greatly modified the algorithms used to treat infertile women. This chapter will focus on the role of surgery and the new thought process that guides surgical treatment decisions in modern infertility care.

Guiding Questions

- How much time does the patient have to achieve a pregnancy?
  - How old is the patient?
  - What are the results of tests of ovarian reserve?
- What other infertility factors exist?
  - Is there a male factor involved?
  - Does the patient have normal ovulation?
  - Is a hydrosalpinx present?
  - Is the uterus normal?

Evaluation

The evaluation of an infertile couple has been discussed extensively in previous chapters. As previously noted, infertility is truly a multifactorial condition and requires a thorough evaluation, for all potential causes, before initiation of any treatment.

HISTORY AND PHYSICAL

Obtaining a patient's history and performing a physical examination remain important parts of the evaluation and decision-making process in assessing the need for surgical intervention. Risk factors for pelvic adhesive disease, or tubal disease, include previous surgeries, both abdominal and pelvic, a history of pelvic inflammatory disease, dyspareunia, and/or dysmenorrhea, a history of endometriosis, ectopic pregnancies, or chronic pelvic pain. A patient with a history of long-standing dysmenorrhea, with a known diagnosis of endometriosis or with a suspicion for endometriosis, may warrant a discussion regarding surgical intervention for pelvic pain in addition to optimization of pregnancy. If there is a history of pelvic inflammatory disease, the number of infections, the mode of therapy, the duration of therapy, and/or the need for hospitalization should be elicited.

A history of previous surgeries, including abdominal surgeries, should be carefully reviewed. For instance, a woman with a history of a ruptured appendix with postoperative peritonitis might have a different outcome compared to a woman with a history of repetitive pelvic infections. For all prior surgeries, a review of the operative report is essential. In the case of prior tubal ligation, not only the operative report, to document the specific type of tubal sterilization, but also the pathology report, should be reviewed. This often proves important since knowing how much of the tube was removed is critical in accurately counseling patients on the expected success with tubal reanastomosis.

Risk factors for defects within the uterine cavity include a history of recurrent pregnancy loss, multiple D&Cs for induced and spontaneous abortions, amenorrhea after surgical manipulation of the uterus, puerperal infection of the uterus, and/or septic abortions. A history of pelvic pain, urinary frequency, pelvic pressure, dyspareunia, menorrhagia, or pelvic mass may suggest the possibility of uterine leoimyomata.

Of equal importance to the review of the patient's history is the physical examination of the patient. Taken together, the surgeon will obtain valuable information that will allow an accurate assessment of risk and the potential benefits of intervention. In performing the examination, the surgeon should note the type of scars and make certain the scars correspond to the history of previous surgeries. Pelvic examination should evaluate the size, position, and mobility of the uterus. Palpation of the adnexa should elicit the presence of pelvic pain and/or any masses or nodularity. Rectovaginal examination should be considered to fully assess the pelvis and evaluate for possible endometriosis.

Pelvic ultrasound examination can prove to be valuable in many situations. Palpated adnexal structures can be further evaluated by this method. The abnormal position of the ovaries or the presence of a dilated tubal structure or persistent ovarian cyst can increase the suspicion for pelvic pathology.

HYSTEROSAL-
PINGOGRAM

Hysterosalpingogram (HSG) is very important in determining whether surgical treatment is appropriate or not. Indications for HSG and the technique of HSG have been discussed in Chaps. 2 and 3. Although most patients who are seeking surgical treatment will most likely have had an HSG, it is important to actually review the films, not just the radiology report. If the procedure has not yet been performed, it is always preferable to perform it yourself. In part, this is due to the fact that HSG is a dynamic test which will yield the most information as the test in being performed. If this is not possible, a review of the films is important. Subtle findings consistent with peritubal adhesions, salpingitis isthmic nodosa (SIN), loculations of dye, delayed spill, and so on should be reviewed by the surgeon prior to scheduling any surgeries.

In summary, HSG is a good nonoperative method of evaluating the uterine cavity and the fallopian tubes. However, one needs to take into account that a high rate of false positives of HSG results has been reported in the literature. False-positive uterine HSG findings have been noted to be as high as 21–57%.[3,4] The report of proximal tubal obstruction also has a high false-positive rate due to tubal spasm and improper technique. Repeat studies, or careful evaluation of the tests previously performed, may allow one to assess risk factors for possible tubal disease and the extent of the disease.

Since most of the HSGs are being performed by radiologists, it is important to specifically request evaluation of the uterine cavity in addition to the assessment of the fallopian tubes. Initial filling of the dye is perhaps the most important part of HSG examination in terms of determining presence or absence of a uterine filling defect. The HSG can also identify the presence of midline uterine defects, but it cannot differentiate between a uterine septum and a bicornuate uterus. Assessment for this type of uterine malformation may require a magnetic resonance imaging (MRI) or a diagnostic laparoscopy at the time of the hysteroscopic procedure.

SALINE SONOGRAPHY

Saline sonography is a relatively new, but important, modality in the evaluation of the uterine cavity. Whether the saline sonography is being performed prior to an IVF cycle or it is being performed as a result of suspicious pelvic ultrasound, real time ultrasound examination of the cavity while the saline is being infused gives you an accurate assessment of the uterine cavity. This will allow one to visualize uterine polyps, submucous leiomyomata, uterine synechaie, and possibly to differentiate between a uterine septum and a bicornuate uterus. The performance of a saline sonogram is critical prior to removal of a submucosal myoma. Determining the appropriate surgical approach requires a knowledge of the size of any fibroid and the extent to which it protrudes into the endometrial cavity. This can best be assessed with the contrast of a saline sonogram. Saline sonography is also quickly becoming an important tool in the evaluation of an infertile woman prior to ART.

SEMEN ANALYSIS

The semen analysis, at quick glance, does not appear to have any relevance to the evaluation of the surgically infertile woman. This is far from true. Prior to surgery on the female partner, evaluation for a possible male factor should be completed. If moderate-to-severe sperm factors are identified, the benefit of a surgical approach may be significantly altered. In those couples with both a male factor and tubal disease, IVF may become the treatment of choice. As stated previously, evaluation of the uterus with a saline sonogram, and correction of any identified abnormalities should be accomplished prior to IVF. The presence of a hydrosalpinx on an ultrasound may also warrant a surgical intervention prior to IVF as discussed in Chap. 13.

AGE

The advanced age of the female partner may also influence decision-making regarding a surgical approach. Risk-to-benefit ratio must be carefully considered prior to undertaking any surgical approach. Thus, a cycle day 3 follicle-stimulating hormone (FSH) and estradiol, and/or an antral follicle count should be performed to assess for possible diminished ovarian reserve. An example of this type of situation is a 40-year-old woman who has a history of bilateral tubal ligation 10 years ago, and is now seeking possible tubal reanastomosis. A woman with an elevated cycle day 3 FSH would have statistically lower chance of success compared to a woman with normal cycle day 3 FSH and estradiol levels. The overall chance of success needs to be compared with the possible morbidity of the procedure and recovery needs of the patient from the surgery. Also, given the time to achieve a pregnancy following a surgical approach, older age, and/or evidence of diminished ovarian reserve may suggest proceeding directly to IVF that offers a greater likelihood for fertility success.

KEY POINT

A complete infertility evaluation, including assessment of the male partner and assessment of ovarian reserve, is required prior to decision-making about surgical treatment for tubal disease.

Treatment

PATIENT SELECTION

Decisions regarding patient selection for infertility surgery, have become very complex. While some situations, as discussed later, seem clear-cut, surgery for patients with pelvic adhesive disease, and distal tubal pathology in particular, face a much more complex decision process. Prior to the development of ART, reconstructive and reparative surgeries were the only option available to these patients. With significant increases in the success rates, IVF has become much more desirable and a more reasonable option compared to surgery. Although no clear randomized trials exist comparing success rates of IVF versus surgical repair, there are sufficient studies (although not randomized and controlled), that indicate treatment through a surgical approach has a relatively low chance of success for distal tubal disease.

Current management of an infertile couple is guided by the principle of optimizing chances for pregnancy in the most expeditious (time matters) and simple manner. If a patient presents to the gynecologist with pelvic pain and evidence of pelvic adhesive disease, the surgeon must then consider how best to address the issue of pain while optimizing attempts for pregnancy. Appropriate management for fertility may be confirmation at the time of diagnostic laparoscopy that IVF is the indicated treatment, or may require salpingectomy of a hydrosalpinx to optimize the pregnancy rate through IVF. However, evaluation of whether surgical management may be possible, via careful salpingolysis or adhesiolysis, may still require an initial diagnostic laparsocopy.

KEY POINT

Prognosis with tubal repair must be contrasted with the success, in the same couple, of IVF.

The patient should be given all the possible scenarios of surgical findings. Careful documentation and an outline of the surgical decision tree should also be part of the preoperative process. Each individual scenario should be discussed in detail. Clear objectives for the surgery should be outlined. If the primary goal of the surgery is to optimize pregnancy versus surgery to alleviate pelvic pain and optimize the chance for pregnancy—each may lead to very different surgical plans. With the availability of IVF as a treatment option, not all infertility surgical cases should aim to restore a woman's pelvic anatomy. And finally, informed consent is a must!

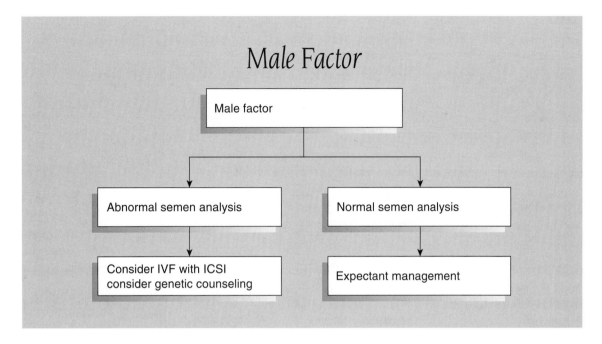

Management of each different factor will be discussed subsequently.

MALE FACTOR Any complete infertility evaluation and treatment includes evaluation of the male partner, which was discussed in Chap. 4. The importance of the evaluation of the male partner is emphasized again as a reminder to always approach infertility treatment globally. A couple who faces severe male factor infertility, as well as tubal disease, should not undergo extensive lysis of adhesions and neopsalpingostomy nor should anyone schedule a tubal reanastomosis surgery without first checking on the ovarian reserve of the woman and the semen parameters of the male partner. Again, risk assessment, as it relates to the eventual goal of pregnancy, should always be considered.

Couples diagnosed with significant male factor infertility should consider *in vitro* fertilization with intracytoplasmic sperm injection (ICSI) as described in Chap. 13. In some cases, the woman may still require surgical intervention for a hydrosalpinx, uterine polyp, or other intracavitary lesions. Thus, a complete and careful assessment is of utmost importance.

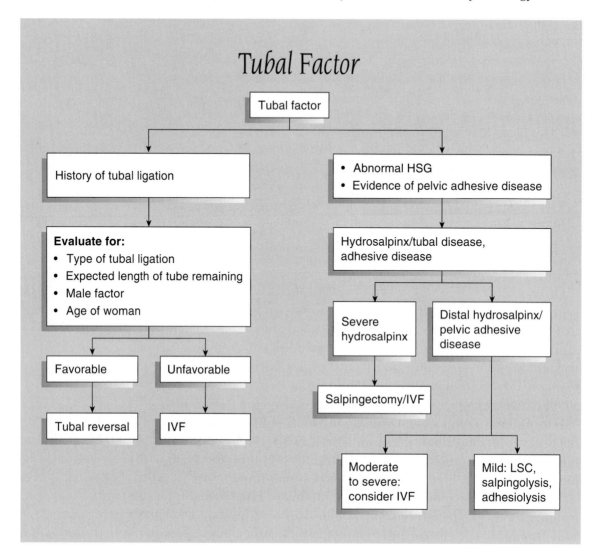

Tubal Factor

TUBAL FACTOR   Reconstructive surgery of the oviduct is applicable to the repair of certain localized or segmental obstructions of the fallopian tube. Consideration for operative intervention is oftentimes the result of findings from the hysterosalpingogram or previous laparoscopy, or based on a previous history of bilateral tubal ligation. A high index of suspicion from the patient's history may also prompt one to consider operative intervention.

TUBAL ANASTOMOSIS   In any reanastomosis, the general principles are the same: adhesiolysis, excision of diseased tissue, hemostasis, and tension-free anastomosis.[5] Pregnancy rates of 50–90% can be achieved by tubal microsurgery for reversal of sterilization with proper patient selection and surgical training.[6]

Variables affecting subsequent pregnancy outcome include the type of sterilization, the segments to be anastomosed, the tubal length, the time interval from sterilization, and the presence of destruction of the intramural segment of fallopian tube. Optimal results require that the remaining fallopian tube length be ≥4 cm after completion of the anastomosis. Anastomoses between isthmic segments will achieve the highest rates of success.

Bipolar coagulation is associated with 3 cm of complete coagulation of the fallopian tube and is currently the most common method of laporoscopic sterilization. Unipolar electrocautery has been associated with a large amount of tubal destruction, especially when the triple burn technique is used. Mechanical methods of sterilization include spring-loaded clips (Hulka-Clemens clips), titanium clips lined with silicone rubber (Filshie clips), and silicone rubber bands (Falope rings). These mechanical approaches destroy less of the fallopian tube (~5 mm for clips and 2 cm for rings) and make microsurgical reversal more likely to succeed. In this setting, a preoperative laparoscopy to assess the remaining distal tube, and a HSG to assess the remaining proximal tube, is often helpful. Destruction of the intramural segment of the oviduct is rarely due to proximal pathologic occlusions, but can result from endometritis, salpingitis, cornual polyps, or salpingitis isthmica nodosa.

Both surgical loupes and the binocular operating microscope are available for magnification. Some studies have demonstrated that the method of magnification did not affect pregnancy rates.[7,8] Another study demonstrated that use of a surgical microscope doubled pregnancy rates from 31 to 64.4% when compared to surgical loupes.[9] Operator comfort is the most important factor in selecting the method of magnification.

Several studies have evaluated suture selection and there is very little difference between synthetic absorbable and nonabsorbable materials. Our preference is the use of 6-0 vicryl to reapproximate the mesosalpinx and eliminate tension at the anastomotic site, and 8-0 vicryl on a 3/8″ circle taper to reapproximate the luminal ends.

The fallopian tube should be kept moist via constant irrigation throughout the surgical procedure. The fallopian tube itself should not be worked on and should remain covered with a moist laparotomy pad in open procedures. The needle should pass through only the muscularis layer of the fallopian tube, and this layer usually requires four interrupted sutures. The sutures should be tied in such a manner that the tissue is reapproximated not strangulated. A second layer of suture is used to reapproximate the tubal serosa.

Techniques may differ slightly depending on the sections of the fallopian tube to be reapproximated. Isthmic-isthmic anastomosis is particularly straight forward due to the fact that there is no difference in luminal size. With isthmic-ampullary and ampullary-interstitial anastomoses, additional steps are needed to overcome the discrepancy in luminal size. Ampullary-ampullary anastomosis is also simpler due to a lack of size discrepancy and also the fact that only a single layer closure is required.

Whether performed by laparoscopy or laparotomy the overall pregnancy rates are similar. A study comparing the two approaches but using the same microsurgical technique of four stitches and two layer closures demonstrated success rates of 80.5% in the laparoscopy group and 80.0% in the laparotomy group. However, the laparoscopy group demonstrated a significantly longer mean operating time and significantly shorter mean hospital stay.[10]

KEY POINT

Prognosis following tubal anastomosis is most dependent on the tubal length at the completion of the anastomosis.

HYDROSALPINX   Hydrosalpinx is a condition where the fallopian tubes become damaged, dilated, and filled with fluid. Management of patients with hydrosalpinx has been a controversial and widely studied phenomenon. Patients with hydrosalpinges who have IVF as a treatment without any intervention experience approximately half the pregnancy rate as patients without hydrosalpinges. The current recommendation for hydrosalpinges is to consider salpingectomy prior to IVF treatment to improve implantation rates, pregnancy rates, and live birth rates.[11,12] However, there is still controversy on whether all patients need salpingectomy or whether less aggressive therapies such as tubal ligation are sufficient. Some clinicians use pelvic ultrasound as a helpful tool. If the hydrosalpinges are visible via pelvic ultrasound, one may consider salpingectomy more aggressively as opposed to a nonvisible hydrosalpinx via ultrasound examination.

The hysterosalpingogram should be evaluated very closely to determine the extent and the nature of the hydrosalpinges. Hydrosalpinges involving both the proximal and the distal aspect of the fallopian tube require minimal thought as opposed to hydrosalpinges that are only apparent at the distal end of the fallopian tubes. Many clinicians are performing pelvic ultrasounds for evidence of persistently filled hydrosalpinges compared to findings of dilation on injection of dye. Often, diagnostic laparoscopy will be necessary to determine the exact nature of the hydrosalpinges. Operative findings will dictate which operative intervention the patient should have. Preoperative discussion of different operative findings and management is required for this type of surgical planning. Findings of severe hydrosalpinges with additional pelvic adhesive disease should prompt the surgeon and the patient to consider bilateral salpingectomies. If the condition is mild to moderate, the patient and the surgeon should have discussed different trigger or decision-making points so that patient's condition can be optimized for pregnancy. With mild-to-moderate hydrosalpinx, one should remember that surgical repairs may lead to a second surgery if the repair is not successful. Thus, factors such as patient's age, semen parameter, previous pregnancy history, and so on, should be considered overall to make the appropriate decision.

Technique The evaluation of hydrosalpinges should be performed laproscopically. Clearly, with prior knowledge of pelvic adhesive disease and/or the presence of hydrosalpinges, one must consider the risk factors for the laproscopic approach. One may consider open laparoscopy depending on the risk factor of the patient. Salpingectomies should always be attempted laproscopically as well. Despite the fact that we do not yet have a randomized studies on simple tubal ligation versus the salpingectomy, morbidity associated with laparotomy may not warrant a microscopic approach but rather a simple tubal ligation can be considered. Further studies do need to be performed to assess the efficacy of the tubal aspirations or proximal tubal ligation.

Tubal Disease/Pelvic Adhesive Disease Tubal disease can be discussed both in terms of location and magnitude. Most tubal diseases are inflammatory in nature; however, conditions such as endometriosis and previous surgical exposure could lead to significant pathology as well. The extent of the disease can usually be evaluated by looking at hysterosalpingogram films or operative reports of previous operations that the patient may have had. A high index of suspicion from the patient's history could be very helpful in preoperative risk assessment. The decision-making process for a patient with tubal disease must again take into consideration the "optimization of pregnancy" and to minimize creation of new pathology such as chronic pelvic pain. An informed decision tree and informed consents are a must when considering tubal disease and treatment options.

PROXIMAL TUBAL OCCLUSION   A diagnosis of tubal occlusion is often derived from the hysterosalpingogram. Evidence of SIN, chronic salpingitis, intratubal endometriosis, and tubal spasm could be some of the etiologies of the proximal tubal occlusion. Management of proximal tubal occlusion is controversial since the diagnosis of proximal occlusion by hysterosalpingogram or diagnostic laparoscopy is unreliable.

A surgical approach to the proximal tubal occlusion using microsurgical technique can be effective but faces possible complications of uterine rupture and varied success rates based on the experience of the surgeon. Since microsurgical training is rarely part of a gynecologic surgical training, a surgical approach to proximal tubal occlusion should be limited to the few experienced centers.[13]

Transuterine catherization of the fallopian tube remains an option for treatment of proximal tubal occlusion. These procedures are typically performed by the interventional radiologic team. This fact often limits one in simultaneously examining the distal tube and any possible peritubal adhesions. Success rates using tubal cannulation are reported to be as high as 50%; however, it is difficult to think that simple cannulation of the tubes will maintain patency in face of SIN, intratubal endometriosis, or chronic salpingitis.[13,14]

DISTAL TUBAL OCCLUSION   Much of the tubal disease one encounters is that of the distal tubal. Tubal damage is often in association with pelvic adhesive disease or other pathology. Trying to work out a decision tree for the management of distal tubal disease is complicated due to lack of properly randomized studies and the difficulty in classifying different degrees of disease.

In reviewing the current literature which consists of, mainly, one nonrandomized observation and a few randomized studies, several conclusions have been reached. Randomized studies have shown that there is no difference in pregnancy rates between the use of CO_2 laser and electrocautery. It is suggested that the instrument that the surgeon feels most comfortable with is the best choice for his or her use. A review of the nonrandomized studies allows us to conclude that there is an advantage in using magnification versus none and that the treatments of adhesions do seem to increase chance of pregnancy. There also appears to be an advantage of open microscopic salpingostomy versus laproscopic salpingostomy. However, the differences appear to be minimal and other risk factors such as length of recovery and rates of postoperative complications make the laproscopic approach a more reasonable one to pursue. Open microsurgical techniques should be used in patients with severe adhesive disease who will not or cannot undergo *in vitro* fertilization.[15]

Patients with fimbrial agglutination with pelvic adhesive disease and distal tubal disease deserve special attention. Again, there is a lack of good data to show which treatment options are best. Isolated distal adhesions without tubal damage (as in a case of ruptured appendicitis that led to pelvic scarring) may have a significantly better chance of pregnancy and a lesser chance of an ectopic pregnancy compared to patient with distal tubal disease with pelvic inflammatory infection as its cause.

Patients with severe distal tubal disease are better served by in vitro fertilization than tubal repair.

Distal tubal disease is often classified as mild, moderate, and severe based on the extent of dilatation, tubal wall thickness, rugal integrity, status of fimbria, and degree of adnexal adhesions. Patients with severe tubal disease have pregnancy rates ranging from 4 to 16% after salpingostomy and lysis of the adhesions. Ectopic pregnancy rates for severe distal tubal disease appear to be around 5%.[16,17] These patients will more than likely fare better moving directly to *in vitro* fertilization. Factors such as hydrosalpinx and age should be considered in the decision-making process. If an attempt is made to repair severely damaged tubes, the patient should be counseled as to the possible need for secondary surgery for the removal of grossly dilated hydrosalpinx (in the case of failed surgical repair) prior to the IVF process.

Patients with mild-to-moderate tubal disease have an option of surgery. Once again, male factor, age, and other fertility issues should be considered prior to taking the surgical approach. These patients can be approached laparoscopically or microsurgically since the pregnancy rates appear to be similar with both techniques. Laparoscopy is associated with less morbidity and less time for recovery. Given this, the laparoscopic approach for mild and

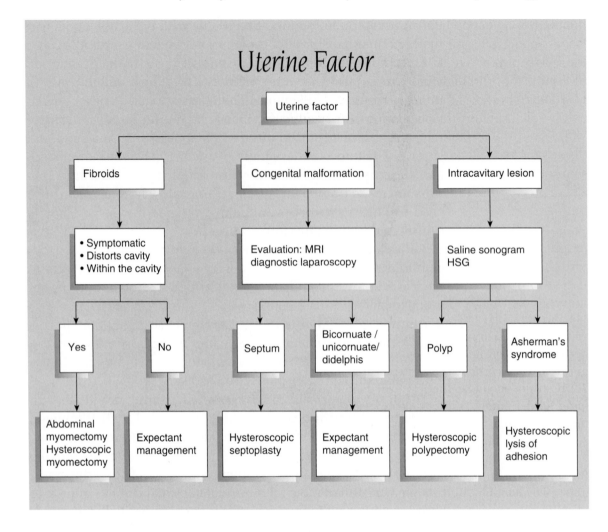

moderate distal tubal disease is reasonable. Pregnancy rates after repair of mildly affected tubes are as high as 70–80%. In moderate cases, the pregnancy rates are 17–30%. All of these patients experience a higher chance of an ectopic pregnancy at a rate of 5–25%.[16,17]

These findings support the notion that patients with distal tubal disease with associated pelvic adhesive disease should undergo a careful preoperative risk factor assessment and a carefully planned operative intervention for different case scenarios.

UTERINE FACTOR   Uterine factor can play a very significant role in fertility. Paying close attention to the history and physical obtained from the patient can yield a significant amount of information regarding potential uterine factors. Imaging studies such as hysterosalpingogram, saline sonography, and MRI can help determine the need for operative intervention. To a great extent uterine surgery is an adjunctive treatment to other infertility treatments and is not necessarily in place of assisted reproductive technologies.

UTERINE MYOMAS A large number of women in their prime reproductive years have uterine myomas (of 20 women in this descriptor, 40% will have myoma); however, most of these are asymptomatic and do not contribute toward infertility. In infertility related myoma, when all other factors have been excluded, the percentage is 2–3% of the cases.[18] Symptomatic fibroids, menorrhagia, pelvic pain, or urinary frequency, lead to as many as 175,000 hysterectomies and 20,000 myomectomies.[19,20] Myomectomy for uterine myoma for symptomatic myoma with infertility should be approached differently to maximize both the outcomes of relieving symptoms and optimizing chances for pregnancy in the patient. Pregnancy rates after myomectomy have been reported to be 40–50%.[21] According to a metaanalysis of abdominal myomectomies performed for infertility between 1982 and 1996, pregnancy rates for intramural myomas were noted to be 58%, subserosal 65%, and submucous 53–70%. The recurrence rate was noted to be 4–47%. Most of these studies in the metaanalysis were neither randomized nor prospective.[22]

The cause of infertility with myoma is not clearly established. However, there are a number of factors that may be responsible for infertility. For instance, anovulatory cycles are more common in women with myomas. Enlargement and deformity of the uterine cavity may interfere with implantation as well as inhibit sperm movement. The increased surface area can cause alteration in the endometrium and lead to menorrhagia, again causing interference with possible implantation. Finally, myoma may also physically impair sperm's ability to enter the cervix, uterine cavity, or the fallopian tube preventing fertilization and pregnancy.

There are no definitive studies that show us what the indicators are for myomectomy for the infertility patient. A patient undergoing IVF treatment who is diagnosed as having submucosal myomas, or myomas distorting the cavity, appears to have a lower pregnancy rate.[23] Thus, current thoughts on myomectomy in asymptomatic patients with infertility is that only patients with submucosal myomas and myomas that are distorting the cavity require myomectomy. Other asymptomatic myomas should be managed expectantly.

The surgical approach to myomectomy depends on the size and the location of the lesion. Myomas which are primarily within the cavity should be approached hysteroscopically using the resectoscope or an equivalent means. Extreme care should be exercised to minimize the fluid overload complication and thus a fluid management system is essential to minimize this risk.

Abdominal myomectomy for infertility follows the same surgical principal as any other myomectomies. Either tourniquets or intramyometrial vasopressin should be used to minimize blood loss. Since postoperative adhesion formation is as high as 94% with a posterior uterine incision and 55% in anterior uterine incision, myomectomies for infertility patients require utmost attention to surgical techniques.[24] Microsurgical principles should be used to keep the bleeding and tissue damage to a minimum. Uterine tissues such as serosa should be handled minimally to decrease the rate of adhesion formation. Dissection of the fibroid should be carried out sharply rather than bluntly. Staining of the uterine cavity with methylene blue using a catheter should be considered as this allows one to minimize the chance of inadvertent entry into the uterine cavity and allows for the proper repair of any defect noted.

KEY POINT

Submucosal fibroids are considered the most relevant to fertility.

Abdominal myomectomy by laparotomy is, in most cases, the method of choice. Although laproscopic myomectomy has become very popular, only pedunculated and serosal fibroids are amenable for the laproscopic approach. Factors such as risk of uterine rupture, incomplete removal of the myoma, prolonged operating time, and inadequate myometrial closure are some of the disadvantages that laproscopic myomectomies face.

UTERINE MALFORMATIONS The expansion of hysteroscopic techniques has simplified the correction of defects such as the uterine septum. Presence of a uterine septum is most often associated with recurrent spontaneous abortion, and rarely with premature labor and late second trimester abortion. Most women with a uterine septum may have no history of obstetrical complications.

Diagnosis is usually by HSG, saline sonography, or diagnostic hysteroscopy. However, differentiation of uterine septum and bicornuate uterus may require diagnostic laparoscopy or MRI.

Uterine malformation, a disorder of lateral fusion, can be classified as unicornuate uterus (a single horn with both a communicating and noncommunicating second horn); uterine didelphus (a complete duplication with two cervices, two uterine cavities, and longitudinal vaginal septum); bicornuate uterus and septate uterus (a symmetric nonobstructed double uterus).[25] There is no need for surgical intervention—for infertility reasons—for unicornuate uterus and uterine didelphus. Resection of the vaginal septum in uterine didelphus may be required for comfort so that the patients are able to have pain free intercourse.

Differentiation of bicornuate uterus and uterine septum is important since bicornuate uterus is associated with minimal early reproductive problems whereas the uterine septum is often associated with early reproductive failures. Among the different types of uterine malformations, septate uterus is the most common and has a spontaneous pregnancy loss rate up to 60%.[26]

In definitively establishing the diagnosis for the surgical approach to the uterine septum, combinations of laparoscopy and hysteroscopy are best used. The repair of a bicornuate uterus via abdominal metroplasty is not routinely performed since the reproductive sequela is minimal and surgical intervention has significant morbidity associated with it. Laparoscopy allows the examination of the outer contour of the uterus thus allowing differentiation between the two types of double uteri. A broad unnotched fundus is typical for the septate uterus as opposed to two separate horns of the uterus, which is a finding consistent for the bicorunate uterus.

The laparoscopic procedure also allows for the evaluation of other infertility factors as well as being an adjunct to the operative treatment for the uterine septum. Concurrent laparoscopy allows the optimal septal incision. Hysteroscopic septal incision can be performed using microscissors, electrosurgery, or laser. The use of microscissors allows for the use of isotonic fluid to minimize complications of fluid overload and the use of a smaller caliber hysteroscope. The choice of resectoscope with electrosurgery is at times convenient since it is readily available, as well as giving improved view with its double lumen for constant irrigation. However, electrosurgery adds the possibility of thermal injury of the myometrium and increases the risk of uterine perforation. In addition, the need to use a larger caliber hysteroscope with resectoscope should be considered in determining the type of system to use for the incision of the uterine septum. Dissection is considered to be complete when the hysteroscope can be moved from one cornua to the other.

Other ways of assessing whether the incision is complete is to look at the light from a laproscopic viewpoint. A significant amount of bleeding is also a sign that the myometrium has been reached and that septum has been incised completely. One may consider leaving <1 cm of the septum if the risk of perforation is deemed to be high.[27]

INTRACAVITARY LESIONS

Polyps Polyps are frequently identified as a filling defect by hysterosalpingogram or by saline sonography. Because of the distortion of the endometrial cavity caused by polyps, they can prevent proper implantation and therefore should be removed prior to *in vitro* fertilization and in the case of unexplained infertility.

Treatment is relatively simple by hysteroscopic technique. The cervix is dilated to accommodate a 5-mm continuous flow system 0° hysteroscope. A variety of fluids including sorbitol or normal saline can be used to distend and visualize the intrauterine cavity. Care should be taken not to over dilate the cervix as this can lead to difficulty in uterine distention. Hysteroscopic scissors are passed through the outer sheath and the polyps may be resected at their base. Special care should be taken when removing polyps near the cornual regions. The use of a resectoscope for uterine polypectomy is often not necessary.

This procedure may be performed with local anesthesia (paracervical block) in an outpatient setting or in the operating room in the case of multiple and larger polyps.

Asherman's Syndrome Asherman's syndrome refers to the formation of intrauterine synechiae. These can lead to secondary amenorrhea, menstrual irregularities, infertility, and recurrent miscarriage. It is well documented that a strong association exists between puerperal D&C and the formation of synechiae in the endometrial cavity. While no prospective studies exist to confirm the incidence, other risk factors to the development of intrauterine synechiae include the development of endometrial infection following D&C, a hypoestrogenic state, and scant endometrium that exposes the basalis to trauma. Rare occurrences of Asherman's syndrome have been documented in the absence of a prior D&C and after severe endometritis, tuberculosis, myomectomy, and cesarean section.[28]

A diagnosis of Asherman's syndrome is made by obtaining a clinical history in conjunction with either hysterosalpingography or saline sonogram, or by direct visualization during hysteroscopy. Surgical management is the appropriate therapy and preferably should be performed by hysteroscopic lysis of adhesions, using either hysteroscopic scissors or KTP laser. Sharp adhesiolysis should be performed by either technique at the point of greatest tension of the adhesion. Conversely, although not preferred, repeat curettage can be performed for management of intrauterine synechiae. With severe Asherman's syndrome, use of laparoscopy or ultrasound guidance should be considered to reduce risk of uterine perforation and surgical correction.

Following either technique, it is important to maintain patency of the uterine cavity. This should be achieved both mechanically and hormonally. An intrauterine device, or balloon catheter inflated with no more than 5 cc of saline (any further inflation results in significant patient discomfort), is placed into the endometrial cavity. When a pediatric foley catheter is used, it may be attached to a leg bag to collect any drainage and left in place for ~7 days. Additionally, the endometrial cavity should be stimulated with oral estrogen therapy. Possible regimens include Estrace 2 mg bid or conjugated estrogen, 2.5 mg qd for 3 weeks, followed by progesterone 10 mg qd for 7 days. At ~6 weeks postoperatively, a saline sonogram or hysterosalpingogram may be performed to confirm patency of the endometrial cavity.

It is important to explain to patients that even with optimal surgical management, the prognosis for pregnancy with significant adhesions is poor. After hysteroscopic lysis of adhesions, pregnancy rates are reported in the range of 40–90%.[29] Likewise, the clinician must consider the significant risks to curettage of the pregnant or infected uterus, and remember that less vigorous scraping should be performed with the goal of minimizing endometrial trauma.[30]

KEY POINT

Intrauterine scarring is most commonly seen following postobstetrical curettage in the face of excessive bleeding and infection.

MANAGEMENT OF SPONTANEOUS ABORTION It is difficult to accurately assess the true incidence of spontaneous abortion, because such a large percentage of these events are unrecognized by the patient. When urine β-human chorionic gonadotropin (β-hCG) samples were monitored in a cohort of women trying to conceive, 62% of fetuses died during the first trimester, and of these 92% of the losses were subclinical without the patient being aware of the pregnancy.[31]

Similar studies have confirmed these findings. However, most studies of spontaneous abortion have addressed only pregnancies recognized by women and these confirm loss rates of 15–17%.[32]

Common risk factors include advancing maternal age, particularly over the age of 35, increasing paternal age, and race. It as been demonstrated that at each stage of pregnancy, minority women have higher rates of spontaneous abortion than do white women with the largest discrepancy occurring at 12–19 weeks gestation.[32]

Surgical intervention is theoretically appropriate in two settings: (1) inevitable abortion and (2) missed abortion. Inevitable abortion refers to the patient with a progressively dilated internal cervical os and no expulsion of products of conception. Missed abortion refers to the presence of a nonviable pregnancy defined as either the absence of fetal heart rate at greater than 6 weeks gestation and/or the presence of no fetal pole growth on consecutive ultrasounds. Usually, ultrasounds are repeated at least once at weekly intervals to confirm this finding. Even at this point, however, it is not unreasonable to observe the patient for a period of 1–2 weeks prior to surgical intervention in light of the risks of endometrial damage in these patients.

Once it has been decided to proceed with some form of evacuation, it is important to consider each patient individually with respect to the selection of treatment location. Outpatient management should be reserved for patients who have tolerated vaginal examinations and ultrasounds well and for gestations of less than 8 weeks. Use of Motrin 800 mg 1 h prior to the procedure is recommended. A tenaculum is gently placed on the anterior lip of the cervix. A paracervical block is placed by instilling ~5 cc of 1% lidocaine at positions 2, 4, 8, and 10 on a clock in the cervicovaginal junction. A flexible Karman cannula with syringe is used as a source of suction, and generally fits into the cervix with minimal, if any, dilatation. Curretage is performed until a uterine crie is achieved and products of conception can be sent for analysis.

If a patient does not seem appropriate for outpatient management, then the procedure may be performed in the operating room under either general anesthesia or preferably, conscious sedation. The procedure is performed after appropriate dilatation of the cervix using a suction curettage.

Knowledge of the patient's Rhesus factor (Rh) type is imperative. Spontaneous abortion can result in sensitization of the

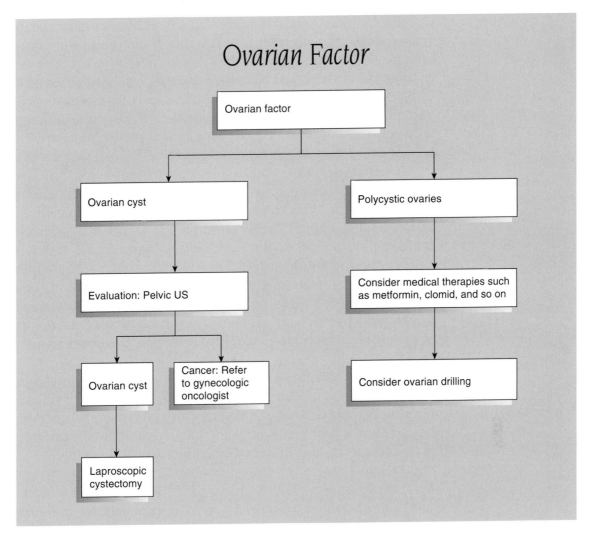

Ovarian Factor

Ovarian factor

Ovarian cyst

Polycystic ovaries

Evaluation: Pelvic US

Consider medical therapies such as metformin, clomid, and so on

Ovarian cyst

Cancer: Refer to gynecologic oncologist

Consider ovarian drilling

Laproscopic cystectomy

Rh-negative woman. Therefore, RhIG candidates at 12 weeks of gestation or less should receive a 50-mcg dose and spontaneous abortions that occur later than that should receive a 300-mcg dose.

OVARIAN FACTOR *OVARY* Ovarian surgery presents a unique challenge because of several anatomic factors, including the ovary's mobility, hard cortex, and rich vascularity. In general, causes for surgery include ovarian cysts, benign ovarian tumors, and endometriomas. The approach can be either laporoscopic or open, but should reflect the skill of the surgeon.

Immobilization should be achieved using either a vascular clamp or an equivalent laporoscopic tool. This stabilization greatly improves the surgeon's ability to work on the ovary. Additionally, in open procedures, the ovary should be surrounded by moist lint-free gauze.

Hemostasis is one of the greater challenges of ovarian surgery, and this should be achieved by exploration of the ovarian stroma with constant irrigation. Precise bipolar coagulation should then be performed covering as minimal a surface as possible.

When suture is used, suture placement should be within the stroma and should not cross into the ovarian cortex. The initial incision into the ovary should be elliptical in an open procedure. Stromal sutures are generally performed in an interrupted fashion using either 4-0 or 5-0 nonreactive sutures on a tapered needle. Again care must be taken to reapproximate the edges without tearing or strangulating the tissue during ligation. The ovarian cortex is then reapproximated using 4-0 or 5-0 sutures to perform either a baseball suture or a subcuticular closure. If at all possible, sutures through the ovarian cortex should be avoided.[33]

Surgery on the ovaries is often done to perform adhesiolysis or to remove surface endometriosis. Adhesions should be excised, not simply divided to ensure that they do not impede future ovulation. This is best achieved using an angled microelectrode or laser and a technique of superficial shaving.[33,34]

POLYCYSTIC OVARIES Polycystic ovaries (PCOS) represent an additional indication for ovarian surgery. The most common presenting feature of patients with PCOS is anovulatory infertility. The first line of treatment for PCOS-related infertility is medical, consisting of clomiphene citrate (CC). Patients who fail to ovulate with CC may be treated with the addition of metformin and gonadotropins. However, this last option (gonadotropins) is associated with disappointing pregnancy rates along with side effects including multiple pregnancy and ovarian hyperstimulation syndrome. As a result, other treatment options such as laparoscopic ovarian drilling have been recommended. This procedure was preceded by the ovarian wedge resection, where 95% of patients undergoing bilateral ovarian wedge resection had normal menstrual cyclicity restored and a pregnancy rate of 85%. The procedure was largely criticized, however, due to reported instances of premature ovarian failure, likely due to excessive tissue loss and interrupted blood supply, and the formation of postoperative scar tissue.

KEY POINT

Ovarian drilling may act in a similar fashion to ovarian wedge resection by decreasing androgen producing stroma within the ovary.

Consequently, a modified version of the ovarian wedge resection, namely, laparoscopic ovarian drilling has been shown to restore ovulation in 92% of patients with a pregnancy rate of 80%.[35] The technique has been performed laparoscopically using either laser or electrocautery and it involves making multiple holes on the surface of the ovary. The procedure involves using an insulated needle unipolar electrode inserted perpendicularly into the ovarian surface. Ten to fifteen punctures were made in each ovary using a 20–30 W coagulating current for 2 s at each point. While the mechanism of such action is unclear, it appears to exert its beneficial effect by destruction of some of the androgen-producing ovarian stroma.[36] This results in a significant reduction in total and free testosterone below preoperative levels. Additionally, after an initial postoperative rise, there appears to be a decrease in luteinizing hormone (LH) pulse amplitudes. Changes in FSH levels are more variable, but overall tend to remain similar. This results in normalization of the FSH:LH ratio. The best prognostic sign of response is a preoperative LH > 10 IU/L. Additionally, poor prognostic signs include grossly obese women, preexisting tubal disease, and >3 years duration of infertility.[37] These were all associated with a less robust response in terms of restoring normal ovulation and pregnancy rates. Several studies have demonstrated that postoperative conception rates continue to rise up to 24 months postoperatively and range from 36% at 6 months to 82% at 24 months.

UNEXPLAINED INFERTILITY Treatment of patients with unexplained infertility has been discussed in previous chapters and will be discussed further in Chap. 12. From a surgical point of view, the issue is whether a diagnostic laparoscopy is indicated in patients with unexplained infertility. Controversy rises out of lack of specificity and sensitivity of hysterosalpingo- gram when finding subtle peritubal disease and/or endometriosis. Patients with a normal hysterosalpingogram with unexplained infertility, who underwent a diagnostic laparoscopy, have been found to have abnormalities in their pelvis up to 50% of the time.[38,39] These data come from nonrandomized trials; however, two randomized trials have been carried out for early stage endometriosis. In one study on endometriosis from a Canadian collaborative group, a multicenter,

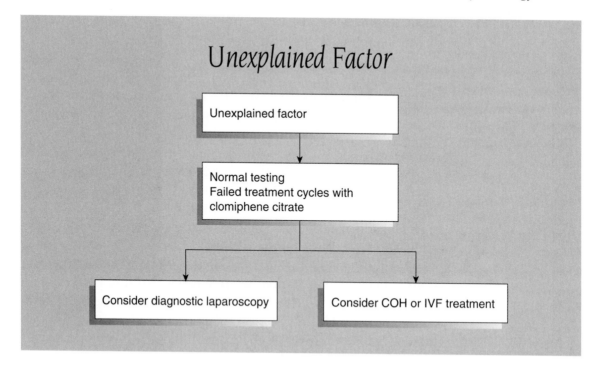

prospectively randomized trial found laparoscopic treatment of the disease to result in a 37.5% conception rate while expectant management produced a pregnancy rate of 22.5%.[40] However, a second randomized trial showed 19.6% live birth rate in group treated for endometriosis and 22.5% rate in the controls within 1 year of surgery.[41] Thus, the value of diagnostic laparoscopy and treatment is unclear.

The current recommendation for unexplained infertility patients is to consider laparoscopy for those patients with an increased risk of pelvic pathology either by their history or by examination. In completely asymptomatic patients, several cycles of ovulation induction with clomiphene citrate and intrauterine insemination and/or controlled ovarian hyperstimulation cycles with intrauterine insemination may be reasonable prior to considering surgery. Patients who cannot or will not proceed to assisted reproductive technology may benefit from the diagnostic laparoscopy.[42] The decision must be weighed by factoring the cost and the invasiveness of the operative intervention. Clearly, further prospective, randomized studies are required to assess whether diagnostic laparoscopy is cost-effective and whether such intervention actually increases the pregnancy outcome.

What's the Evidence?

- False-positive rate with HSG may be as high as 21–57%.[3,4] Repeat studies or careful review of prior studies may prevent unnecessary surgical intervention.
- General principles of adhesiolysis, excision of disease tissue, hemostasis, and tension-free anastomosis is important in all surgical interventions.[5]
- Patients with severe distal tubal disease have pregnancy rates of only 4–16% after salpingostomy and lysis of adhesions.[16,17] These patients are better served by IVF.
- Evidence supports the removal of a hydrosalpinx prior to IVF.[11,12]
- Evidence supports attempted repair of mild disease where success rates may be as high as 70–80%. But all patients have an increased risk of ectopic pregnancy.[16,17]
- Evidence supports a lowered chance for pregnancy in IVF with submucosal fibroids.[23]

Discussion of Cases

CASE 1

A 39-year-old woman, G3 P3 who has her fallopian tubes tied with her last pregnancy presents with request for tubal reanastomosis. Her pregnancies were uncomplicated and all births were vaginal. She had her tubes "tied" 6 weeks postpartum. She is in a relationship with a new partner and would like to consider another pregnancy.

What other information is necessary in proper counseling of this patient?

- **Menstrual history (frequency of menses, amount of menses, history of vaginal dryness, history of hot flushes)**
- **Ovarian reserve: cycle day 3 FSH and estradiol and/or antral follicle count by pelvic ultrasound**
- **Partner's semen parameters: semen analysis is absolutely required even with evidence of prior paternity**
- **Operative report from the surgery (tubal ligation)**
- **Pathology report (if applicable)**

She reports her menstrual cycles have become more frequent, decreasing from a prior 28-day interval to every 21–24 days. In addition, she reports the need for lubricants on occasion due to vaginal dryness. The semen analysis on her new partner is normal. The operative report from the surgery indicates that she had laproscopic tubal fulguration of the fallopian tubes with "triple burn." Lastly, her cycle day 3 FSH and estradiol level returned in the normal ranges. Her pelvic ultrasound showed a total antral follicle count of 10 in her ovaries.

What are her treatment options?

- **Bilateral tubal reanastomosis**
- ***In vitro* fertilization**

What factors should be considered in counseling the patient?

- **Age**
- **Change in menstrual frequency**
- **Vaginal dryness**
- **Type of tubal ligation**

This is a typical patient who seeks out information about tubal reversal. Many patients are not aware of what type of tubal ligation they had and frequently are under the misperception that they are different from other infertile patients and can achieve pregnancy easily. It is important to counsel the patient regarding the effects of age on pregnancy rates. In addition, type of tubal ligation is very important.

Typically, fallopian tubes that are "burned" either by bipolar or unipolar cautery have less chance of success due to the shortness of the total viable tubes. Dissipated heat damage could often extend through the tubes. The types of tubal ligation which enjoys the best success in reversal include fallop ring, Hulka clips, or the postpartum pomeroy styled tubal ligation. In the later type, pathology report with the total length of tube removed is helpful in the decision-making process. It is also important to assess the ovarian reserve of the patient. If she exhibits signs of perimenopause, such as more frequent cycles, vaginal dryness, one would be less likely to expose the patient to the operative risks of tubal reversal. Evaluation of her ovarian reserve with cycle day 3 FSH and estradiol, or counting the number of antral follicles, may help determine the woman's ovarian status.

In this particular patient with an unfavorable type of tubal ligation and her advancing age with some initial signs of perimenopause, she may not be the best candidate for the tubal reversal. Given that her cycle day 3 FSH and estradiol and the antral follicle counts are reasonable, she may be a candidate for *in vitro* fertilization.

CASE 2

Twenty-eight-year-old woman, G0, P0 with primary infertility of 16 months duration. Her infertility evaluations have included

- **TSH, PRL: normal**
- **Semen analysis: normal**
- **Menstrual history: normal 28-day cycle with positive results using ovulation predictor kits**

- **Hystersosalpingogram: normal uterine cavity, bilateral fill of the fallopian tubes with delayed spill of dye on the left and loculation of dye on the right fallopian tube**

The patient has undergone three failed cycles of ovulation induction with clomiphene citrate with intrauterine insemination. The couple is seeking counseling on the next course of therapy.

What other information is necessary in proper counseling of this patient?

- **History of pelvic inflammatory disease**
- **History of previous surgeries (ruptured appendix)**
- **History of dysmenorrhea, dyspareunia, pelvic pain**
- **History or evidence of endometriosis**

The patient denies any history of pelvic infections. She reports that all of the cultures of infections have been negative. She does recall having an appendectomy as a child. She does not remember much of the care given. She denies any significant dysmenorrhea, or pain with intercourse or pelvic pain in general. No one has ever mentioned the word endometriosis to her before.

What are her treatment options?

- **Diagnostic laparoscopy**
- **Controlled ovarian hyperstimulation with intrauterine inseminations**
- ***In vitro* fertilization**

What factors should be considered in counseling the patient?

- **History of previous surgery**
- **Hysterosalpingogram results**
- **Patient's concerns with each treatment options**

The operative report for the appendectomy was not available. The hysterosalpingogram films when reviewed were consistent with the report. Given her young age, lack of history of pelvic infection, and pain, it was agreed that diagnostic laparoscopy was a reasonable course of action.

Findings at the time of laparoscopy included a normal left fallopian tube and some peritubular adhesions of the right tube with minimal scarring. Lysis of adhesion was carried out.

Postoperatively, patient decided to proceed with the controlled ovarian hyperstimulation with intrauterine insemination as a treatment course.

REFERENCES

1 Jones HW. Evolving aspects of reparative surgery. In: Rock JA, Thompson JD (eds.), *Te Linde's Operative Gynecology.* Philadelphia, PA: Lippincott-Raven, 1997, pp. 445–452.

2 Baggish MS. Operative hysteroscopy. In: Rock JA, Thompson JD (eds.), *Te Linde's Operative Gynecology.* Philadelphia, PA: Lippincott-Raven, pp. 415–442, 1997.

3 Siegler AM. Hysterography and hysteroscopy in the infertile patient. *J Reprod Med* 18:143, 1977.

4 Valle RF. Hysteroscopy in the evaluation of female infertility. *Am J Obstet Gyncol* 137:425, 1980.

5 Hunt RB. Tubal anastomosis. In: Hunt RB (ed.), *Text and Atlas of Female Infertility Surgery.* St. Louis, MO: Mosby, 1999, pp. 287–306.

6 Murphy AA. Reconstructive surgery of the oviduct. In: Rock JA, Murphy AA, Jones HW (eds.), *Female Reproductive Surgery*. Baltimore, MD: Williams & Wilkins, 1992, pp. 146–169.

7 Rock JA, Bergquist CA, Kimball AW Jr, Zacur HA, King TM. Comparison of the operating microscope and loupe for microsurgical tubal anastomosis: a randomized clinical trial. *Fertil Steril* 41:229–232, 1984.

8 Rock JA, Guzick DS, Katz E, Zacur HA, King TM. Tubal anastomosis: pregnancy success following reversal of Falope ring or monopolar cautery sterilization. *Fertil Steril* 48:13–17, 1987.

9 Gomel V. Microsurgical reversal of female sterilization: a reappraisal. *Fertil Steril* 33:587–597, 1980.

10 Cha SH, Lee MH, Kim JH, Lee CN, Yoon TK, Cha KY. Fertility outcome after tubal anastomosis by laparoscopy and laparotomy. *J Am Assoc Gynecol Laparosc* 8:348–352, 2001.

11 Zeyneloglu HB, Arici A, Olive DL. Adverse effects of hydrosalpinx on pregnancy rates after in vitro fertilization-embryo transfer. *Fertil Steril* 70:492–499, 1998.

12 Johnson NP, Mak W, Sowter MC. *Surgical treatment for tubal disease in women due to undergo in vitro fertilisation (Cochrane Review)*. The Cochrane Library, Issue 4. Chichester, UK: John Wiley & Sons, 2003.

13 Jones HW. Evolving aspects of reparative surgery. In: Rock JA, Thompson JD (eds.), *Te Linde's Operative Gynecology*. Philadelphia, PA: Lippincott-Raven, 2003, p. 452.

14 Honore GM, Holden AEC, Schenken RS. Pathophysiology and management of proximal tubal blockage. *Fertil Steril* 71:785, 1999.

15 Watson A, Vandekerckhove P, Lilford R. *Techniques for pelvic surgery in subfertility (Cochrane Methodology Review)*. The Cochrane Library, Issue 4. Chichester, UK: John Wiley & Sons, 2003.

16 Rock, JA, Katayama KP, Martin EJ, et al. Factors influencing the success of salpingostomy techniques for distal fimbrial obstruction. *Obstet Gynecol* 52:591, 1978.

17 Schlaff WD, Hossiokos D, Damewood MD, et al. Neosalpingostomy for distal tubal obstruction: prognostic factors and impact of surgical techniques. *Fertil Steril* 54:984, 1991.

18 Buttram VC Jr, Reiter RC. Uterine leiomyomata: etiology, symptomatology, and management. *Fertil Steril* 36:433–445, 1981.

19 Dicker RC, Greenspan JR, Strauss LT, et al. Complications of abdominal and vaginal hysterectomies among women of reproductive age in the United States. The Collaborative Review of Sterilization. *Am J Obstet Gynecol* 144:841–848, 1982.

20 Gambone JC, Reiter RC, Lench JB, Moore JG. The impact of a quality assurance process on the frequency and confirmation rates of hysterectomy. *Am J Obstet Gynecol* 163:545–550, 1990.

21 Verkauf BS. Myomectomy for fertility enhancement and preservation. *Fertil Steril* 58:1–15, 1992.

22 Vercellini P, Maddaleana S, DeGiorgi O, et al. Abdominal myomectomy for infertility: a comprehensive review. *Hum Reprod* 13(4):873–879, 1998.

23 Surrey ES, Lietz AK, Schoolcraft WB. Impact of intramural leiomyomata in patients with a normal endometrial cavity on in vitro fertilization-embryo transfer cycle outcome. *Fertil Steril* 75:405–410, 2001.

24 Tulandi T, Murray C, Guralnick M. Adhesion formation and reproductive outcome after myomectomy and second-look laproscopy. *Obstet Gynecol* 82:213–215, 1993.

25 Damewood MD, Rock JA. Uterine reconstructive surgery. In: Hunt RB (ed.), *Text and Atlas of Female Infertility Surgery*. St. Louis, MO: Mosby, 1999, pp. 268–286.

26 Heinonen PK, Saarikoski S, Pystynen P. Reproductive performance of women with uterine anomalies. *Acta Obstet Gynecol Scand* 61:157–160, 1982.

27 Homer HA, Li TC, Cooke ID. The septate uterus: a review of management and reproductive outcome. *Fertil Steril* 73:1–14, 2000.

28 Winkel CA. Lesions affecting the uterine cavity. In: Keye, Chang, Rebar, Soules (eds.), *Infertility: Evaluation and Treatment*. Philadelphia, PA: W.B. Saunders, 1995, pp. 435–438.

29 Rock JA. Uterine reconstructive surgery. In: Rock JA, Murphy AA, Jones HW (eds.), *Female Reproductive Surgery*. Baltimore, MD: Williams & Wilkins, 1992, pp. 128–135.

30 Butler WJ. Normal and abnormal uterine bleeding. In: Rock JA, Thompson JD (eds.), *Te Linde's Operative Gynecology*. Philadelphia, PA: Lippincott-Raven, 1997, pp. 453–475.

31 Edmonds DK, Lindsay KS, Miller JF, et al. Early embryonic mortality in women. *Fertil Steril* 38:447, 1982.

32 Grimes DA. Management of abortion. In: Rock JA, Thompson JD (eds.), *Te Linde's Operative Gynecology*. Philadelphia, PA: Lippincott-Raven, 2003, p. 483.

33 Murphy AA. Reconstructive surgery of the ovary. In: Rock JA, Murphy AA, Jones HW (eds.), *Female Reproductive Surgery*. Baltimore, MD: Williams & Wilkins, 1992, pp. 190–204.

34 Cohen BM. Surgery of the ovary, including anatomic derangements of the fimbrial-gonadal ovum-capture mechanism. In: Hunt RB (ed.),

Text and Atlas of Female Infertility Surgery. St. Louis, MO: Mosby, 1999, pp. 322–333.

35 Donesky BW, Adashi EY. Surgically induced ovulation in the polycystic ovary syndrome: wedge resection revisited in the age of laparoscopy. *Fertil Steril* 63:439, 1995.

36 Sanfilippo JS, Rock JA. Surgery for benign disease of the ovary. In: Rock JA, Thompson JD (eds.), *Te Linde's Operative Gynecology.* Philadelphia, PA: Lippincott-Raven, 2003, pp. 653–654.

37 Amer SA, Banu Z, Li TC, et al. Long-term follow up of patients with polycystic ovary syndrome after laproscopic ovarian drilling: endocrine and ultrasonographic outcomes. *Hum Reprod* 17:2851–2857, 2002.

38 Belisle S, Collins JA, Burrows EA, Wilan AR. The value of laparoscopy among infertile women with tubal patency. *J SOGC* 18:326–336, 1996.

39 Al-Badawi IA, Fluker MR, Bebbington MW. Diagnostic laparoscopy in infertile women with normal hysterosalpingograms. *J Reprod Med* 44(11):953–957, 1999.

40 Marcoux S, Maheux R, Berube S. Laparoscopic surgery in infertile women with minimal or mild endometriosis. Canadian Collaborative Group on Endometriosis. *N Engl J Med* 337:217–222, 1997.

41 Parazzini F. Ablation of lesions or no treatment in minimal-mild endometriosis in infertile women: a randomized trail. Gruppo Italiano per lo Studio dell'endometriosi. *Hum Reprod* 14:1332–1334, 1999.

42 Fatum M, Laufer N, Simon A. Investigation of the infertile couple: should diagnostic laparoscopy be performed after normal hysterosalpingogram in treating infertility suspected to be of unknown origin? *Hum Reprod* 17:1–3, 2002.

Medical and Surgical Management of Male Infertility

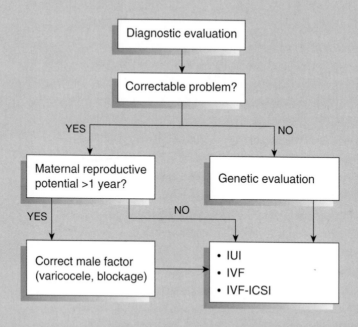

11

Medical and Surgical Management of Male Infertility

Paul J. Turek

Findings from Male Diagnostic Evaluation

As discussed earlier (Chap. 4), the male infertility evaluation is performed to systematically acquire information from the patient's history, physical examination, semen quality, and hormone tests. In conjunction with the female evaluation, this is used to choose one or more of the following clinical pathways: treat male factor, treat female factor, or proceed to assisted reproductive technology (ART).

The Decision to Treat Male Factor

Male infertility is caused by definable disease in half of cases. In addition, 1–2% of male infertility is due to significant or life-threatening disease.[1] There is no question that life-threatening diseases should be treated (Table 11-1). However, because of revolutionary advances in assisted reproduction [including intracytoplasmic sperm injection (ICSI)], there has been a recent trend to avoid specific male factor treatments that are not life threatening in favor of assisted technologies. This is unfortunate, as many such male factor treatments may actually help infertile couples conceive without assisted reproduction.[2]

**Table 11-1. SIGNIFICANT MEDICAL CONDITIONS PRESENTING
AS MALE INFERTILITY**

Diabetes	Prostate cancer
Hemochromatosis	Retroperitoneal tumors
Hypopituitarism	Spinal cord tumors
Klinefelter's syndrome	Testis cancer
Multiple sclerosis	Thyroid disease
Pituitary adenoma	Urinary tract infection

KEY POINT

*If maternal
reproductive
potential is
determined to be
relatively stable for
1 year, then
treatments to
improve
spermatogenesis in
the male are almost
always warranted.*

Certainly, maternal reproductive potential should be considered before treatment of non-life-threatening male factors. This reasoning becomes obvious when one considers that spermatogenesis and sperm maturation within the epididymis require 80–90 days to complete. Therefore, one might expect the effects of most medical or surgical treatments that seek to improve spermatogenesis to result in changes in semen quality 3–4 months after initiation. These physiologic variables actually play out in clinical experience: the average time to conception after varicocele repair and vasectomy reversal is 9 and 12.4 months, respectively.[2,3] Thus, if the goal of treating the infertile couple is pregnancy, then an important guiding principle in the decision to treat male factor infertility is to first determine whether or not the female partner has 1 year of relatively stable reproductive potential. If so, then correcting male infertility is almost always warranted. Examples of correctable male infertility factors follow this discussion.

Guiding Questions

**MALE INFERTILITY
TREATMENT**

- Is there a life-threatening medical condition causing the infertility?
- Is there a correctable medical or surgical problem causing the infertility?
- Is there adequate female reproductive potential to allow the necessary time for male factor treatments to work?
- Does the couple's cultural agenda and timeline for pregnancy have sufficient space to allow the value of male infertility treatment to be realized?

Correctable Male Factor Diagnoses

COITAL THERAPY	Simple counseling on issues of coital timing, frequency, and gonadotoxin avoidance can improve fertility. Coital lubricants should be avoided if possible. If necessary, vegetable oils, olive oil, and petroleum jelly are the safest. Although scarcely published, heat exposure from hot baths, Jacuzzis, and hot tubs are very detrimental to sperm production. Avoidance of tobacco, marijuana, excessive alcohol, and other recreational drugs is mandatory. In summary, it is good to emphasize to couples to "treat their bodies like a temple" as they try to conceive.
EJACULATORY DYSFUNCTION	Men can also have problems with ejaculation. Low ejaculate volumes (<2.0 mL) can be associated with retrograde ejaculation, which results from a failure of the bladder neck to close during ejaculation. Diagnosed by the finding of sperm within the postejaculate bladder urine, it is treated with sympathomimetic medications. Approximately 30% of men will respond to treatment, but the side effects of medications usually limit the efficacy of therapy. For medication failures, sperm can be harvested from the bladder and used with intrauterine insemination (IUI) to achieve a pregnancy. Premature ejaculation occurs when men ejaculate before their partner is ready. Although not a formal cause of infertility, premature ejaculation can cause significant relationship stress. Sexual counseling combined with tricyclic antidepressants or serotoninergic uptake inhibitors can be very effective treatment. Ejaculatory failure or anejaculation is the inability to ejaculate. It has a variety of causes that include pelvic nerve damage from diabetes mellitus, multiple sclerosis, or abdominal-pelvic surgery and spinal cord injury. Vibratory stimulation and rectal probe electroejaculation are two commonly performed techniques that may enable anejaculatory patients to conceive.[4]
PYOSPERMIA	Elevated leukocytes in semen is termed pyospermia or leukocytospermia and has been associated with[1] subclinical genital tract infection,[2] elevated reactive oxygen species, and poor sperm function and infertility.[3] However, one must not confuse the presence of immature germ cells with white blood cells in the ejaculate. Among asymptomatic, infertile men, elevations in seminal round

cells are usually (70%) immature germ cells and should raise no concern. If, however, special stains confirm that leukocytes are elevated, then an evaluation is in order. Sperm are highly susceptible to the effects of oxidative stress induced by leukocytes because they harbor little cytoplasm and therefore little antioxidant activity. The treatment of pyospermia is controversial in the absence of overt bacteriologic infection. It is important to evaluate the patient for sexually transmitted diseases, penile discharge, prostatitis, or epididymitis. An expressed prostatic secretion is examined for leukocytes, and urethral cultures are obtained for chlamydia and mycoplasma. When appropriate, the limited use of broad-spectrum antibiotics such as doxycycline and trimethoprim-sulfamethoxazole has been shown to reduce seminal leukocyte concentrations, improve sperm function, and increase conception. Generally, the female partner is also treated.

IMMUNOLOGIC INFERTILITY

Antisperm antibodies are a complex problem that can underlie male infertility.[5] Available treatment options include corticosteroid suppression, sperm washing, IUI, in vitro fertilization (IVF), and ICSI. Steroid suppression is based on the concept that an overactive immune system can be weakened to reduce sperm antibodies. Intrauterine insemination places more sperm nearer the ovulated egg to optimize the sperm-egg environment. IVF and ICSI are very effective in overcoming infertility due to antisperm antibodies. In general, >50% of sperm bound with antibodies is considered significant and merits treatment. In addition, head-directed or midpiece-directed sperm antibodies may cause more dysfunction than tail-directed antibodies. Since the presence of antibodies is associated with obstruction in the genital tract, such lesions should be sought and corrected. There is renewed interest in the causes and possible treatments of this interesting problem, as several animal models exist that mimic the human condition.

VARICOCELE

The varicocele is elongated, dilated, and tortuous spermatic veins within the scrotum, and is basically a consequence of man's upright posture. It is found in 40% of infertile men and is associated with infertility. These lesions can cause scrotal discomfort or infertility in adults. Although eternally debated by clinicians in the field, there is substantial evidence to support the value of varicocele repair in male infertility. The most convincing evidence of a cause-effect relationship between varicocele and infertility was reported in a prospective, randomized, cross-over study in which 60% of men conceived within 1 year after varicocele repair ($n = 20$) compared to 10% in an untreated control group ($n = 25$). During the second year of the study, the control group underwent varicocele repair and after that year, 44% of this group conceived.[6] Female factors were well-controlled in this study. In general, semen quality will improve in two-third of men after varicocele repair; the associated pregnancy rate is approximately 35%, with pregnancies occurring an average of 9 months after surgery.[2]

WHAT'S THE EVIDENCE? In addition to clinical care arguments that suggest varicocele repair is beneficial for infertility, economic analyses also support this concept. Cost-benefit arguments have shown that varicocelectomy is more cost-effective than ART procedures.[7] In fact, on average, the delivery rate achieved after varicocele treatment (30%) is actually higher than that obtained with a single cycle of IVF-ICSI.[7] More recently, it has been demonstrated in "shift of care" analyses that as many as 30–50% of couples who would only be candidates for ART procedures due to low semen quality can be "rescued" from such procedures and conceive naturally with varicocelectomy.[2] On the contrary, it has also become apparent that oligospermic men with varicocele might not respond as well to repair in the presence of coexisting genetic factors compared to men without coexisting genetic infertility.[8]

Several modalities are available for varicocele treatment, including incisional ligation of the veins through retroperitoneal, inguinal, or subinguinal approaches, percutaneous transvenous embolisation, and laparoscopic varicocelectomy. The overall complication rate ranges from 1% for the incisional approach to 4% for laparoscopy. The most significant complication with radiologic occlusion is the 10–15% technical failure rate (inability to access and occlude the culprit veins). Return to activity is relatively quick after varicocele repair, especially with the subinguinal, muscle-sparing approach.

EJACULATORY DUCT OBSTRUCTION

Ejaculatory duct obstruction is the cause of infertility in 5% of azoospermic men, but is often overlooked in the male evaluation. Ejaculatory duct obstruction is clinically suspected if the ejaculate volume is <2.0 mL with pH <7.2 and no sperm or fructose is present. Low ejaculate volume in combination with low sperm motility may also represent partial ejaculatory duct obstruction. Clinical suspicion can be confirmed by transrectal ultrasound (TRUS) demonstration of dilated seminal vesicles (>1.5 cm width) or dilated ejaculatory ducts (>2.3 mm) in association with a cyst, calcification, or stones along the duct. A 20–30% pregnancy rate can be expected from surgical treatment in which the obstruction is removed endoscopically, and 70% of men who undergo the procedure will achieve a significant improvement in semen quality.[9]

VASOVASOSTOMY

The male reproductive tract is basically one long and very thin tube. Infection or trauma can result in scarring and blockage within this tube. A classic example is a vasectomy. Approximately 7% of men who have a vasectomy undergo a vasectomy reversal. The success of a vasectomy reversal depends on many factors, the most important of which are the skill of the surgeon and the findings at the time of surgery. Since this is a microsurgical procedure, experienced surgeons use a microscope.

Findings before and at the time of surgery correlate with the success rate of vasectomy reversal. Evidence of inflammation or infection after the vasectomy and a long interval from vasectomy-to-reversal are both associated with a decrease in surgical success.[3] If sperm are found at the cut edge of the vas during surgery, then 85–99% of patients can be expected to have a return of sperm after vasovasostomy (vas to vas connection). With a healthy female partner, this is associated with a pregnancy rate of 60–65%. If the vas fluid is of poor quality (thick, creamy) or scant in amount and sperm are not present, the primary procedure involves connecting the vas to the epididymis in a procedure termed epididymovasostomy. In this case, approximately 80% of men will have sperm in the ejaculate and a 30–35% pregnancy rate can be expected. Operating time for a vasovasostomy or epididymovasostomy is approximately 2.5–3.5 h and a general anesthetic or local anesthesia with sedation is most commonly used. The surgery is performed as an outpatient and the patient is generally able to return to work in 3–4 days.

WHAT'S THE EVIDENCE?   There is a building body of literature suggesting that vasectomy reversal may be more cost-effective in achieving pregnancies than IVF and ICSI. This may be true, in fact, even in cases of older (>15 years old) vasectomies and in advanced maternal age couples.[10] There have also been several recent innovations in urologic microsurgery, including invagination epididymovasostomy, that appear to be associated with improved patency and pregnancy rates after vasectomy reversal. Interestingly, we have applied decision analysis modeling to compare vasectomy reversal to IVF-ICSI.[11] In this model in which at least 10 clinical variables were included, microsurgical skill was the single most important factor in determining which approach was the most cost-effective: if a patency rate (rate of sperm in ejaculate) of >74% can be obtained after reversal surgery, then reversal surgery is less expensive than IVF-ICSI for pregnancy.[11] This finding was independent of age-related changes in maternal reproductive potential.

In addition to vasectomy, male infertility can also result from idiopathic obstruction. In such cases, a blockage can be found in the epididymis in 65% of cases, in the vas deferens 30% of the time, and in the ejaculatory duct in 5% of cases. The clinical triad of obstructive azoospermia, chronic sinusitis, and bronchiectasis is a particular form of epididymal obstruction termed Young's syndrome. In most cases of idiopathic obstruction, the actual location of the blockage can be pinpointed with microsurgery and surgery can be performed at most sites to repair the blockage in an approach similar to that used for vasectomy. To distinguish obstructive azoospermia from that due to a sperm production problem in the absence of obstruction, a testis biopsy and hormonal analysis [testosterone and follicle-stimulating hormone (FSH)] are necessary.

HORMONAL OR OXIDATIVE DYSFUNCTION

Effective hormone therapy can be offered to patients with diseases that predispose to infertility. Treating these problems is aimed at reversing specific abnormalities. Other less effective treatments are those that seek to overcome conditions that are not well understood or those that have no well-proven treatments. Examples of treatable conditions include hyperprolactinemia, hypothyroidism, congenital adrenal hyperplasia, and testosterone excess or deficiency due to steroids or conditions like Kallman's syndrome. Examples of medical treatments that may not work in all men include clomiphene citrate, tamoxifen, human chorionic gonadotropin (hCG) therapy, ProXeed, and antioxidant and herbal therapy.

Although there have been over 30 published trials on clomiphene citrate since 1964, only a few include control arms. In general, an improvement in the semen analysis is noted in approximately 50% of well-selected patients and pregnancies occurring in 25–30% of patients in such studies. Men with low-normal testosterone and FSH levels may be the best responders to this therapy. ProXeed, a form of L-carnitine, is a supplement given to improve sperm motility. The rationale for its use is based on the fact that this amino acid is found in high concentrations in the normal epididymis. Again, no rigorous, placebo-controlled trials exist to support its use in the treatment of male infertility. Finally, there is evidence that up to 30% of infertile men have increased levels of reactive oxygen species in the reproductive tract. These oxidative species (OH, O_2 radicals, and hydrogen peroxide) can cause lipid peroxidation damage to sperm membranes. Treatment with scavengers of these radicals may protect sperm from oxidative damage: glutathione, 600 mg daily, or vitamin E, 400–1200 U/day may be useful in a subgroup of infertile men with elevated levels of seminal reactive oxygen species. Currently, smokers are the best candidates for antioxidant therapy.

Noncorrectable Male Factor Diagnoses

CONGENITAL ABSENCE OF THE VAS DEFERENS

Among infertile males, 1–2% have congenital absence of the vas deferens (CAVD) which is considered a genital form of cystic fibrosis (CF). Affected patients exhibit the same spectrum of Wolffian duct defects as patients with CF, but generally lack the severe pulmonary, pancreatic, and intestinal problems. It is thought that CAVD is based on similar allelic patterns (homozygous and compound heterozygous) as that observed in typical CF but involves less severe mutations. Predictably then, CF mutations are found very frequently (up to 80%) in men with CAVD. Fortunately, sperm can be retrieved from the epididymis or testes of men with CAVD and used with ICSI for pregnancy.[12] Epididymal sperm aspiration can be performed either microsurgically (MESA)

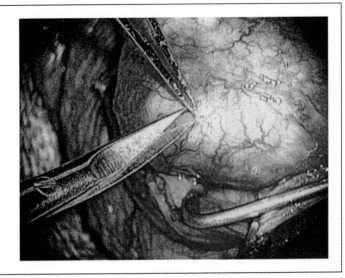

Figure 11-1: Microscopic epididymal sperm retrieval. The epididymis is about to be opened with microscissors.

or percutaneously (PESA) and has been used since 1988 for sperm retrieval (Fig. 11-1). Epididymal sperm is much less motile than ejaculated sperm and fertilizes human eggs in about a third as well. This is why ICSI is needed with epididymal sperm (Table 11-2). Testis sperm retrieved by needle (TESA) or biopsy (TESE) can also be used to achieve pregnancies in CAVD men (Fig. 11-2). Originally, it was thought that sperm from the testis were not capable of egg fertilization; indeed this has only become possible with ICSI (Table 11-2). Indeed, normal oocyte fertilization rates of 70–80% are routinely achieved with testis sperm and IVF-ICSI.

Importantly, all patients with CAVD or idiopathic obstruction should be screened for CFTR gene mutations. An analysis of the

Table 11-2. **SOURCES OF SPERM FOR ASSISTED REPRODUCTIVE PROCEDURES**

PROCEDURE	SOURCE	IVF	ICSI	CRYOPRESERVATION
Vasal aspiration	Vas deferens	Yes	Maybe	Yes
Epididymal aspiration	Epididymis	Yes	Yes	Yes
Testis extraction	Testis	Yes	Yes	Yes

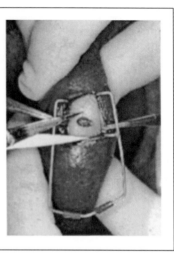

Figure 11-2: Sperm retrieval by testis biopsy (TESE) to be used with IVF-ICSI.

5T, 7T, or 9T variants should also be included in this testing. In addition, renal ultrasounds should be performed on all men with CAVD to evaluate for renal hypoplasia or agenesis, findings that have implications for the likelihood of associated CFTR mutations and general health issues. Finally, female partners of affected men should also be tested for CFTR mutations to fully inform the couple about all phenotypic possibilities in offspring. This is also discussed below.

NONOBSTRUCTIVE AZOOSPERMIA

Azoospermia is the complete lack of sperm in the ejaculate. It occurs in approximately 5–10% of infertile men. Based on the male infertility evaluation, azoospermic men are categorized as either obstructed or nonobstructed based on whether spermatogenesis is normal within the testis. Men with nonobstructive azoospermia generally have testis atrophy, an elevated FSH level, and azoospermia. The definitive diagnosis of nonobstructive azoospermia requires that the testis biopsy show abnormal or absent spermatogenesis. The etiology of this condition varies widely from gonadotoxin exposure to underlying genetic abnormalities and it occurs in about 1–5% of all infertile men.

Since 1995, testis sperm has been used with ICSI to help infertile men achieve paternity. With experience, it is now clear that testis sperm retrieval in obstructed men with normal sperm production is not difficult. However, there is a failure to obtain sperm for ICSI in 25–50% of men with nonobstructive azoospermia. In addition, clinical features including testicular size, history of ejaculated sperm, serum FSH level, or biopsy histology, do not accurately predict whether or not sperm will be recovered during testicular exploration. Because of this, strategies have been developed to more accurately determine which men with failing testes are candidates for ICSI and surgical techniques refined to minimize trauma to the testis during sperm harvest procedures. This kind of thinking is important to minimize the emotional and financial costs associated with cancelled IVF cycles.

One of the first strategies developed, the multibiopsy TESE, involves taking as many biopsy samples as needed at the time of egg retrieval for ICSI. Another approach involves taking testis tissue by biopsy for both diagnosis (histology) and sperm retrieval simultaneously. This procedure is performed *in advance* of ICSI to avoid cancellation of cycles if sperm harvest fails. Multiple biopsies are taken from the testis and all sperm are cryopreserved and then thawed for the future IVF cycles. Microdissection TESE involves microsurgical exploration of the widely opened testis to look for pockets of sperm. Finally, we have found that performing a fine needle aspiration (FNA)"map" (Fig. 11-3) in the office under local anesthesia helps determine the patient's candidacy for future sperm retrieval.[13] Using this information, at the time of egg retrieval for IVF, we then "direct" biopsies to testis locations informed by the map. By having a "map" ahead of time, fewer and

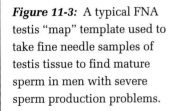

Figure 11-3: A typical FNA testis "map" template used to take fine needle samples of testis tissue to find mature sperm in men with severe sperm production problems.

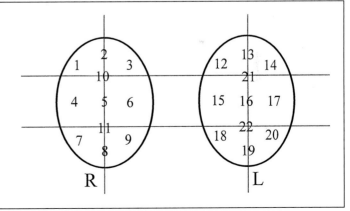

smaller biopsies are required to harvest sufficient sperm for ICSI. We have also found that having prior knowledge of sperm location with FNA mapping helps achieve high sperm retrieval success rates on repeat attempts at sperm retrieval during subsequent IVF cycles. Regardless of approach, most men with nonobstructive azoospermia will have usable sperm within the testis with a comprehensive evaluation as described.

Genetic Evaluation

KEY POINT

Genetic conditions causing male infertility, known or not, are likely to be transmitted to offspring with ICSI.

High technology solutions to pregnancy, including ICSI, are now known to be a two-edged sword. On the one hand, these technologies are very enabling and allow men who would otherwise have no chance for paternity the opportunity for genetic fatherhood. On the other hand, since man and not nature selects sperm for ICSI, how the processes of natural selection are altered is not clear. In addition, the safety profile of ICSI was not determined by fundamental research in clinically relevant models before it was introduced clinically. Thus, with ICSI it is likely that genetic conditions are being passed on that might not be sustained naturally. Furthermore, it is also conceivable that the male offspring of subfertile men will inherit larger or more severe genetic defects that may lead to complete sterility.

We have taken this concept very seriously and have initiated a genetic counseling and testing program at the University of California, San Francisco (UCSF) (Fig. 11-4). Initially, all infertile men are seen by a urologist for thorough medical evaluation. Patients deemed "at risk" for genetic infertility are then seen by a genetic counselor for nonprescriptive or classic counseling in which patients at risk for genetic conditions meet with a genetic counselor prior to laboratory testing[14] (Fig. 11-4). During that visit, the risks and benefits of laboratory testing are discussed with the patient and the couple then decides whether or not to proceed with formal testing. Subsequent to testing, patients are counseled regarding the results, whether positive or negative. This approach has added value in clinical disciplines like infertility in which the complete spectrum of genetic conditions that cause the problem is incompletely understood. In other words, it is important to counsel patients that although formal testing may reveal no definable genetic abnormality, they may still be at risk for other,

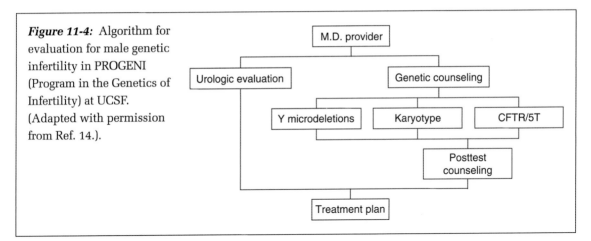

Figure 11-4: Algorithm for evaluation for male genetic infertility in PROGENI (Program in the Genetics of Infertility) at UCSF. (Adapted with permission from Ref. 14.).

currently undefined types of genetic infertility. In addition, formal genetic counseling can also procure information about family history or pedigree that can lead to further diagnoses or testing that may have clinical relevance in the setting of IVF and ICSI.

A remarkably large proportion of male infertility is currently unexplained. It is likely that advances in molecular genetics and discovery will reveal that the vast majority of unexplained male infertility is genetic in origin. What we currently understand about genetic infertility is likely only the tip of the iceberg. Genetic risk is currently defined for many cases of poor sperm production. In 6–8% of men with low sperm counts and 15% of men with no sperm counts, there may be mutations in a small region of the Y chromosome that explain the infertility. These mutations, termed Y chromosome microdeletions, can be passed to offspring with ICSI. Similarly, 2% of men with low sperm counts and 15% of men with no sperm counts can have an abnormality in the structure or number of any one of 23 pairs of chromosomes (karyotype) that can both lead to infertility and be passed to offspring with a risk for developmental problems. Therefore, karyotype and microdeletion of the Y chromosome testing is recommended in men with low (<10 million/mL) or no sperm counts and small testes.

Another group of men with low or no sperm counts may be missing the vas deferens on physical examination, referred to earlier as CAVD. As discussed above, the genetic mutations found in CAVD patients are similar to those detected in patients with cystic fibrosis. Approximately 80% of men with CAVD will harbor a cystic fibrosis gene mutation or gene variant. A blood test that examines cystic fibrosis genetic mutations and gene variants is indicated for CAVD patients.

Discussion of Cases

CASE 1

A 29-year-old man and his 28-year-old partner present with 1 year of infertility. Her evaluation revealed a prior terminated pregnancy at age 25, regular ovulatory cycles, no history of endometriosis, and a normal hysterosalpingogram. His evaluation has demonstrated no prior paternity, triweekly use of Jacuzzis after working out in the gym, and a physical examination showing a large left varicocele and a smaller left than right testis. His semen analyses show normal volumes, and low sperm concentrations and motilities of 16×10^6 sperm/mL and 35%, respectively. Serum FSH and testosterone levels are normal.

What other tests, if any, would you recommend at this point?

Consider a strict morphology in addition to a semen analysis, as varicoceles and Jacuzzis can both heat the testis and produce a characteristic (but not pathognomic) "stress" pattern. Obviously, also consider referral to a urologist for a complete evaluation of the varicocele.

What is your initial management?

Assuming the varicocele and the Jacuzzis are the only male-factor problems uncovered, one could consider discontinuing the Jacuzzi exposure, encouraging timed intercourse, and repeating a semen analysis in 3 months. If semen quality shows no improvement, then varicocele repair should be considered. IUI and IVF-ICSI are always possible, depending on the couple's resources and timeline, but may actually not be needed here especially given the female partner's young age.

CASE 2

A 45-year-old man and his 39-year-old partner would like to conceive. He had a vasectomy 10 years prior after conceiving three children unremarkably in another marriage. Her evaluation has revealed no prior pregnancies, regular ovulatory cycles, no history of endometriosis, a normal hysterosalpingogram, and an elevated day 3 cycle FSH.

What are the reproductive options for this couple?

Proceed with vasectomy reversal and attempt to conceive naturally or attempt sperm aspiration from the epididymis or testis (MESA or TESA) with IVF and ICSI. Donor sperm insemination and adoption are other alternatives.

What issues should be discussed with the couple to help them decide on a treatment plan? How many children do we want?

Sperm aspiration may be a better fit for the couple who wants only one child, as the man gets to keep his vasectomy after the procedure.

Are we comfortable with dealing with birth control issues again?

Birth control may be required again after a vasectomy reversal is performed. This is an argument in favor of sperm aspiration and IVF-ICSI.

Are we comfortable with assisted reproductive technology?

It is important that the couple think about (and agree upon) how they feel about children conceived with the help of technology. Other issues include: How does the couple feel about multiple gestations? Freezing embryos? Many unusual ethical and moral decisions are handled in cases of sperm aspiration and IVF and patient comfort with these decisions is important.

Do we have 1 year of reproductive potential?

This is likely to be the question with the highest impact on their decision. Remember that the average time to pregnancy after vasectomy reversal is 12 months. If female reproductive time is very limited, a reversal may not be in their best interest. On the contrary, a vasectomy reversal in this setting may allow the couple to conceive as often as possible at home, despite the lower monthly fecundity rate associated with her age.

REFERENCES

1 Honig SC, Lipshultz LI, Jarow JP. Significant medical pathology uncovered by a comprehensive male infertility evaluation. *Fertil Steril* 62:1028, 1994.

2 Cayan S, Erdemir F, Ozbey I, et al. Can varicocelectomy significantly change the way couples use assisted reproductive technologies? *J Urol* 167:1749, 2002.

3 Belker AM, Thomas AJ Jr, Fuchs EF, et al. Results of 1,469 microsurgical vasectomy reversals by the Vasovasostomy Study Group. *J Urol* 145:505, 1991.

4 Masters V, Turek PJ. Ejaculatory physiology and dysfunction. *Urol Clin North Am* 28:363, 2001.

5 Turek PJ. Immunopathology and infertility. In: Lipshultz LI, Howards SS (eds.), *Infertility in the Male*, 3rd ed. Philadelphia, PA: Mosby Year Book, p. 305, 1997.

6 Madgar I, Korasik A, Weissenberg R, et al. Controlled trial of high spermatic vein ligation for varicocele in infertile men. *Fertil Steril* 63:120, 1995.

7 Schlegel PN. Is assisted reproduction the optimal treatment for varicocele-associated male infertility? A cost-effectiveness analysis. *Urology* 49:83, 1997.

8 Cayan S, Lee D, Black LD, et al. Response to varicocelectomy in oligospermic men with and without defined genetic infertility. *Urology* 57:530, 2001.

9 Turek PJ, Magana JO, Lipshultz LI. Semen parameters before and after transurethral surgery for ejaculatory duct obstruction. *J Urol* 155:1291, 1996.

10 Fuchs EF, Burt RA. Vasectomy reversal performed 15 years or more after vasectomy: correlation of pregnancy outcome with partner age and with pregnancy results of in vitro fertilization with intracytoplasmic sperm injection. *Fertil Steril* 77:516, 2002.

11 Meng MV, Turek PJ. Vasectomy reversal or intracytoplasmic sperm injection: a decision analysis of cost-effectiveness. *Fertil Steril* 74:P405A, 2000.

12 Turek PJ, Nudell DM, Conaghan J. Methods of epididymal sperm retrieval: a urologic perspective. *Assist Reprod Rev* 9:60, 1999.

13 Turek PJ, Givens C, Schriock ED, et al. Testis sperm extraction and intracytoplasmic sperm injection guided by prior fine needle aspiration mapping in nonobstructive azoospermia. *Fertil Steril* 71:552, 1999.

14 Turek PJ, Reijo Pera RA. Current and future genetic screening for male infertility. *Urol Clin North Am* 29:767, 2002.

Unexplained Infertility

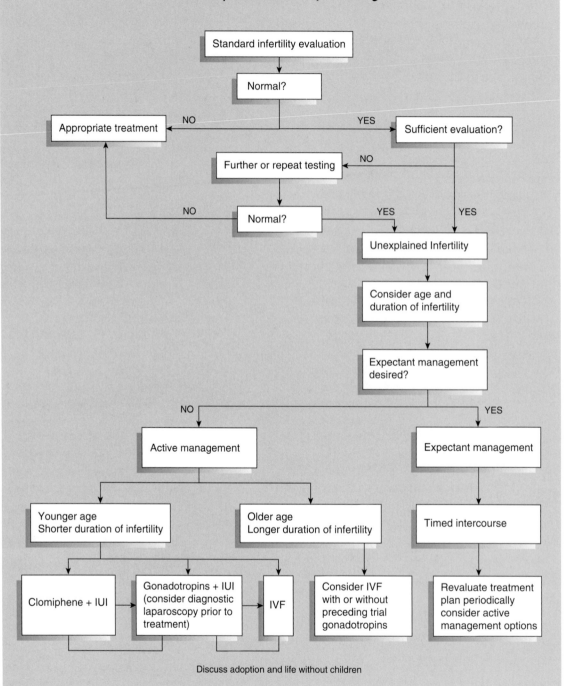

Standard infertility evaluation

↓

Normal?

NO → Appropriate treatment

YES → Sufficient evaluation?

NO → Further or repeat testing

YES → Unexplained Infertility

Further or repeat testing → Normal?

Normal? — NO → Appropriate treatment

Normal? — YES → Unexplained Infertility

Unexplained Infertility

↓

Consider age and duration of infertility

↓

Expectant management desired?

NO → Active management

YES → Expectant management

Active management:
- Younger age / Shorter duration of infertility
- Older age / Longer duration of infertility

Expectant management:
- Timed intercourse

Younger age / Shorter duration of infertility:
- Clomiphene + IUI
- Gonadotropins + IUI (consider diagnostic laparoscopy prior to treatment)
- IVF

Older age / Longer duration of infertility:
- Consider IVF with or without preceding trial gonadotropins

Timed intercourse:
- Revaluate treatment plan periodically consider active management options

Discuss adoption and life without children

12

Unexplained Infertility

David Guzick

Introduction

Unexplained infertility is a common and challenging diagnosis for both patients and physicians. In approximately 15% of infertile patients, a standard infertility evaluation will fail to identify a likely etiology. Once assigned a diagnosis of unexplained infertility, patients may be overwhelmed by a sense of futility—they might think that if there is no identifiable cause for the infertility it follows that there can be no effective treatment. In reality, the majority of these patients will be able to conceive, either spontaneously or with treatment.

Guiding Questions

APPROACHING A COUPLE WITH UNEXPLAINED INFERTILITY

- Has the patient had a satisfactory infertility evaluation warranting the diagnosis of unexplained infertility?
- Would any other tests be useful?
- Should any tests be repeated?
- Given the likelihood of spontaneous conception, does the patient desire an expectant or proactive approach at this time
- If the former, when is a more active approach warranted?
- What treatment options are available?
- What is the initial treatment of choice?
- What is the cost-effectiveness of treatments for unexplained infertility?
- How does cost impact a couple's treatment plan?

Diagnosis

The diagnostic workup of infertility has been discussed previously (see Chaps. 1–4) and has also been delineated by the American Society for Reproductive Medicine.[1] Evaluation should be thorough but focused. Prior to labeling infertility as unexplained, the presence of male, uterine, tubal, or ovulatory factors should be excluded. The evaluation is tailored to the specific patient but typically will include semen analysis, documentation of ovulation, examination of the uterus, and assessment of tubal patency. Laparoscopy can be considered in women with symptoms or history suggestive of adhesions or endometriosis.

When seeing a patient in consultation, prior diagnostic tests should be examined critically. In some situations, such tests may need to be repeated. This may be true if significant time has passed, if there are discrepancies between tests, or if the results are unclear. However, the impulse to repeat multiple tests should be tempered by good judgment. The risk of a type I error—a false positive result—increases as tests are repeated or added. A false positive result may expose the patient to potentially harmful and ultimately useless interventions.

Moreover, interpretation of diagnostic infertility test results must be balanced with the knowledge that the ability of many components of the standard infertility tests to discriminate between infertile and fertile patients is not consistently evident. In a small case-control study comparing fertile patients undergoing tubal ligation with infertile patients, two-thirds of fertile patients were found to have an abnormality of at least one infertility test.[2] In a recent study of a large sample of infertile women, the prevalence of out-of-phase endometrial biopsies among the infertile women was no different than that in a matched group of fertile women.[3]

Additional tests beyond the standard evaluation have *not*, in general, proven to be useful. Tests that are poor or inconsistent predictors of subsequent pregnancy include the postcoital test, screening for chlamydia/mycoplasma/ureaplasma, varicocele identification, immunologic testing, tests of sperm function, identification of antisperm antibodies, and assessment of antiphospholipid antibodies.

KEY POINT

Prior to a diagnosis of "unexplained infertility," a basic infertility evaluation should confirm ovulation, tubal patency, a normal uterine cavity, and a normal semen analysis.

Expectant Management

When counseling couples with unexplained infertility, it is important to inform them of the likelihood that they have a reasonable chance of conception without treatment. As an estimate of this baseline (treatment-independent) pregnancy rate, couples with unexplained infertility assigned to the control (no treatment) group of randomized clinical trials have been found to have a pregnancy rate of about 3–4% per month.[4,5] While infertile couples who present for consultation for infertility generally wish to proceed directly with treatment, the knowledge that the diagnosis of unexplained infertility is not a sentence of sterility can be reassuring. Indeed, some younger patients may decide not to pursue more invasive treatments for a period of time after appropriate counseling.

Patients should also be aware that the likelihood of spontaneous conception is influenced by the woman's age, duration of infertility, and prior pregnancy history. It has been demonstrated in many different populations over many years that fertility is inversely related to age (Fig. 12-1).[6] Moreover, as seen in Fig. 12-1, the decline in natural fertility with age becomes accelerated when a woman reaches her late thirties.

As applied to unexplained infertility, it is not surprising, therefore, that treatment yields a higher cumulative pregnancy rate among younger women than older women (Fig. 12-2).[7] The likelihood of pregnancy also decreases with increasing duration of infertility (Fig. 12-3).[7] This may be due to a combination of increasing age and dropout of those with subfertility across time. Prior pregnancy history is also important. Couples with secondary infertility have a higher rate of spontaneous pregnancy than those with primary infertility.

Treatment

Over the years, many empiric treatments of unexplained infertility have been attempted, including bromocriptine, thyroid hormone, danazol, and antibiotics. None of these treatments has been shown to be effective.

Beginning in the mid-1980s and continuing to the present, there has been a marked increase in the use of superovulation,

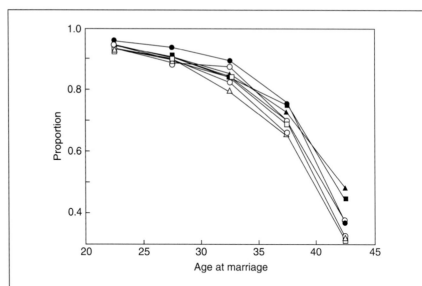

Figure 12-1: Proportions having at least one child by 5-year age group at marriage and estimated typical pattern.[5] The populations (in descending order at age 35–39) are Germany, 14 village genealogies, marriages 1750–1899 (●); England, family reconstitution of 16 rural parishes (midsixteenth to early nineteenth centuries) by the Cambridge Group for the History of Population and Social Structure (■); Ireland, 1911 census (▲); typical pattern (▬); England, family reconstitution for Quakers (O); Quebec, rural women born before 1876 (□); Scotland, 1911 census (○); and Quebec, 1946 census, rural women born 1876–1885 (Δ).

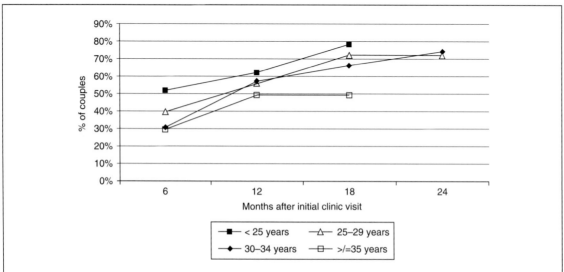

Figure 12-2: Cumulative rates of conception related to age of women. (Adapted with permission from Ref. 7.)

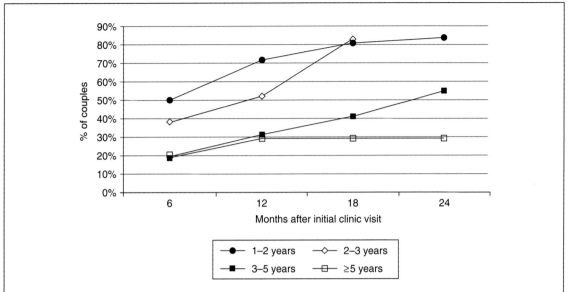

Figure 12-3: Cumulative rates of conception related to duration of infertility. (Adapted with permission from Ref. 7.)

with or without intrauterine insemination (IUI), in the treatment of unexplained infertility. Both clomiphene citrate (CC) and gonadotropins have been used for superovulation.

Clinicians involved with infertility patients often provide anecdotal examples from their own practices of women with unexplained infertility who conceive "on their own" between cycles of ovarian stimulation and/or IUI, while on a waiting list for assisted reproduction, or after all treatment has failed. Of course, many conceptions also occur while on "treatment." This raises the central issue of coincidence versus consequence. In any individual case, it is impossible to establish causality. The important question is whether superovulation/IUI treatment, in general, provides an increase in the expectancy of pregnancy above the baseline rate.

What might be the rationale for administering costly and potentially dangerous medication to stimulate ovulation in women who already have regular menstrual periods and normal ovulatory function? And why introduce washed sperm into the uterine cavity in situations where the semen analysis is normal and there is no cervical factor present?

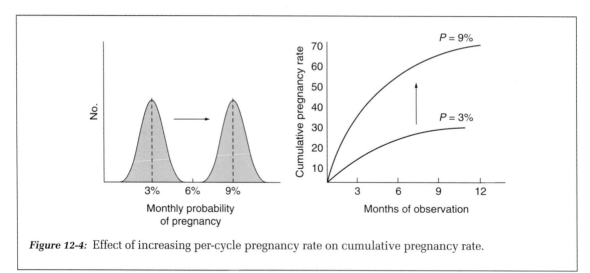

Figure 12-4: Effect of increasing per-cycle pregnancy rate on cumulative pregnancy rate.

With respect to ovarian stimulation, there has been some argument to the affect that such treatment can overcome a subtle defect in ovulatory function not uncovered by conventional testing. There are few data, however, to support this view. Rather, it appears likely that superovulation enhances the likelihood of pregnancy by simply increasing the number of eggs available for fertilization. Thus, if the pregnancy rate in unexplained infertility is 3% per month with ovulation of a single oocyte, as has been suggested from control group results in randomized trials, then perhaps this rate could be increased several-fold with ovarian stimulation and the ovulation of several oocytes.

Along similar lines, increasing the density of motile sperm available to these eggs through the use of IUI might further increase the monthly probability of pregnancy. To the extent that superovulation and/or IUI results in an increase in the monthly pregnancy rate, this has a cumulative impact across treatment cycles, as shown in Fig. 12-4.

What's the Evidence?

A sizable literature has evolved on the treatment of unexplained infertility with superovulation (using clomiphene citrate or gonadotropins) and/or intrauterine insemination.

A literature review on unexplained infertility through 1996 found pregnancy rates associated with CC of 5.6% without IUI and

8.3% with IUI.[5] A 2002 systematic review analyzed the use of clomiphene as identified in six randomized-controlled trials.[8] The odds ratios (confidence intervals) for pregnancy in relation to CC treatment were 2.37 (1.22–4.62) per patient and 2.5 (1.35–4.62) per treatment cycle.

CC is attractive because of its ease of use and relative low cost. Thus, it may be considered a first-line agent for many patients, especially younger women. However, patients should be informed of possible complications with its use, including multiple pregnancies (8–10%), development of ovarian cysts, and occasional side effects such as hot flashes, headache, rash, and mood change.

If CC is unsuccessful, the next step is often injectable gonadotropins. A recent systematic review examined trials that compared the efficacy of CC and gonadotropins.[9] Five randomized-controlled trials with a total of 231 couples were identified as appropriate for inclusion. After analysis, the authors stated that there was insufficient evidence to conclude that oral agents were either inferior or superior to injectables. An earlier retrospective analysis[5] (Table 12-1) calculated the pregnancy rate per cycle with clomiphene citrate to be 5.6% and the rate with human menopausal gonadotropins (hMG) to be 7.7%. This was not a direct comparison and had the bias that many couples that are treated with hMG

Table 12-1. AGGREGATE DATA FOR VARIOUS TREATMENTS OF UNEXPLAINED INFERTILITY

TREATMENT	STUDIES (#)	PREGNANCIES PER INITIATED CYCLE (%)	QUALITY-ADJUSTED PREGNANCIES PER INITIATED CYCLE (%)
Control groups	11	64/3539 (1.8)	1.3
Control groups, randomized studies	6	23/597 (3.8)	4.1
IUI	9	15/378 (4)	3.8
CC	3	37/617 (6)	5.6
CC + IUI	5	21/315 (6.7)	8.3
HMG	13	139/1806 (7.7)	7.7
HMG + IUI	14	139/1806 (18)	17.1
IVF	9	378/683 (22.5)	20.7
GIFT	9	158/607 (26.0)	27.0

SOURCE: With permission from Ref. 5.

have already had unsuccessful attempts with clomiphene citrate. When intrauterine insemination was added to hMG, the pregnancy rate of 17.1% did appear to represent a marked improvement over CC alone, CC with IUI, and hMG alone.

The National Cooperative Reproductive Medicine Network conducted the only large-scale, controlled, randomized trial of the effectiveness of gonadotropins with or without insemination.[4] Nine hundred and thirty-two couples were randomized to undergo following treatments for up to four cycles: IUI, superovulation with follicle-stimulating hormone (FSH), FSH plus IUI, or control (timed intracervical insemination). The mean female age was 32 and the mean duration of infertility was 44 months. Results are shown in Table 12-2. Couples treated with FSH plus IUI were 1.7 times as likely to become pregnant as IUI alone (95% confidence interval 1.2–2.6) and 3.2 times as likely as controls (95% confidence interval 2.0–5.3). Those who underwent IUI alone were 1.9 times (95% confidence interval 1.1–3.2) as likely to conceive as control couples, and those receiving FSH alone were 1.8 times (95% confidence interval 1.0–3.0) as likely to conceive as controls. This suggests that superovulation and IUI have a separate and additive effect on conception. It should be noted that the couples in this study included men with any motile sperm on semen analysis and women with a prior diagnosis by laparoscopy of mild endometriosis. This study is highly relevant to couples with unexplained infertility, but due to its heterogeneity with respect to male factor infertility, the quantitative estimates of success rates may not be directly applicable to pure unexplained infertility.

It is evident that the use of gonadotropins with IUI does improve outcomes. However, costs of injectable agents are considerable, as are the potential adverse effects, including multiple gestations and ovarian hyperstimulation syndrome (see Chap. 9).

Patients with unexplained infertility may consider *in vitro* fertilization (IVF) if several cycles of superovulation are not successful. Composite data from studies in the 1980s and 1990s suggested a pregnancy rate of 20.7%[5] (Table 12-1). However, in light of the significant improvement in pregnancy and live birth rates after IVF over the last 10 years, IVF may be recommended earlier in the management algorithm, especially for older women.

KEY POINT

Superovulation with clomiphene citrate or gonadotropins plus IUI improves pregnancy outcome over continued timed intercourse, IUI alone, and/or superovulation alone.

Table 12-2. PREGNANCY RATES WITH ARTIFICIAL INSEMINATION AND SUPEROVULATION

TREATMENT	COUPLES (#)	INSEMINATION CYCLES (#)	PREGNANCIES (#)	PREGNANCY RATE PER COUPLE (%)	PREGNANCY RATE PER CANCELLED OR REST CYCLE (%)	PREGNANCY RATE PER INSEMINATION CYCLE (%)
Intracervical insemination	233	706	23	10	3.1	2.0
Intrauterine insemination	234	717	42	18	2.4	4.9
Superovulation and intracervical insemination	234	637	44	19	2.4	4.1
Superovulation and intrauterine insemination	231	618	77	33	3.4	8.7

SOURCE: With permission from Ref. 4.

313

In the most recent report from the CDC (2001 data), the national pregnancy rate per IVF egg retrieval was 32.8%.[10]

Genetic testing in couples with repeated implantation failure after IVF is gaining interest. Repeated implantation failure may be viewed as part of a continuum with recurrent miscarriage after IVF. A number of chromosomal abnormalities were present in a select group of patients with multiple implantation failures (6 or more IVF trials involving 15 or more total embryos).[11] Of 65 women who were karyotyped, 15% were found to have abnormalities, including 6 translocations. Certainly, this is a highly selected population and a small sample. Pregnancy outcomes over the year following karyotyping were not different among those with normal karyotypes and the 16 women with abnormal karyotypes. Depending on the exact chromosomal abnormality, recommendation of donor eggs or preimplantation genetic diagnosis may be appropriate in some cases. More data will be needed to determine if karyotyping should become a routine part of the infertility workup.

Finally, it is important to discuss other options with couples such as adoption or living without children. Some couples may need this permission to consider alternatives and find relief that they can stop treatments for their infertility.

Cost-Effectiveness of Treatment Options

The cost-effectiveness of various treatments for unexplained infertility has not been extensively studied. The Practice Committee of the American Society for Reproductive Medicine calculated the number of additional pregnancies achieved with various treatments compared to untreated controls based on a literature review of available studies.[12] For IUI one additional pregnancy in 37 cycles would be achieved compared with untreated controls. With clomiphene there would be one additional pregnancy in 40–76 cycles and with clomiphene in conjunction with IUI, one additional pregnancy in 16 cycles. Gonadotropins with IUI would lead to an increase of one additional pregnancy in 15 cycles. Randomized-controlled data were not available to calculate the benefit of IVF compared to controls. As these treatments are not without significant costs, they may impact both the order of treatments and the number of cycles undertaken with a particular treatment.

Table 12-3. ESTIMATED INCREMENTAL IMPROVEMENTS IN PREGNANCY RATES ABOVE BASELINE AND COST PER PREGNANCY[a]

TREATMENT	1.3% INCREMENT IN PREGNANCY RATE OVER BASELINE	4.1% INCREMENT IN PREGNANCY RATE OVER BASELINE	COST PER INCREMENTAL PREGNANCY (1.3%)	COST PER INCREMENTAL PREGNANCY (4.1%)
CC + IUI	7.0	4.2	$7143	$11,905
HMG + IUI	15.8	13.0	$15,823	$19,230
IVF	19.4	16.6	$46,391	$54,217

[a]Cost data based on the following average 1998 costs: CC + IUI ($500), hMG + IUI ($2500), IVF ($9000).
SOURCE: With permission from Ref. 5.

Obviously, expectant management is without monetary cost and may be worthwhile in situations where the duration of infertility is less than 2 years and in women below the age of 35. The results of a 1998 analysis of cost per incremental pregnancy are shown in Table 12-3.[5] Cost for each pregnancy achieved above the baseline rate was estimated to be $10,000 for clomiphene plus IUI, $17,000 for gonadotropins plus IUI, and $50,000 for IVF. As pregnancy rates from IVF increase, assuming a less-than-proportional increase in costs, the cost per pregnancy from IVF should decline. Moreover, to the extent that improved technology allows for fewer embryos per transfer, the multiple pregnancy rate from IVF should be less than that from treatment with gonadotropins plus IUI.

Clearly, there are substantial costs involved in achieving a pregnancy after the diagnosis of unexplained infertility. Recognizing the occurrence of spontaneous abortion and multiple pregnancies, the costs of achieving the live birth of a healthy baby are even more considerable.

Conclusions

Unexplained infertility is a common and potentially frustrating diagnosis. Expectant management should be encouraged for younger patients and those with a short duration of infertility. Other treatments may be offered with consideration given to the balance between success and risk as well as the cost. In general, simple and cost-effective treatments such as clomiphene and IUI are recommended before more invasive and expensive procedures such as

IVF. If initial treatments do not result in pregnancy, a dialogue about adoption and living without children should be opened with the couple. Hopefully, as our understanding of ovulation, conception, and implantation improve we will be able to reduce the number of couples labeled as having unexplained infertility and develop effective treatments for identified etiologies.

Discussion of Cases

CASE 1

A 28-year-old G0P0 presents to the office with her husband to discuss their inability to conceive after 14 months of unprotected intercourse. She and her husband are anxious about this delay and feel they may never be able to have children. Both are healthy and neither has had any previous children.

What is the initial workup of this couple's infertility?

- Semen analysis
- Documentation of ovulation
- Documentation of tubal patency
- Examination of the uterine cavity

The patient has regular menstrual cycles every 28–30 days. (This strongly suggests ovulation unless proven otherwise. If there is any question about the cyclicity of menstruation, ovulation can be confirmed with a midluteal phase progesterone determination.) A hysterosalpingogram demonstrates a normal uterine cavity and with free spill of contrast from both fallopian tubes. The husband's semen analysis is within reference values.

Are any further tests necessary?

Traditionally, diagnostic laparoscopy would complete the workup of this patient to rule out endometriosis or adhesions as a cause of infertility. This patient gives no history of pelvic pain or prior surgeries so the presence of severe endometriosis or adhesions is unlikely. A prospective cohort study compared the pregnancy rates after expectant management in women with minimal or mild endometriosis and women with unexplained infertility.[13] These rates were not significantly different. Even if minimal or mild endometriosis were found at laparoscopy, it is controversial as to whether surgical ablation enhances subsequent fertility. Thus, this couple with unexplained infertility is unlikely to benefit from immediate laparoscopy.

What is the appropriate treatment to begin?

Expectant management is reasonable in this couple, given the age of the woman and the relatively short duration of infertility. Although the couple's fecundity may be reduced compared to the general population, they are likely to achieve a spontaneous pregnancy given further time. Recommendation of timed intercourse for 6 or more months is safe, inexpensive, and often successful.

In general, in a woman younger than 35 years old the first treatment of choice is superovulation with clomiphene citrate plus intrauterine insemination. For the treatment of unexplained infertility the dose of CC should be such that two or more mature follicles are seen by ultrasound prior to ovulation. The cost per pregnancy of CC is much less than other ovulation induction agents and the risks and side effects are fewer. The increased occurrence of multiple gestations (8–10%) should be discussed with the couple at this point. It is recommended that treatment with CC should continue for up to four to six cycles before proceeding to other treatments.

The couple returns after six cycles of clomiphene plus IUI are unsuccessful. Preovulatory ultrasounds documented two or more follicles and semen analyses were normal. The couple is anxious to explore other treatment options. What recommendations are appropriate at this point?

There are several acceptable treatment strategies at this point (see algorithm). The patient may consider superovulation with gonadotropins combined with IUI, or they may proceed directly to IVF. Diagnostic laparoscopy to rule out anatomic causes of infertility might be considered again if the patient desires gonadotropins, especially if there are symptoms of significant dysmenorrhea. If the patient elects to proceed to IVF, laparoscopy would be unnecessary.

The patient decides to undergo laparoscopy while considering other options. Tubal patency is again documented and there is no evidence of endometriosis or adhesions. What treatment should be offered at this point?

Several cycles of injectable gonadotropins in conjunction with IUI would often be the next treatment option. The risks and benefits of this intervention should be discussed with the couple. The high rate of multiple gestations along with the cost and inconvenience of injectable medications should be clearly stated.

The couple has several friends who have had twins after gonadotropins and ask if there is less risk of multiple gestations with IVF. How does the rate of multiple gestations compare?

Multiple gestations are a concern after both ovulation induction and IVF but are more common with ovulation induction. Additionally, high-order gestations are much more common with ovulation induction. The risk of preterm labor and delivery are increased with multiple gestations, contributing to increased morbidity and mortality for the infants. Maternal complications are also more frequent, including the development of gestational diabetes and preeclampsia.

It is reasonable to discuss IVF as an option at this point, allowing the couple to weigh their options. In 2000, 35% of IVF cycles resulted in multiple-infant births; 30.7% resulted in twins, while 4.3% resulted in triplets or greater.[10] Risk of multiple gestations can be reduced in this young woman by limiting the number of embryos transferred if IVF is chosen.

The couple decides to undergo IVF and two good quality embryos are transferred. The patient becomes pregnant after the first cycle and carries a singleton gestation to term.

CASE 2

A 39-year-old G3P2012 presents with her 39-year-old husband to discuss their inability to conceive after 14 months of unprotected intercourse while using luteinizing hormone (LH) kits to time intercourse. She and her husband are anxious and feel they may never be able to have children together. Both are healthy and have children from prior marriages. The woman had no difficulty conceiving her children when she was 25 and 29 with one intervening spontaneous abortion at 7 weeks. She has had no prior surgeries and no symptoms consistent with endometriosis. She has regular menstrual cycles every 30–32 days.

What is the workup of this couple's infertility?

- **Semen analysis**
- **Documentation of ovulation**
- **Documentation of tubal patency**
- **Examination of the uterine cavity**

Semen analysis is within normal limits. As the patient has regular menstrual cycles, ovulation is presumed. A hysterosalpingogram demonstrates patent fallopian tubes and a normal uterine cavity. Transvaginal ultrasound is unremarkable.

Are any further tests warranted in this patient?

In the older patient, a day 3 FSH level should be drawn as part of the initial workup to document the presence of ovarian reserve. An elevated FSH would explain, at least in part, the couple's reduced fecundity. In our practice, an FSH value above 10 mIU/mL would trigger a clomiphene challenge test of ovarian reserve, and a value above 13 mIU/mL would

trigger a discussion of donor oocytes. However, FSH assays vary, and each center must titrate cutoffs for such recommendations against its own assay.

The patient's FSH level is eight (within normal limits) and the couple is presumed to have unexplained diagnosis. The patient returns to the office to consider her options. What treatments can be offered?

In this 39-year-old patient, it is reasonable to forego the use of clomiphene for ovulation induction and instead consider gonadotropins with intrauterine insemination, or progressing directly to IVF.

What are risks of injectable gonadotropins and IVF for this patient?

A major concern is the risk of multiple gestations with either of these modalities. In the older patient, who is more likely to have reduced fecundity based on age, this may be less of a concern. Nonetheless, with IVF there is more control via the number of embryos replaced.

What are the costs of these treatments?

Costs vary significantly depending on region and the presence or absence of mandated infertility coverage. Also, costs are greater for both treatments if more gonadotropins are needed for ovarian stimulation due to age. A rough estimate of costs would be $3000 for a cycle of gonadotropins plus IUI and about $10,000 for a cycle of IVF. Additional costs also may be incurred with multiple gestations not just due to the delivery of multiple infants but also because of the increase in preterm delivery and resulting costs of caring for premature infants.

The couple opts to attempt IVF. The patient is unsuccessful in the first cycle after transfer of three embryos but has a live birth of twins after the second IVF cycle with transfer of four embryos.

REFERENCES

1 Optimal evaluation of the infertile female: a practice committee report. *Am Soc Reprod Med* 2000.

2 Guzick DS, Grefenstett I, Baffone K, et al. Infertility evaluation in fertile women: a model for assessing the efficacy of infertility testing. *Hum Reprod* 9(12):2306–2310, 1994.

3 The Reproductive Medicine Network. The endometrial biopsy as a diagnostic tool in the evaluation of the infertile patient. Abstract presented at the ASRM Annual Meeting. *Fertil Steril* 76(3S):S2, 2002.

4 Guzick D, Caron S, Coutifaris C, et al. Efficacy of superovulation and intrauterine insemination in the treatment of infertility. *N Engl J Med* 340(3):177–183, 1999.

5 Guzick D, Sullivan M, Adamson D, et al. Efficacy of treatment of unexplained infertility. *Fertil Steril* 70(2):207–213, 1998.

6 Menken J, Trussell J, Larson U. Age and infertility. *Science* 233:1389–1394, 1986.

7 Hull R, Glazener C, Kelly N, et al. Population study of causes, treatment and outcome of infertility. *Br Med J* 291:1693–1697, 1985.

8 Hughes E, Collins J, Vanderkerckhove P. Clomiphene citrate for unexplained subfertility in women. Cochrane Database Syst Rev 4, 2002.

9 Athaullah N, Proctor M, Johnson N. Oral versus injectable ovulation induction agents for unexplained subfertility. *Cochrane Database Syst Rev* (3):CD003052, 2002.

10 CDC website: cdc.gov/nccdphp/drh

11 Raziel A, Friedler S, Schachter M, et al. Increased frequency of female partner chromosomal abnormalities in patients with high-order implantation failure after in vitro fertilization. *Fertil Steril* 78(3):515–519, 2002.

12 Effectiveness and treatment for unexplained infertility: a practice committee report. *Am Soc Reprod Med* 2000.

13 Berube S, Marcoux S, Langevin M, et al. Fecundity of infertile women with minimal or mild endometriosis and women with unexplained infertility. *Fertil Steril* 69(6):1034–1041, 1998.

13

In Vitro Fertilization

Heather Hoddleston
Mark D. Hornstein

Introduction

The birth of Louise Brown, the first child born as a result of an *in vitro* fertilization (IVF) cycle, galvanized the world in 1978.[1] In the past two decades, the technology and pregnancy rates with IVF have improved dramatically. As a result, thousands of pregnancies have been achieved through this technology. Registry data for the United States in 2000 indicated that a total 99,639 cycles were performed that year and that these cycles resulted in 35,025 live born babies.[2]

Indications and Selection of Patients

KEY POINT

IVF is currently used in couples with all causes of infertility who fail simpler modalities.

IVF is generally indicated for cases of severe infertility, including tubal factor, endometriosis, and male factor infertility.[3] Increasingly, however, IVF is being recommended for all refractory infertility conditions, including unexplained infertility that has not responded to other therapies. A typical infertility workup includes history, physical examination, documentation of ovulation, day 3 level of follicle-stimulating hormone (FSH), hysterosalpingogram (HSG), and semen analysis. Those diagnosed with oligomenorrhea, amenorrhea, mild male factor infertility, mild endometriosis, cervical factor, or unexplained infertility may be candidates for several cycles of ovulation induction with intrauterine inseminations (IUI). Women with a diagnosis of severe endometriosis may be candidates for surgical resection of endometriosis while those with a diagnosis of tubal occlusion may first be candidates for a tuboplasty. Those couples that fail to conceive following such therapies will generally be offered IVF.

IVF is most successful for couples in which the female partner has an adequate ovarian follicular pool, often referred to as ovarian reserve. Ovarian reserve is closely tied to age, with the ovarian follicular pool declining rapidly as a woman approaches 40 years of age.

Another predictor of ovarian reserve is the measurement of FSH level on cycle day 3.[4] Elevated day 3 FSH levels can be an indicator of diminished ovarian reserve that is detectable before a woman has experienced any changes in menstrual pattern. Additional information on ovarian reserve can be obtained through the use of a clomiphene citrate challenge test (CCCT). A CCCT involves the measurement of serum FSH on cycle day 3 and then on day 10, following administration of 100 mg of clomiphene on cycle days 5 through 9. Women with a normal day 3 FSH level and an abnormal day 10 level following a CCCT appear to have diminished ovarian reserve and lower pregnancy rates with IVF than patients with normal values at both time points (see Fig. 13-1).[5]

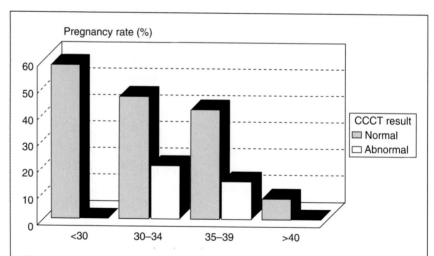

Figure 13-1: Clinical pregnancy rates as function of age and response to clomiphene citrate challenge test (CCCT) in a general infertility population. In women with abnormal CCCT results, pregnancy rates are low regardless of age. (Adapted with permission from Ref. 7.)

What's the Evidence?

- In a study of 431 women aged ≥41 undergoing IVF, women aged 41–43 had a 2–7% chance of delivery/oocyte retrieval. In this group, there were no clinical pregnancies among women older than 45 and no deliveries for women over 44.[6]
- In a retrospective study of 758 IVF cycles, Scott et al. found that pregnancy rates decreased markedly as FSH levels rose. Ongoing pregnancy rates were 25% for women with a day 3 FSH <15 mU/mL, while those who had an FSH value over 25 mU/mL had less than a 5% chance of achieving an ongoing pregnancy. The differences in pregnancy rates would not have been predicted by age alone.[7]

Guiding Questions

PATIENT UNDERGOING
IN VITRO
FERTILIZATION

- What success rate can be expected?
- How is the best superovulation strategy selected?
- Is the semen analysis adequate for standard insemination?
- How many embryos should be transferred?

Clinical Components of IVF

OVARIAN
STIMULATION

Several techniques are available for preparing the ovary for oocyte retrieval. For those women who ovulate regularly, the most conservative method is the monitoring of a natural cycle. This involves monitoring follicle size through ultrasound and serum hormone and gonadotropin levels through frequent blood tests. Monitoring of a natural cycle for IVF can lead to the aspiration of a lead follicle and retrieval of a single fertilizable oocyte. While the implantation rate per embryo is equivalent to that obtained through other stimulation methods, the small number of embryos produced results in an extremely low clinical pregnancy rate and a high rate of cancellation due to early ovulation. As a result, nearly all programs use techniques designed to stimulate the ovary and thus increase the number of oocytes retrieved. This technique may be referred to as superovulation or controlled ovarian stimulation (COS).

KEY POINT

IVF involves the superovulation of the ovaries to increase the number of embryos available for transfer.

Currently in the United States most IVF cycles involve the use of injectable gonadotropins to stimulate follicular growth in the ovary. A variety of gonadotropin preparations have been developed over the years. All are administered daily, either subcutaneously or intramuscularly. The use of injectable medications in this fashion requires that the patient and her partner undergo significant education and training in injection techniques before start of a cycle. Human menopausal gonadotropin (hMG), extracted from the urine of menopausal women, was the first gonadotropin product to be used. It was quickly found that doses of hMG capable of superovulating the ovary increased the number of oocytes retrieved and thus increased the number of embryos produced. Recently, a recombinant form of FSH (rFHS) has become available. A significant difference between the preparations is the complete lack of luteinizing hormone (LH) in the rFSH formulation. Recombinant FSH appears to be more efficacious than hMG: a metaanalysis of eight randomized studies comparing rFSH with hMG demonstrated a significantly higher pregnancy rate in the rFSH group.[8]

KEY POINT

The use of GnRH agonists (agonist and antagonist) prevent premature luteinization and ovulation.

Many centers combine the administration of gonadotropins and a gonadotrophin-releasing hormone (GnRH) agonist or antagonist. The addition of a GnRH agonist serves to increase cycle control by preventing premature LH surges and reducing the chance of premature luteinization of granulosa cells and premature ovulation. Importantly, prevention of an LH surge allows further maturation of the follicle, which has been shown to increase clinical success rates.[9] The clinical effect of the GnRH agonist can vary depending on the timing and dose of GnRH given, with GnRH given as part of a "long protocol" or "short protocol." In the long protocol, the GnRH agonist is started in the luteal phase of the cycle preceding the start of gonadotropins. The short protocol calls for the use of smaller doses of GnRH agonist in conjunction with gonadotropins at the start of the treatment cycle. This protocol may induce a "flare" effect, in which the agonist initially stimulates pituitary release of gonadotropins to augment the exogenous gonadotropins. This protocol is therefore used in women with decreased ovarian reserve. Another advance in ovarian stimulation regimens is the use of gonadotropin antagonists. GnRH antagonists cause a more rapid and complete pituitary suppression than do GnRH agonists. In addition, antagonists, unlike the agonists do not induce a flare effect. The antagonist is usually started after the patient has been administering gonadotropins for several days.

OOCYTE RETRIEVAL

For several reasons, women undergoing ovarian stimulation undergo frequent monitoring of serum levels of hormones and follicular development as defined by transvaginal ultrasound. The monitoring is useful in identifying patients who require changes in medication dosage. For example, a patient showing a limited response to her stimulation protocol, as manifested by a low estradiol level and/or minimal follicular development, might require an increase in the dose of her medication. In contrast, a patient whose estradiol level rises rapidly might need to have her medication dose reduced. Ultrasound and serum hormone monitoring is also critical for identifying the optimal time for oocyte retrieval. In general, oocytes can be retrieved with a high rate of success from follicles with a mean diameter of 16–18 mm. Once it has been determined that an adequate number of appropriately sized follicles has been produced, patients are instructed to administer human chorionic gonadotropin (hCG). Generally, 10,000 units of hCG is administered subcutaneously or intramuscularly. This dose of hCG mimics an LH surge and induces final maturation of the oocyte. To maximize oocyte maturation while minimizing the chance of spontaneous ovulation, oocyte retrieval is generally scheduled for 34–36 h after hCG administration.

KEY POINT

Ultrasound-guided transvaginal aspiration decreases the risk of oocyte retrieval.

Oocytes are retrieved through the aspiration of ovarian follicles. Oocyte retrieval was once carried out via the laparoscopic approach; however, today oocytes are typically retrieved through a transvaginal ultrasound-guided approach. Intravenous analgesia and/or light sedation generally provide sufficient comfort during the procedure. A 16 or 17 gauge long needle is placed in a sterile needle guide that is attached to the vaginal ultrasound transducer. The transducer is then placed in the vagina and manipulated until the ovary is in view. The needle is then introduced into the ovary with care to avoid the surrounding organs and vessels. One needle stick per ovary usually allows for sequential aspiration of all follicles. The transvaginal technique is appropriate for most patients. Rarely, however, the ovaries are not accessible through the transvaginal route. In these cases, transabdominal aspiration may be most appropriate.

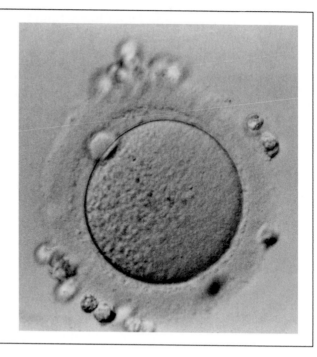

Figure 13-2: Mature oocyte. Note first polar body at 10 o'clock position. (Courtesy of Katharine Jackson, BS, Brigham and Women's Hospital ART Embryology Laboratory, Boston, MA.)

During the retrieval, oocytes are collected in sterile containers and are brought to the embryology laboratory for further assessment. Oocytes, surrounded by their cumulus masses, are identified under a microscope and isolated. Care is taken to limit their exposure to ambient temperature and light. Oocytes may be retrieved at different stages of maturation; those that have completed metaphase 1 have the highest rate of successful fertilization (see Fig. 13-2).

INCUBATION OF OOCYTES AND SPERM

Detailed information regarding the embryology laboratory is covered in Chap. 14. Briefly, sperm are generally added to the eggs for insemination about 4–6 h following oocyte retrieval. Semen is generally collected by masturbation. Techniques of sperm preparation may vary according to laboratory. In general, the semen is allowed to liquefy at room temperature for approximately 30 min. Sperm are then counted and washed on a gradient to allow removal of debris. The sperm are then centrifuged, washed, and recentrifuged.

Roughly 4 h after oocyte retrieval, approximately 150,000 sperm/oocyte are added to dishes containing the oocytes. The

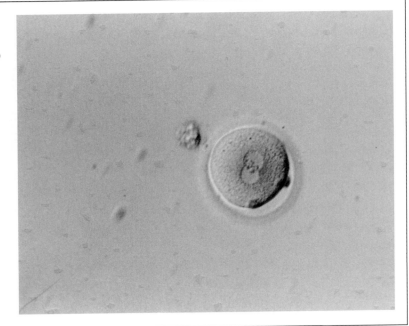

Figure 13-3: Zygote. Note two polar bodies in the perivitelline space and two pronuclei in the middle of the zygote. (Courtesy of Katharine Jackson, BS, Brigham and Women's Hospital ART Embryology Laboratory, Boston, MA.)

following day, the oocytes are examined for evidence of successful fertilization. The presence of two pronuclei and two polar bodies is evidence of fertilization and the creation of a zygote. Approximately 65–80% of mature oocytes will be fertilized (see Fig. 13-3).

INTRACYTOPLASMIC SPERM INJECTION

Male factor infertility may be due to a variety of semen abnormalities, including low sperm concentration (oligospermia), poor sperm motility (asthenospermia), and abnormal sperm morphology (teratospermia). While there are few treatment options for male factor infertility outside of IVF (See Chap. 11), severe abnormalities of the semen may be overcome with adjunctive assisted reproductive techniques. First reported in 1992, intracytoplasmic sperm injection (ICSI) is a micromanipulation technique that involves the placement of a single spermatozoan into the cytoplasm of the oocyte, thus bypassing the zona pellucida and perivitelline space.[10] ICSI is most beneficial for men who have severe oligospermia, obstructive azoospermia, or asthenospermia. Increasingly, ICSI has been combined with surgical harvesting of epididymal or testicular sperm in men who have no sperm in their ejaculate. ICSI does

Figure 13-4:
Intracytoplasmic sperm injection. (Courtesy of Katharine Jackson, BS, Brigham and Women's Hospital ART Embryology Laboratory, Boston, MA.)

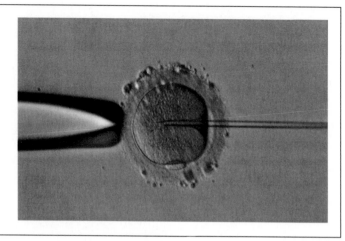

not appear to offer an advantage to couples in which the male's sperm parameters are normal (see Fig. 13-4).

EMBRYO TRANSFER

KEY POINT

By increasing the number of embryos transferred, the pregnancy rate is increased. However, so is the rate of twins and higher-order multiple gestation.

Following fertilization, the embryos are kept in culture for a variable amount of time. Although pregnancies have been shown to occur after transfer of embryos at any stage of development, most programs transfer embryos 3 days after oocyte retrieval, at which time the embryos are optimally at the eight-cell stage. An attempt is made to transfer embryos that have the best chance of achieving a pregnancy. Embryos are evaluated by microscopy and scored along morphologic criteria that may indicate the overall quality of the embryo and its chance for implantation. Criteria often used include cell number, degree of fragmentation, and symmetry of individual blastomeres. Fragmentation refers to small areas of blebbing of cytoplasm visualized in the embryo. Embryos that have reached the eight-cell stage by day 3, appear symmetrical, and have minimal fragmentation are thought to have a better chance of implantation than embryos without these characteristics (see Fig. 13-5). The chance of achieving a pregnancy can also be increased by increasing the number of embryos transferred; however, increasing the number of embryos transferred can also dramatically increase the risk of a multiple gestation. Factors taken into consideration when deciding how many embryos to transfer include age of the female partner and the overall quality of the embryos. In the United States, typically two, three, or four embryos are transferred.

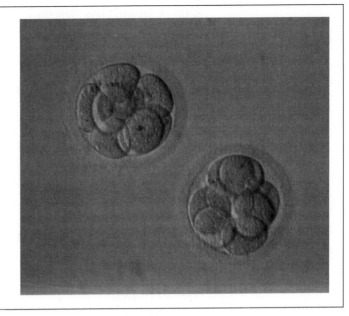

Figure 13-5: Two eight-cell embryos (day 3 after egg retrieval). Both embryos show minimal fragmentation and a high degree of symmetry. (Courtesy of Katharine Jackson, BS, Brigham and Women's Hospital ART Embryology Laboratory, Boston, MA.)

Recently, many IVF programs have begun transferring embryos 5 days after oocyte retrieval as a method of decreasing the overall number of embryos transferred. Following 5 days in culture, only the hardiest of embryos will develop into blastocyts (see Fig. 13-6). The theory is that by allowing an additional

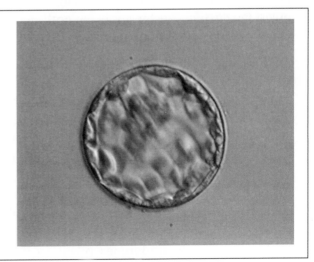

Figure 13-6: Blastocyst (5 days after egg retrieval). (Courtesy of Katharine Jackson, BS, Brigham and Women's Hospital ART Embryology Laboratory, Boston, MA.)

2 days in culture, the embryos of superior quality will emerge as blastocysts. As a result, fewer embryos need to be transferred to achieve the same pregnancy rate and the risk of multiple gestation is lower.

Once it has been decided how many embryos will be transferred, the embryos are transferred transcervically with the use of a soft, flexible catheter. Typically, a patient will have undergone a "mock transfer" prior to embryo transfer. A mock transfer helps the clinician obtain information to plan the transfer. Information typically gathered includes the depth of the uterine cavity and angle of cervix and/or uterus. Attempt is made to transfer embryos above the level of the cervical internal os, but below the uterine fundus. Great care is taken by clinicians to achieve an efficient and nontraumatic transfer of embryos. A difficult or traumatic transfer may decrease the chance of a successful implantation, possibly due to effects on the endometrium or on the embryos themselves.

LUTEAL PHASE SUPPORT

Endometrial receptivity plays a critical role in the implantation of an embryo in an IVF cycle. Because aspiration of follicles at the time of oocyte retrieval may result in the removal of granulosa cells, there is concern that luteal phase progesterone may be inadequate to support the endometrium and possible early pregnancy. Thus, supplemental progesterone is commonly given. This therapy is initiated after oocyte retrieval and may be given as an intramuscular injection or a vaginal suppository. For ongoing pregnancies, progesterone is generally continued until the 8th or 10th week of the pregnancy.

KEY POINT

Progesterone, and oftentimes estradiol, is given following egg retrieval to support the possible early pregnancy.

OVUM DONATION

Older women, women with premature ovarian failure, or women who have failed all other IVF attempts, may be candidates for ovum donation. Ovum donors are typically women younger than 33 years of age who may or may not be known to the recipient. Following identification of an oocyte donor, the donor is screened for both physical and psychologic health and her genetic history is recorded. She then undergoes a standard ovarian stimulation protocol as described above; the recipient simultaneously prepares her uterus for embryo transfer. Generally, the recipient undergoes pituitary downregulation with a GnRH agonist and then takes estradiol until the ultrasound indicates adequate endometrial development (endometrial lining thickness) and the oocyte donor is ready for retrieval. Progesterone will be added to the recipient's regimen to prepare the endometrium for implantation. The success rate for ovum donation approaches 50% in many centers (see Chap. 16 for further information).

OTHER ASSISTED REPRODUCTIVE TECHNOLOGY (ART) TECHNIQUES
In addition to IVF, several other ART techniques are available to overcome infertility. In gamete intrafallopian transfer (GIFT), oocytes generally are obtained through transvaginal aspiration. After oocytes are identified in the embryology laboratory they are placed in a transfer catheter that contains concentrated, motile sperm. A transcervical technique or laparoscopy is used to place the transfer catheter into the distal 4 cm of fallopian tube, where the contents are gently discharged.

In zygote intrafallopian transfer (ZIFT), a zygote, or one-cell embryo, is transferred into the fallopian tube by the GIFT technique. GIFT and ZIFT are more invasive than standard IVF. Because of the increasing efficiency, safety, and success rates of IVF, GIFT and ZIFT play increasingly smaller roles in ART. Nevertheless, there are rare instances in which the intratubal techniques may be superior. An example of an indication for ZIFT is when a patient's cervix is severely scarred, making an efficient, nontraumatic transcervical transfer impossible. GIFT may be used when a couple's religious beliefs prohibit extracorporeal fertilization.

PREIMPLANTATION GENETIC DIAGNOSIS Historically, couples at high risk of passing a genetic disorder to their progeny had to wait until the second trimester before the woman could undergo amniocentesis, or the late first trimester for chorionic villus sampling, to determine if their offspring would be affected. If this testing revealed the presence of the disorder, couples were then faced with the decision of whether or not to continue the pregnancy. Preimplantation genetic diagnosis (PGD) refers to the diagnosis of a genetic disorder in an embryo before its transfer. The term PGD refers to several different methods that may be used to gather genetic information about an embryo. The first technique involves the removal of one polar body. Each polar body contains only one copy of a gene. However, if a normal copy is found, it can be presumed that the oocyte contains a normal copy. This method is technically difficult and may be in error if crossing over has occurred and both copies are present in the polar body. A second method involves sampling cells that are destined to become the placenta. This requires culture of an embryo to the blastocyst stage and has been shown to result in a lower implantation rate when the embryo is transferred.

The final technique is the blastomere biopsy, which involves removal of a single cell from the six to eight cell embryo. The genetic material from the cell is then analyzed for chromosomal abnormalities, such as trisomy or translocation by fluorescent *in situ* hydridization (FISH). FISH may be used for sex selection for couples at risk for transmitting an X or Y linked disorder. In addition, several single gene defects, such as cystic fibrosis, sickle cell anemia, or Duchene's muscular dystrophy, can now be detected using PGD. When information on a single gene is sought, DNA from the embryo can be amplified with the polymerase chain reaction (PCR) and probed with fluorescent-labeled probes for these genes. The blastomere biopsy technique has not been shown to affect development of the embryo.

RISKS AND COMPLICATIONS OF IN VITRO FERTILIZATION   The risks of an IVF cycle can be divided into those associated with ovarian stimulation, oocyte retrieval, and pregnancy.

OVARIAN STIMULATION   The major risk of ovarian stimulation with exogenous gonadotropins is ovarian hyperstimulation syndrome (OHSS), a potentially life-threatening complication (see Chap. 9). In mild cases, patients may develop ovarian enlargement, abdominal distention, and weight gain. In severe cases, however, patients may become critically ill, presenting with ascites pleural effusion, electrolyte imbalance, hypovolemia, and possibly oliguria. Patients presenting with severe OHSS require hospitalization and supportive care.

Patients with mild or moderate symptoms may be monitored closely as outpatients. Severe OHSS may occur in as many as 1% of women undergoing an IVF cycle. Patients with an exuberant

KEY POINT

The major risk of ovarian stimulation is ovarian hyperstimulation syndrome.

response to gonadotropin stimulation, as evidenced by high estradiol levels and the production of a greater-than-average number of follicles are at an elevated risk of acquiring this disorder. Younger patients and/or patients who carry the diagnosis of polycystic ovarian syndrome (PCOS) are at increased risk.

The detailed pathophysiology of OHSS is still unclear; however, the disorder appears to stem from increased capillary permeability triggered by vasoactive substances, such as vascular endothelial growth factor (VEGF), that are released by the stimulated ovary.[11] While the stimulated ovary may lay the groundwork for OHSS, the administration of hCG may play a role in triggering this disorder. An increase in OHSS symptoms is seen several days following the administration of hCG in susceptible patients. Moreover, patients at risk for OHSS, based on their ovarian response, often first manifest symptoms at the time of the initial rise of hCG from a pregnancy.

To date, there is no effective cure for OHSS. Treatment is supportive and designed to reduce symptoms and risk of complications. Women with severe cases may require hospital admission for administration of parenteral fluids, electrolyte replacement, supplemental oxygen, and possibly prophylactic antithromboembolic medications such as subcutaneous heparin. In cases in which ascites accumulation prevents adequate respiratory effort, therapeutic paracentesis may make the patient more comfortable. Eventually OHSS symptoms begin to resolve spontaneously, although this may be as long as several weeks following its initial presentation. Given the lack of effective treatment for this complication, prevention is critical. Techniques for prevention include the judicious use of gonadotropin in patients likely to have exuberant responses, such as young women or those with PCOS. Cycle cancellation may be necessary in the patient who develops an exuberant ovarian response despite low doses of medication. Another frequently used option to reduce the risk of OHSS is to proceed with egg retrieval but then to cryopreserve all embryos. By preventing the chance of pregnancy, which would increase circulating hCG levels, a patient's chance of a protracted course of OHSS will be reduced. Thawed embryos can then be transferred several months later after OHSS has resolved.

OOCYTE RETRIEVAL Transvaginal ultrasound-guided oocyte retrieval is a procedure with a low rate of complications but is not without its risks. There is a small risk of infection; however, the incidence is extremely rare with the use of prophylactic antibiotics. Bleeding complications also are encountered, but only rarely require further surgery or transfusion. Finally, the risk of injury to bowel, bladder, or blood vessels exists, although it is rare in common practice.

KEY POINT

The greatest risk of an IVF pregnancy is the risk of multiple birth.

PREGNANCY A major risk of pregnancy occurring from IVF is the risk of multiple gestations. The risk of prematurity in twin and triplet pregnancies is increased compared with singletons. National registry data published for 2000 indicated that of all IVF cycles that year, 74,957 involved fresh, nondonor eggs that yielded 23,042 pregnancies. Of these 58.1% were singletons, 28.4% were twins, 7.7% were triplets, and 5.8% could not be determined due to miscarriage.[2] Whether or not IVF children have a higher rate of congenital malformations than their naturally conceived peers is an area of ongoing debate. The baseline risk for malformations of all births is approximately 2–4%. Most studies have not shown an increased risk of malformations associated with IVF.

IVF Results

In 1992, the Congress passed the Fertility Clinic Success Rate and Certification Act was passed. This law mandated that all IVF clinics report their IVF success rates to the Centers for Disease Control and Prevention (CDC) annually and these data are available to the public. The CDC reports overall success rates for the United States as well as for individual clinics. Data for 2000 reveal that 99,639 cycles of IVF were initiated. Of these, 75.2% involved fresh nondonor cycles. These cycles yielded a live birth per cycle rate of 25.4%. Not unsurprisingly, success rates vary by age. For the youngest patient group (women <35 years of age), the success rate (rate of live birth per cycle) was 33%. For women 38–40 years old, the success rate was 18%, while for those 41–42 years old, the success rate was 10%. Importantly, overall success rates appeared to be increasing over the past 4 years. For example, for the youngest patient group, success rates were 28.4% in 1996 and 33% in 2000.[2]

Discussion of Cases

CASE 1

A couple presents for evaluation of infertility. The woman is 34 years old and her husband is 39. They report attempting pregnancy using ovulation indicator kits for the past 15 months without success. She reports regular menses since the age of 13 and reports that they are accompanied by minimal pain. She has no history of abnormal pap smears. Her husband has never fathered any children. He is otherwise healthy with no prior surgeries. He drinks alcohol socially and does not smoke cigarettes.

The woman's physical examination reveals the following:

Ht. 5′3″, wt. 134 lb, BMI 23.7
Abdomen: Soft, nontender, no masses
Bimanual examination: Mobile, anteverted uterus, no masses, no cervical motion tenderness
External genitalia, vagina, and cervix within normal limits

What other testing would you recommend at this point?

- **Clomid challenge test:**
  - **Day 3 FSH: 12 mU/mL**
  - **Day 10 FSH: 9 mU/mL**

- **Hysterosalpingogram: No uterine cavity abnormalities noted. Spill from both tubes.**
- **Semen analysis: WNL**

What is your recommendation for further management?

The woman's workup is significant for slightly elevated FSH levels on a CCCT, suggestive of borderline ovarian reserve. This may indeed be the root cause of this couple's infertility. HSG results do not reveal a tubal obstruction. The semen analysis is within normal limits. She does not have a history consistent with endometriosis; thus a laparoscopy is not necessarily indicated.

Does she require any further testing to initiate management?

No further testing is recommended.

What is your recommendation for initial management?

Given that this couple does not appear to have a tubal factor or a male factor etiology to explain their infertility, an initial management plan would likely start with IUIs. Because of her reduced ovarian reserve, stimulation with gonadotropins is recommended.

This couple undergoes three cycles of gonadotropins and IUIs. The woman is initially started on a GnRH agonist in the luteal phase of her cycle. After menses occurs, gonadotropin stimulation with rFSH is started on the second day of her cycle. Unfortunately, she fails to become pregnant through these three cycles.

What is the next step in management?

Given the failure of three gonadotropin-stimulated IUIs, this couple would next be offered IVF.

CASE 2

A 28-year-old woman who has recently undergone an IVF cycle presents with abdominal pain. She underwent oocyte retrieval 12 days previously. A review of this patient's record reveals a history of oligomenorrhea/polycystic ovary disease. Her cycle was notable for achieving a high peak estradiol level of 3700 pg/mL following stimulation with recombinant FSH. She had 28 eggs retrieved. The patient has noted increasing abdominal distention associated with vague abdominal discomfort over the past several days. She has a decreased appetite and has had several episodes of emesis. She has not noted any fevers or localized pain.

Her physical examination reveals the following:

Afebrile
Ht. 5'5", wt. 180 lbs (baseline of 170 lbs)
HR: 110 bpm, BP 105/70 mmHg, RR 20 breaths/min
Lungs: Dullness at bases of both lungs, otherwise, no wheezes, rubs, or crackles.
CV: Regular rhythm, tachycardic
Abdomen: Softly distended throughout, (+) fluid wave, no tenderness to deep palpation
Extremities: No edema, no tenderness, no Hohmann's sign

What testing would be useful for guiding management of this patient?

- **CBC: Hematocrit 52, white blood cell count 11,000/L platelets 340**
- **Electrolytes: Na^+ 136, K^+ 3.7, bicarbonate 105, Cl^- 111, BUN 11, Creatinine 0.9**
- **Ultrasound: Moderate ascites, right ovary 12 × 11 cm, left ovary 11 × 9 cm, both with multiple cysts. Small bilateral pleural effusions**

What is the next step in management of this patient?

This patient has several risk factors for OHSS, including young age, diagnosis of PCOS or oligoovulation, and exuberant response to gonadotropin stimulation. Indeed, the patient's physical examination and laboratory findings are most consistent with a diagnosis of OHSS. Other diagnoses to exclude would be pelvic infection (unlikely without fever or localized pain) and ovarian torsion (relatively benign abdominal examination makes this unlikely). The history of distention, poor oral intake, weight gain, and the findings of ascites, hemoconcentration, and pleural effusions are of particular concern for OHSS. Indeed, the degree of hemoconcentration and the presence of ascites and pleural effusions indicate

that this patient meets criteria for severe OHSS. Particularly in light of her evidence of hemoconcentration, she would benefit from hospital admission for supportive care.

The patient is admitted and started on intravenous fluids. Given her increased risk for thrombo-embolic events, she is started on prophylactic subcutaneous heparin. Her urine output is maintained at greater than 50 cc/h. On hospital day 2, she is noted to have gained 2 lb. Her abdomen continues to be distended; however, she is having no difficulty breathing and is tolerating a small amount of food taken orally.

What further management is necessary?

A therapeutic paracentesis can be considered in some patients with OHSS, depending on the degree of the patient's discomfort. Given that this patient is able to tolerate some oral intake and is not dyspneic, this intervention is not absolutely necessary at this time. Continued supportive measures, however, will be important until her symptoms begin to gradually resolve.

REFERENCES

1 Steptoe P, Edwards R. Birth after the reimplantation of a human embryo. *Lancet* 2:366–368, 1978.

2 www.cdc.gov.nccdphp/drh/art00.

3 Hull M. Infertility treatment: relative effectiveness of conventional and assisted conception methods. *Hum Reprod* 7:785–792, 1992.

4 Toner J, Philput CB, GS J, Muasher SJ. Basal follicle stimulating hormone level is a better predictor of in vitro fertilization performance than age. *Fertil Steril* 55:784–791, 1991.

5 Scott RT, Hofmann GE. Prognostic asessment of ovarian reserve. *Fertil Steril* 63(1):1–11, 1995.

6 Ron-El R, Raziel A, Strassburger D, et al. Outcome of assisted reproductive technology in women over the age of 41. *Fertil Steril* 74:471–480, 2000.

7 Scott R, Toner J, Muasher SJ, Ochninger S, Robinson S, Rosenwales Z. Follicle-stimulating hormone levels on cycle day 3 are predictive of in vitro fertilization outcome. *Fertil Steril* 51:651–654, 1989.

8 Daya S, Gunby J, Hughes E. Follicle stimulating hornmone versus human menopausal gonadotropin for in vitro fertilization cycles: a meta-analysis. *Fertil Steril* 64:347–351, 1995.

9 Hughes E, Fedorkow M, Daya S. The routine use of gonadotropin releasing hormone agonists prior to in vitro fertilization and gamete intrafallopian tube transfer: a meta-analysis of randomized controlled trials. *Fertil Steril* 58:888–796, 1992.

10 Palermo G, Joris H, Devroey P, Van Steirteghem A. Pregnancies after intracytoplasmic injection of a single spermatozoon. 340:17–21, 1992.

11 Elchalel U, Rosen G, Cassidenti D. Role of vascular endothelial cell growth factor in ovarian hyperstimulation syndrome views and ideas. *Hum Reprod* 12:1129, 1997.

14

The IVF Laboratory

Nancy L. Bossert
Christopher J. DeJonge

Introduction

The *in vitro* fertilization (IVF) laboratory has a critical and integral role in the success of an assisted reproductive technology (ART) program. The birth of Louise Brown in 1978 was the culmination of years of scientific advances using mostly animal models.[1,2] At the time of the first IVF birth, comprehensive scientific descriptions of the living human oocyte and the dynamic events of human fertilization and early development were still at an embryonic stage of development. Likewise, understanding of the elements and conditions necessary for a functional, much less optimized, human IVF laboratory was not clear.

Pioneering embryologists (many of whom still practice today) came from an array of clinical and basic science research laboratories and they had backgrounds in embryology, tissue culture, agricultural science, genetics, microbiology, and clinical chemistry. As a consequence, many individual styles evolved for performing the various IVF techniques, and different laboratories often use slightly different procedures, materials, and equipment to get the job done. It is now 25 years since the birth of Louise Brown and as she has matured, so has the IVF laboratory. Standardization has become more the order of the day via training and implementation of quality control (QC) and quality assurance (QA) practices. This chapter will highlight current philosophical and functional practice in today's IVF laboratory.

Quality Control

KEY POINT

> *The development of a quality control program is essential for the function of an IVF laboratory.*

One element that successful IVF laboratories have in common is a QC program. The goal of any QC program is to provide routine inspection of a system's components in order to ensure that a product or service is delivered under optimal conditions. A QC program for the laboratory has several components, including personnel qualifications and training, instrumentation and equipment, disposable supplies such as culture media and plasticware, procedures and policies, patient specimen management, documentation and record-keeping, and a corrective action system.[3,4] The QC program can then serve as a cornerstone for a QA program, the goal of which in an IVF laboratory is to provide optimal care to the patient by constant surveillance of the system in which the patient's care is delivered.[5]

LABORATORY PHYSICAL PLANT

The IVF laboratory physical plant should be carefully designed to enhance efficiency and traffic flow, and it should have adequate space for equipment and instruments, separation of tasks, and storage of supplies.[6] Ideally, the procedure room(s) for egg retrievals and embryo transfers should be adjacent to the laboratory. Air quality in the laboratory is also important and it can be improved with positive pressure ventilation and high efficiency particulate air (HEPA) filtration. Access to the laboratory should be limited to essential personnel. In order to minimize access of unauthorized personnel into the laboratory and to ensure the products used for cleaning are compatible with the conduct of the laboratory, cleaning should only be performed by laboratory personnel. For the same reasons, maintenance and repair should be scheduled in advance to avoid disruption of laboratory function and to minimize the potential for contamination. The providers of environmental services, engineering services, and security should be notified in writing regarding special requirements and conditions for the laboratory.

PERSONNEL QUALIFICATIONS AND TRAINING

Arguably, the single most important attribute for someone working in an IVF laboratory is elegant psychomotor skills, i.e., hand-to-eye coordination. Other important attributes include orientation to detail and a sound knowledge of embryology. Minimum standards for assisted reproductive technology practices have been developed[7] and they include qualification guidelines for IVF laboratory personnel. The minimum standards also recommend a backup system for all personnel essential to a program. Training of IVF laboratory staff mostly occurs through mentoring by an experienced embryologist. Formal courses that offer a combination of didactic and hands-on training have recently become available and include more advanced IVF procedures, e.g., micromanipulation techniques such as intracytoplasmic sperm injection (ICSI), assisted zona hatching (AH), and blastomere biopsy. In any case, the completion of training and the ability of the staff member to work unsupervised in the IVF laboratory is determined and documented by the laboratory director. Continuing education for IVF laboratory staff can be attained and documented by attendance at formal courses, annual professional society meetings, and participation in intramural journal clubs. Documentation of a laboratory staff member's proficiency in performing clinical procedures should be recorded and updated as necessary.

INSTRUMENTATION AND EQUIPMENT

Essential elements in equipping an IVF laboratory include an incubator, dissecting and inverted microscopes, a micromanipulator, a cell freezer, a liquid nitrogen storage tank, a centrifuge, heating units such as stage warmers or temperature blocks, a pH meter, an osmometer, and pipettors. Duplication of essential instruments and equipment represents an effective safety plan but is sometimes financially unattainable. However, a written backup plan for each instrument and piece of equipment in the case of failure is essential. Regular cleaning and preventative maintenance should be performed and documented on all instruments and equipment. Any corrective maintenance should also be documented. All instruments and equipment should be monitored every day that they are in use. For example, an incubator should be monitored daily for temperature, atmospheric gas (e.g., % CO_2), and relative humidity in the chamber as well as gas (e.g., CO_2) level in the supply tank(s). Independent monitors such as certified thermometers and infrared CO_2 detectors must verify digital displays on the incubator itself. Any monitoring that is performed should be documented.

CULTURE MEDIA AND CONTACT MATERIAL

A current inventory of disposable supplies and culture media is essential to a quality control program. The disposable supplies that are especially important are those that come in direct or indirect contact with gametes and embryos. For each contact material or culture medium, the inventory should include the date it is received in the laboratory, the expiration date, and the date it is put into use. The contact material and culture media must undergo rigorous testing to ensure that they will provide an environment that will optimally support fertilization and early embryo development.

Since the culture media and contact material must provide immaculate culture conditions, they must be free from toxins and contaminants. Endotoxin levels in culture media and water can be determined using the limulus amoebocyte lysate (LAL) test.[8] The bioassays that are commonly used to detect other embryotoxins include those that examine *in vitro* development of mouse embryos to the blastocyst stage (the mouse 1-cell embryo assay[9] or the mouse 2-cell embryo assay[10]) or those that examine the *in vitro* survival of sperm motility and forward progression (the hamster sperm motility assay[11] or the human sperm survival assay[12]).

Individual IVF laboratories choose among the assays based on convenience, cost, and assay sensitivity. Most of the culture media and some of the contact materials that can be purchased commercially for use in an IVF laboratory are tested during the manufacturing process and are delivered with certificates of analysis that include assay results. An IVF laboratory can then accept the results at face value or run their own bioassays. However, most of the contact material purchased commercially has not been tested prior to its arrival in the laboratory, and it should be tested prior to being put into use.

PROCEDURES AND POLICIES

The IVF laboratory must have a written procedure manual in which each procedure has a list of media, supplies, and instruments or equipment necessary to perform the procedure along with a detailed step-by-step description of the procedure itself. The procedure can also contain a section describing quality control elements for that procedure, e.g., the use of aseptic technique throughout or the verification of patient identification (ID) for an oocyte retrieval. A written procedure manual for all procedures in the IVF laboratory will help ensure consistent and reproducible results. It can also serve as a training tool for new laboratory staff prior to hands-on mentoring. A written policy manual is also essential for the IVF laboratory. In addition to ensuring consistent and reproducible results, written policies will aid in decision-making processes, e.g., what happens to immature oocytes. Both the policy manual and procedure manual should be updated as necessary and reviewed by the laboratory director or their designee at least annually.

PATIENT SPECIMEN MANAGEMENT

Patients want assurance and ongoing reassurance that the sperm and eggs used to create their embryos came from them. Fueling their insecurity are news media reports of children born which were visibly distinct from their parents. Thus, chain of specimen custody with accurate patient identification is a critical and essential element in the quality control program for an IVF laboratory. To accomplish this goal, the IVF laboratory staff must initially verify and document the identity of the patient providing the gametes and maintain the identity of the gametes and embryos throughout handling and culture until the final disposition of all gametes and embryos, whether it be embryo transfer, cryopreservation, or disposal.

The ID of any patient providing a semen specimen should be verified and documented with a photo ID, and the labeling on the container should be checked with the patient for accuracy and completeness. Once the specimen is transferred from the original container, the new container (whether it is a centrifuge tube or a counting chamber) should be labeled with the patient's name and unique ID number. Thus, a chain of custody is established from the time the patient brings the specimen to the IVF laboratory until the sperm is combined with the appropriate oocytes.

The ID of the patient undergoing the oocyte retrieval should also be verified and documented. A unique ID number should be assigned to the cohort of oocytes from the patient, and all culture dishes and laboratory records should be labeled with the patient's name and unique ID number. The laboratory staff member responsible for performing each procedure should also be documented. A chain of custody is then established from the time the oocytes are retrieved until the final disposition of all oocytes and embryos.

DOCUMENTATION AND RECORD-KEEPING

Written records serve as a permanent history of a patient's treatment, and the IVF laboratory chart documents the identity of the patient, the date and type of procedures performed, the identity of the laboratory staff member who performed the procedures, and the results of the procedures. These results would include the number of oocytes retrieved, inseminated, and fertilized; the semen analysis of the specimen provided for IVF; the numbers of embryos cryopreserved and transferred; and the final disposition of each oocyte and embryo. The IVF laboratory chart might also include information on the types of culture media that were used for that particular patient. This information would be useful in the event of a product recall for a culture medium or supplement. A final reminder of the significant role that documentation has in any QC program is the adage: "If it wasn't documented, then it didn't happen."

CORRECTIVE ACTION SYSTEM

While it is important to document the performance of components in the QC program, it is imperative to have a system to appraise the documentation so that any deficiencies in the system or its components can be corrected and improvements can be implemented. For example, temperature and atmospheric gas are measured daily in an incubator. If either of these measurements is out of range, then it should be noted on the record along with any corrective action that is taken. The laboratory director or their designee should regularly review QC records (including any corrective action taken) to determine whether the same problem repeats itself frequently, and if so, what actions to take in order to improve the system.

Embryo Culture Systems

Methods for embryo culture and media composition have changed greatly over the last quarter century.[13–15] While the various culture media used for IVF differ in composition, there appears to be little difference in their ability to support human embryo development. The same can be said with respect to the different culture vessels available and the methods by which media and vessels are collaboratively used.

EMBRYO METABOLIC REQUIREMENTS AND CULTURE MEDIA

Basic scientific research in early embryo physiology and metabolism suggested that human embryos are metabolically dynamic and their metabolic requirements change in a stage-dependent manner during development. Data from several laboratories demonstrate that early embryos undergo a shift in their requirement for energy substrates.[2,16] Embryos under maternal genetic control prefer pyruvate and lactate as substrates while embryos with activated embryonic (zygotic) genomes use a glucose-based metabolism.[17] An additional stage-specific requirement occurs at the onset of transcription, immediately after zygotic genome activation (around day 3), when essential and nonessential amino acids are needed to serve as the building blocks for further protein synthesis. This pivotal information has been used by several laboratories to formulate embryo culture media that are used sequentially to specifically address the changing metabolic requirements of the embryo.[18,19]

Media used to culture human preimplantation embryos generally fall into one of three categories. One category is simple salt solutions with added energy substrates. Examples of media in this category are T6, Earle's, human tubal fluid (HTF) medium, and P1. These media are usually supplemented with whole serum or serum albumin. A second category is complex tissue culture media that were originally formulated to support somatic cell growth *in vitro*. An example of this type of medium is Ham's F-10, and it is also usually supplemented with whole serum or serum albumin. The third category is sequential media, which take into account the changing requirements of the developing embryo. Examples of sequential media are G1/G2 and P1/blastocyst medium.

TYPES OF CULTURE SYSTEMS

Embryo culture systems can differ based on the type of culture vessel used, the use of an oil overlay, and the use of coculture with helper cells. The choice of which to use is made by each IVF laboratory based on experience, success, convenience, safety, and cost.

Human embryos can be cultured in a variety of vessels. In the early days, embryos were cultured in glass test tubes[20]; hence the "test tube baby" moniker. While some IVF laboratories continue to culture in test tubes (the original glass tubes having been replaced by plastic tubes), other laboratories use plastic culture dishes, organ culture dishes, or 4-well tissue culture plates. Another option commonly used in embryo culture is to overlay the culture medium with equilibrated mineral (paraffin) oil in an attempt to control for potential fluctuations in pH and temperature.

Oil overlay can be used with the larger volumes of culture medium in organ culture dishes and 4-well plates or it can be used with microdrops of culture medium. In the case of microdrops, the oil overlay helps to prevent evaporation of the medium, which would cause a catastrophic change in medium osmolarity (salt content).

Coculture of human embryos with helper cells is used by some IVF laboratories in the belief that the helper cells exert a beneficial influence by either releasing embryotrophic factors or detoxifying the culture medium by removing inhibitory or toxic products. The type of cells that have been used as helper cells include heterologous donor cells from human (tubal epithelial, endometrium), bovine (fetal uterine, oviductal epithelial, Madin-Darby kidney epithelial), and monkey (Vero) as well as autologous cells from the patient (granulosa, cumulus, endometrium). While some reports of coculture with human embryos demonstrate improved embryo quality and increased implantation and ongoing pregnancy rates,[21] other reports question whether coculture offers any real benefit.[22]

BLASTOCYST CULTURE The availability of a number of successful sequential media culture systems has led many ART programs to perform blastocyst stage embryo transfers (Fig. 14-1), usually on day 5 or day 6 after fertilization. Since blastocysts usually implant with higher frequency than day 3 embryos, the primary advantage of blastocyst transfer is the improved ability for embryo selection so that fewer embryos can be transferred, thus reducing the potential for high order multiple gestation. Approximately 40–60% of fertilized

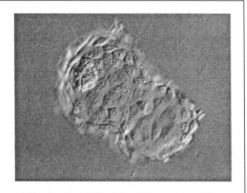

Figure 14-1: Blastocyst-stage human embryo.

oocytes reach the blastocyst stage when cultured in sequential media.[19,23] Yet one risk of attempting blastocyst transfer is the possibility that no embryos will be available for transfer due to failure to develop to the blastocyst stage. As a consequence, ART programs performing blastocyst transfers usually have rigorous criteria for the minimum number of fertilized oocytes and/or defined developmental criteria (e.g., cell number and embryo quality) for cleavage stage (day 3) embryos before patients are allowed to continue as candidates for blastocyst transfer. If the criteria are not met, then the embryos may be transferred on day 3.

The procedure for extended culture simply involves transferring the embryos to the appropriate sequential medium that is tailored for their stage-specific metabolic requirements. This transfer usually takes place on day 3, although some IVF laboratories prefer to move the embryos in the morning of day 4. The embryos are put back in the incubator until day 5 when they are examined and their developmental quality assessed using several parameters, including blastocoel (central fluid-filled cavity in the embryo) expansion, and the number of cells in both the inner cell mass (future fetus) and the trophectoderm (future extraembryonic structures).[17] One or two blastocysts are usually transferred on day 5, although some ART programs prefer to transfer on day 6.

Laboratory Procedures

Clearly defined and documented laboratory procedures serve as a critical backbone to ensure successful IVF laboratory performance. Quality control (e.g., temperature control, pH control, and aseptic technique) is an essential partner for ensuring optimized performance. For example, working quickly and carefully with gametes and embryos outside of the incubator is one way to minimize changes in their culture conditions (i.e., temperature and pH).

OOCYTE IDENTIFICATION AND ISOLATION

During oocyte retrieval, the IVF laboratory receives test tubes of follicular aspirates containing follicular fluid, the cumulus-oocyte complex (COC), differentiated and nondifferentiated granulosa cells, theca cells, and red blood cells. Each test tube is decanted into a large petri dish and the contents of the dish are viewed at

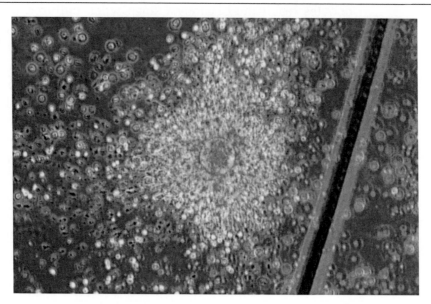

Figure 14-2: Human cumulus-oocyte complex.

10× magnification using a dissecting stereomicroscope. A cumulus mass, easily seen with the naked eye, is a cluster of differentiated granulosa cells held together by an extracellular matrix of hyaluronic acid. Once a cumulus mass is identified, it is microscopically examined for the presence of an oocyte centered in that mass. If an oocyte is present, the mass is referred to as the cumulus-oocyte complex (Fig. 14-2), and the tightly packed ring of cells immediately surrounding the oocyte is called the corona radiata.

The COC is then aseptically and carefully aspirated and transferred from the petri dish to a culture dish containing culture medium buffered appropriately to maintain pH. Once all of the tubes of follicular fluid have been examined, all of the COCs are transferred to culture dishes containing a bicarbonate-based medium (to help maintain pH) and placed in an incubator at 37°C and 5–6% CO_2 atmosphere.

OOCYTE MATURITY ASSESSMENT AND INSEMINATION

The stage of oocyte maturity is assessed prior to insemination because it provides an indication of the relative fertilizing potential of the oocyte. The COCs are removed from the incubator and each COC is quickly observed at 40× magnification using a dissecting stereomicroscope to determine the stage of oocyte nuclear maturity.[24] The three stages of oocyte nuclear maturity are prophase I (PI), metaphase I (MI), and metaphase II (MII).

The PI oocyte is immature, in part because it is tetraploid (4N). The PI oocyte matures in response to gonadotropin surges and a reduction in follicular maturation-inhibiting factors. The germinal vesicle, the enlarged nucleus of an oocyte before meiotic division is completed, begins its progression to germinal vesicle breakdown (GVBD) simultaneous with oocyte enlargement. More than 80% of oocytes have succeeded in passing through PI and MI to ultimately reach MII by the time of oocyte retrieval.

Microscopically, the PI oocyte is characterized by a distinct germinal vesicle with a refractile nucleolus and an irregularly shaped centrally dark and granular ooplasm (Fig. 14-3). Attached cumulus cells may be compact and multilayered or may be luteinized. PI oocytes with very mature characteristics generally represent arrested maturation and fail to undergo GVBD.

The MI oocyte is intermediate in maturation. The oocyte has completed the prophase of meiosis I, whereby the germinal vesicle and its nucleolus have disappeared. Microscopically, the MI oocyte is characterized by the absence of both the germinal vesicle and the first polar body (Fig. 14-4). A late MI oocyte is round and even in form, with homogeneously granular and light-colored ooplasm. Early MI oocytes may display minor central granularity. Luteinized cumulus cells are usually associated with late stages.

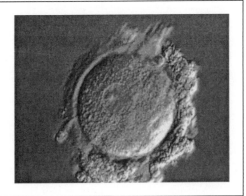

Figure 14-3: Prophase I (PI) human oocyte.

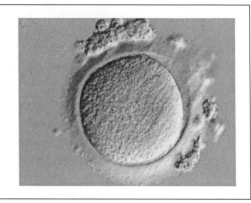

Figure 14-4: Metaphase I
(MI) human oocyte.

The MII oocyte is mature. This oocyte is at a resting stage of meiosis II after extrusion of the first polar body and direct passage to metaphase II. The first polar body contains half of the oocyte DNA, and the oocyte is now diploid (2N). Microscopically, the MII oocyte is characterized by a round, even shape, and ooplasm of light color and homogeneous granularity (Fig. 14-5). It is usually associated with an expanded, luteinized cumulus, and a "sunburst" corona radiata.

KEY POINT

Assessment of sperm and egg prior to fertilization yields valuable information.

After all oocytes have been assessed for nuclear maturity, the COCs are returned to the incubator. Under most circumstances oocytes will be inseminated approximately 4–6 h postaspiration. If an oocyte is judged to be immature, then the timing for insemination can be delayed for several hours. As a general rule, approximately 50,000–500,000 progressively motile sperm are used for

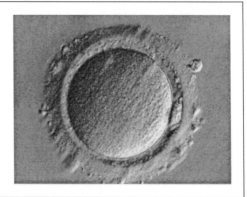

Figure 14-5: Metaphase II
(MII) human oocyte.

insemination of each mature oocyte. Factors that can influence the insemination concentration include sperm motility and morphology as well as the presence of sperm agglutination or aggregation. At the time of insemination, an appropriate number of sperm are added to each culture dish containing COCs, which are then returned to the incubator.

FERTILIZATION ASSESSMENT

Oocytes incubated with sperm need to be examined within 15–18 h in order to determine whether normal fertilization has occurred. At the time of fertilization check, inseminated oocytes are still surrounded by the cumulus and corona, but the cellular associations are weakened due to the action of hyaluronidase, an enzyme carried by sperm that acts on the hyaluronic acid holding cumulus cells together. Mechanical removal of the cumulus and coronal cells, usually by repeat pipetting using a small bore pipet, facilitates the examination of the oocyte for evidence of fertilization. Cumulus cell removal is performed at 10x magnification using a dissecting microscope, and the denuded oocytes are then examined at 40× magnification for the presence of pronuclei. If too many coronal cells are left attached to the oocyte, then they can obscure viewing of pronuclei.

A normally fertilized oocyte has two pronuclei and two polar bodies (Fig. 14-6).[25] The second polar body is formed as a consequence of sperm-initiated oocyte activation. The two pronuclei are formed from sperm and oocyte chromatin, respectively, and are

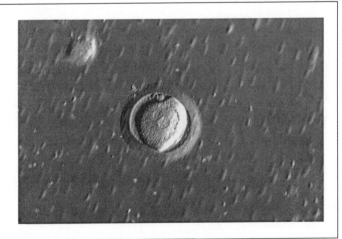

Figure 14-6: Normally fertilized human oocyte with two pronuclei and two polar bodies.

referred to as the male pronucleus and the female pronucleus. The stage at which the pronuclei are visible is termed the pronuclear stage. Early after their formation, pronuclei may be seen distant from each other and later they migrate together centrally. By 15 h after insemination, pronuclei are most often observed lying close to one another, and one to nine nucleoli will be observed in each pronucleus. The pronuclei ultimately fuse in a process called syngamy and the new genome is created.

Normally fertilized oocytes are transferred to fresh culture medium and returned to the incubator. Oocytes with one pronucleus or with more than two pronuclei are abnormally fertilized and they are discarded. Unfertilized oocytes and degenerate/nonviable oocytes are also discarded.

EMBRYO QUALITY ASSESSMENT

Embryo quality is assessed on day 3 prior to embryo transfer. The culture dish containing embryos is removed from the incubator and placed on the stage of an inverted microscope with modulation contrast optics. Each embryo is observed at 200× to determine the number of cells comprising the embryo (blastomeres), the symmetry of the blastomeres, and the amount (if any) of cytoplasmic fragmentation. These criteria are then used to assign a grade to each embryo.[24]

Regularly cleaving 2-cell embryos are usually observed 22–24 h after insemination and may be seen up to 44 h postinsemination. Four-cell embryos are routinely observed 36–50 h postinsemination. Eight-cell embryos are not commonly seen until after 48 h but are usually noted before 72 h. Commonly, 3-, 5-, and 7-cell stages are interposed between these divisions, especially if examination is carried out during mitotic cell division. Typically, the length of embryo culture prior to embryo transfer is between 64 and 68 h postinsemination.

UTERINE EMBRYO TRANSFER

Embryos generated during an IVF cycle are usually replaced in the patient's uterus on day 3 postaspiration. The number of embryos to be transferred is based on the patient's wishes, the physician's recommendation, and the embryo quality. Once the patient is in position for the transfer, the culture dish containing the embryos to be transferred is removed from the incubator to the stage of a dissecting stereomicroscope. The transfer catheter is rinsed with culture medium and the embryos are aspirated into the catheter in a small volume of medium. The physician gently passes the catheter through the cervix and into the uterus so that the embryos can be atraumatically expelled near (but not touching) the uterine fundus. The catheter is then withdrawn from the uterus and rinsed and examined under the microscope for the presence of retained embryos. If retained embryos are seen, then the transfer is repeated until the embryos are in the uterus.

Micromanipulation

There are several types of micromanipulation techniques applied to oocytes and embryos, including partial zona dissection (PZD), subzonal sperm insertion, and blastomere or polar body biopsy for preimplantation genetic diagnosis. The two most common micromanipulation techniques are intracytoplasmic sperm injection and assisted zona hatching.

INTRACYTOPLASMIC SPERM INJECTION

Intracytoplasmic sperm injection is a laboratory procedure developed to help infertile couples undergoing IVF due to male factor infertility. ICSI is a micromanipulation technique in which a single spermatozoon is injected directly into the cytoplasm of a mature (MII) oocyte using a glass micropipette.[26] This assisted fertilization technique increases the likelihood of fertilization when there are abnormalities in the number, quality, or function of the sperm.

Male infertility can be caused by a variety of abnormalities. Sperm can be completely absent from the ejaculate (azoospermia), present in low concentrations (oligozoospermia), have poor motility (asthenozoospermia), or have an increased percentage of abnormal shapes (teratozoospermia). There may also be functional abnormalities that prevent sperm from binding to and/or fertilizing the oocyte. ICSI bypasses several of the steps in the fertilization process, i.e., sperm binding to and penetrating through the zona pellucida and fusion of the spermatozoon with the oolemma. Because of this bypass, ICSI may facilitate fertilization by a spermatozoon with deficient motility parameters or anomalies of the acrosome.[27] Other indications for ICSI include the presence of antisperm antibodies, prior or repeated fertilization failure with standard IVF, use of frozen sperm, and obstruction of the male reproductive tract not amenable to surgical repair. In the latter instance, sperm may be obtained from the epididymis by a procedure called microsurgical epididymal sperm aspiration (MESA) or from the testis by testicular sperm extraction (TESE).

The ICSI procedure requires an inverted microscope with modulation contrast optics and a pair of micromanipulators. ICSI is commonly performed using a shallow petri dish in the center of which is a small drop of 7–10% polyvinylpyrrolidone (PVP) surrounded by six to eight drops of appropriately buffered culture medium. PVP is a viscous substance that is used to slow the sperm so that they can be examined for morphology, coat the inside of the glass micropipette to prevent the sperm from sticking to the glass during the procedure, and give more control over the fluid dynamics in the micropipette.[28] A small drop of sperm is placed in the PVP drop, and the oocytes to be injected are placed in the drops of buffered culture medium surrounding the PVP.

The glass micropipette on the right side of the microscope serves as the injection pipette. Using the micromanipulator, the injection pipette is lowered into the PVP drop and a small volume of PVP is aspirated. Subsequently, a morphologically normal spermatozoon displaying any motion is located in the PVP drop. A slight slashing motion is made with the injection pipette across the top of the tail to immobilize the spermatozoon and to induce intracellular changes that will contribute to the normal progression of fertilization events, e.g., oocyte activation and spermatozoon nuclear decondensation. The immobilized spermatozoon is aspirated tail first until it is completely inside the injection pipette. The injection pipette is then moved to one of the drops containing an oocyte.

The glass micropipette on the left side of the microscope serves as the holding pipette. Using the micromanipulator, the holding pipette is lowered into one of the oocyte drops and moved so that the opening of the pipette is adjacent to the mature oocyte. Gentle suction is applied using a microsyringe and the oocyte becomes affixed to the pipette. The oocyte is then rotated and positioned such that the polar body is at the 12 or 6 o'clock position while the holding pipette is at the 9 o'clock position. Continued gentle aspiration to the holding pipette keeps the oocyte in a fixed position. The injection pipette is moved to the 3 o'clock position at the equator of the oocyte, the aspirated spermatozoon is slowly moved to the distal tip of the pipette, and the pipette is then slowly inserted through the zona into the oocyte. Once the injection pipette is about halfway through the oocyte, a small volume of ooplasm is gently aspirated into the injection pipette until evidence of oolemma breakage, and the aspirated ooplasm and the spermatozoon are deposited in the center of the oocyte. The injection pipette is withdrawn slowly to ensure that the spermatozoon remains in the oocyte, pressure is released from the holding pipette, both the injection and holding pipettes are removed from the oocyte drop, and the entire process is repeated until all of the oocytes have been injected.

Fertilization occurs on average in 50–80% of injected oocytes. The ICSI process may infrequently cause mechanical damage to the oocyte, the likelihood of which may be influenced by characteristics of the injection pipette or the ICSI technique itself. Alternatively, the oocyte may possess innate characteristics that make it less resilient to the ICSI procedure, perhaps revealing a vulnerability that might otherwise have been expressed later in development. In addition, in a small percentage of cases, the fertilized oocyte may fail to divide or the embryo may arrest at an early stage of development. Whether the ICSI procedure is the cause of either type of failure cannot reliably be determined. Approximately 30% of all ICSI cycles performed in the United States in 2000 resulted in a live birth, which is comparable to rates seen with standard IVF.[29] Factors such as poor egg quality and advanced maternal age may result in lower rates of success while younger patients may achieve greater rates of success.

Because ICSI is a relatively new technique, long-term data concerning the future health and fertility of children conceived with ICSI are not yet available. Some studies have demonstrated that children conceived with ICSI did not perform differently on developmental tests at 2 years of age than those conceived following standard IVF, and that both groups performed better than the fertile control population.[30,31]

KEY POINT

ICSI is a major advance for IVF allowing fertilization even in the face of severe sperm deficiencies. Potential risk to the offspring appears minimal but is currently under investigation.

Current data do not support that ICSI carries an increased risk of genetic disorders in the offspring.[32] However, men with (severely) compromised semen parameters have a higher frequency of chromosomal abnormalities in their somatic cells and sperm, and current data show a slight but significant increase in sex chromosome abnormalities in offspring.[33] Further, since pregnancy can be achieved in couples where the man has Y-chromosome microdeletions (a cause of male infertility), it is likely that any male offspring will have similar Y-chromosome deletions and reproductive problems at adulthood. While these concerning issues merit continued monitoring, ICSI is still a major advance in the treatment of severe infertility.

ASSISTED ZONA HATCHING

The zona pellucida is an extracellular glycoprotein matrix surrounding oocytes/embryos that serves as a species-specific filter for fertilization and also as a protective barrier during early embryonic development. However, once a preimplantation stage embryo reaches the blastocyst stage, one of the last hurdles prior to implantation is hatching out of the zona pellucida. Failure of the embryo to hatch out of its encasing zona pellucida may be one of the factors that limit human reproductive efficiency.

AH has been hypothesized to increase implantation and pregnancy rates after IVF. Early studies by Cohen[34] found that mechanically opening the zona by PZD resulted in an increased implantation rate, and they suggested that opening the zona might facilitate the hatching process. A subsequent randomized, prospective study of AH using zona drilling with acidified Tyrode's medium demonstrated an increase in implantation rate when the procedure was selectively applied to embryos with a poor prognosis.[35]

Since these early reports, many ART programs have implemented AH in an attempt to improve implantation and pregnancy rates for their patients. The AH procedure is usually performed on day 3 postfertilization, and it involves the creation of a gap in the zona by either PZD with a glass micropipette, drilling with acidified Tyrode's medium, laser photoablation,[36] or use of a piezomicromanipulator.[37] The pregnancy success rates after using AH in different ART programs vary considerably. At a minimum, it appears that AH is beneficial to patients with two or more failed IVF attempts.[37–39]

Summary

IVF laboratories have come a long way since the birth of Louise Brown. Improvements in culture conditions and quality control as well as advancements in laboratory technology have made it possible for more patients than ever to have children. However, the IVF laboratory does not exist in a vacuum and it takes the collaboration and support of the entire team (physicians, nursing staff, clerical and administrative staff, and laboratory staff) to achieve success in an ART program.

REFERENCES

1 Bavister BD. Early history of in vitro fertilization. *Reproduction* 124:181, 2002.

2 Bavister BD. How animal embryo research led to the first documented human IVF. *Reprod Biomed Online* 4(Suppl. 1):24, 2002.

3 Go K. Quality control: a framework for the ART laboratory. In: Keel BA, May JV, DeJonge CJ (eds.), *Handbook of the Assisted Reproduction Laboratory.* Boca Raton, FL: CRC Press, 2000, p. 253.

4 Hill DL. Role of the in vitro fertilization laboratory in a negative pregnancy outcome. *Fertil Steril* 75:249, 2001.

5 Byrd W. Quality assurance in the reproductive biology laboratory. *Arch Pathol Lab Med* 116:418, 1992.

6 Ball GD. ART laboratory organization: size, layout, personnel and equipment. In: May JV (ed.), *Assisted Reproduction: Laboratory Considerations.* Philadelphia, PA: W.B. Saunders, 1998, p. 275.

7 Revised minimum standards for practices offering assisted reproductive technologies. *Fertil Steril* 80:1556, 2003.

8 Bongso A. *Handbook on Blastocyst Culture.* National University of Singapore Department of Obstetrics and Gynaecology, 1999.

9 Fleetham JA, Pattinson HA, Mortimer D. The mouse embryo culture system: improving the sensitivity for use as a quality control assay for human in vitro fertilization. *Fertil Steril* 59:192, 1993.

10 Ackerman SB, Swanson GK, Stokes RJ, et al. Culture of mouse preimplantation embryos as a quality control assay for human in vitro fertilization. *Gamete Res* 9:145, 1984.

11 Gorrill MJ, Rinehart JS, Ramhane AC, et al. Comparison of the hamster sperm motility assay to the mouse one-cell and two-cell embryo bioassays as quality control tests for in vitro fertilization. *Fertil Steril* 55:345, 1991.

12 Critchlow JD, Matson PL, Newman MC, et al. Quality control in an in vitro fertilization laboratory: use of human sperm survival studies. *Hum Reprod* 4:545, 1989.

13 Pool TB. Development of culture media for human assisted reproductive technology. *Fertil Steril* 81:287, 2004.

14 Pool TB, Atiee SH, Martin JE. Oocyte and embryo culture: basic concepts and recent advances. In: May JV (ed.), *Assisted Reproduction:*

Laboratory Considerations. Infertility and Reproductive Medicine Clinics of North America, vol. 9. Philadelphia, PA: W.B. Saunders, 1998, p. 181.

15 Quinn P. The development and impact of culture media for assisted reproductive technologies. *Fertil Steril* 81:27, 2004.

16 Hardy K, Hooper MAK, Handyside AH, et al. Non-invasive measurement of glucose and pyruvate uptake by individual human oocytes and preimplantation embryos. *Hum Reprod* 4:188, 1989.

17 Gardner DK, Lane M. Embryo culture systems. In Trounson A, Gardner DK (eds.), *Handbook of In Vitro Fertilization,* 2nd ed. Boca Raton, FL: CRC Press, 2000, p. 205.

18 Gardner DK. Mammalian embryo culture in the absence of serum or somatic cell support. *Cell Biol Int* 18:1163, 1994.

19 Behr B, Pool TB, Milki AA, et al. Preliminary clinical experience with human blastocyst development in vitro without co-culture. *Hum Reprod* 14:454, 1999.

20 Steptoe PC, Edwards RG. Birth after the reimplantation of a human embryo. *Lancet* 2:366, 1978.

21 Wiemer KE, Cohen J, Wiker SR, et al. Coculture of human zygotes on fetal bovine uterine fibroblasts: embryonic morphology and implantation. *Fertil Steril* 52:503, 1989.

22 Bongso A, Sakkas D, Gardner DK. Coculture of embryos with somatic helper cells. In: Trounson A, Gardner DK (eds.), *Handbook of In Vitro Fertilization,* 2nd ed. Boca Raton, FL: CRC Press, 2000, p. 181.

23 Gardner DK, Schoolcraft WB, Wagley L, et al. A prospective randomized trial of blastocyst culture and transfer in in-vitro fertilization. *Hum Reprod* 13:3434, 1998.

24 Veeck LL. *Atlas of the Human Oocyte and Early Conceptus*, vol. 2. Baltimore, MD: Williams & Wilkins, 1991.

25 Guelman V. Fertilization and cleavage. In: Patrizio P, Tucker MJ, Guelman V (eds.), *A Color Atlas for Human Assisted Reproduction: Laboratory and Clinical Insights*. Philadelphia, PA: Lippincott Williams & Wilkins, 2003, p. 49.

26 Lanzendorf SE, Malony MK, Veeck LL, et al. A preclinical evaluation of pronuclear formation by microinjection of human spermatozoa into human oocytes. *Fertil Steril* 49:835, 1988.

27 Palermo G, Joris H, Devroey P, et al. Pregnancies after intracytoplasmic injection of single spermatozoon into an oocyte. *Lancet* 340:17, 1992.

28 Palermo G, Joris H, Derde MP, et al. Sperm characteristics and outcome of human assisted fertilization by subzonal insemination and intracytoplasmic sperm injection. *Fertil Steril* 59:826, 1993.

29 Society for Assisted Reproductive Technology and the American Society for Reproductive Medicine: Assisted Reproductive Technology in the United States: 2000 results generated from the American Society for Reproductive Medicine/Society for Assisted Reproductive Technology Registry. *Fertil Steril* 81:1207, 2004.

30 Bonduelle M, Joris H, Hofmans K, et al. Mental development of 201 ICSI children at 2 years of age. *Lancet* 22:1553, 1998.

31 Bonduelle M, Canus M, De Vos A, et al. Seven years of intracytoplasmic sperm injection and follow-up of 1987 subsequent children. *Hum Reprod* 14(Suppl I):243, 1999.

32 American Society for Reproductive Medicine Practice Committee: Does intracytoplasmic sperm injection (ICSI) carry inherent genetic risks? Birmingham, AL: American Society for Reproductive Medicine, 1994.

33 Bonduelle M, Wilikens A, Buysse A, et al. Prospective follow-up study of 877 children born after intracytoplasmic sperm injection (ICSI), with ejaculated, epididymal and testicular spermatozoa and after replacement of cryopreserved embryos obtained after ICSI. *Hum Reprod* 11(Suppl. 4):131, 1996.

34 Cohen J. Zona pellucida micromanipulation and consequences for embryonic development and implantation. In: Cohen J, Malter HE, Talansky BE, et al. (eds.), *Micromanipulation of Human Gametes and Embryos.* New York, NY: Raven Press, 1991, p. 191.

35 Cohen J, Alikani M, Trowbridge J, et al. Implantation enhancement by selective assisted hatching using zona drilling of human embryos with poor prognosis. *Hum Reprod* 7:685, 1992.

36 Obruca A, Strohmer H, Sakkas D. Use of lasers in assisted fertilization and hatching. *Hum Reprod* 9:1723, 1994.

37 Nakayama T, Fujiwara H, Yamada S, et al. Clinical application of a new assisted hatching method using a piezomicromanipulator for morphologically low-quality embryos in poor-prognosis infertile patients. *Fertil Steril* 71:1014, 1999.

38 Chao KH, Chen SU, Chen HF, et al. Assisted hatching increases the implantation and pregnancy rate of in vitro fertilization-embryo transfer but not that of IVF-tubal embryo transfer in patients with repeated IVF failures. *Fertil Steril* 67:904, 1997.

39 Magli MC, Gianaroli L, Ferraretti AP, et al. Rescue of implantation potential in embryos with poor prognosis by assisted zona hatching. *Hum Reprod* 13:1331, 1998.

15

Assisted Reproductive Technologies: Oocyte and Embryo Cryopreservation

Shehua Shen

Introduction

Cryopreservation of embryos has become a standard procedure in assisted reproductive technology (ART) services. In order to maximize the chances of the pregnancy, a large number of embryos are generated for the purpose of embryo selection; on the other hand, the number of embryos transferred is typically minimized in order to avoid high-order multiple pregnancies. Routinely, there are many leftover embryos available for cryopreservation.

With cryopreservation of embryos, there are several immediate benefits:

1. Frozen embryo transfer (FET) can be used to greatly enhance the cumulative pregnancy rate for a single ovarian stimulation cycle.

2. Severe, prolonged ovarian hyperstimulation syndrome (OHSS) can be prevented by avoiding fresh embryo transfer (ET) altogether, if there is a high risk of OHSS in a cycle.
3. The implantation can be postponed if the uterine environment is not optimal, including bleeding and unfavorable endometrium with intracavitary fluid and/or polyps not previously identified.

According to the 2000 data from Center for Disease Control (CDC) Society for Assisted Reproductive Technology (SART), the live birth rate per ET was 31.6%. This data also recorded 13,083 cycles using frozen embryos. The live birth rate per thaw was 19.5% and the live birth rate per FET was 20.3%. Although the success rate from FET is lower than that from fresh ET, the procedure is less expensive and less invasive. FET has become widely accepted by both *in vitro* fertilization (IVF) programs and patients to augment the opportunity for pregnancy from a single ovarian stimulation cycle.

Clinically, endometrial preparation for the FET cycle includes two major approaches: a natural cycle or a controlled cycle with complete hormonal replacement. In a natural cycle, endogenous follicular growth and luteinizing hormone (LH) surge levels are monitored to predict a suitable day for transfer. Such cycles can be modified or more controlled by the use of clomiphene citrate, human menopausal gonadotropin (hMG), or human chorionic gonadotropin (hCG). A controlled cycle, with or without gonadotropin-releasing hormone analog to downregulate endogenous follicle-stimulating hormone (FSH)/LH, involves the use of exogenous replacement with estradiol and progesterone.[1]

KEY POINT

Cryopreservation has become an important tool to improve ART outcome and reduce multiple gestation.

It is noted, however, implantation potential is largely determined by embryo quality. The clinical outcome of FET relies highly on the optimal embryo culture system, cryopreservation technique including the type of cryoprotectant, the freezing protocol, and the embryo selection. Obviously, freezing poor quality embryos will lead to poor cryosurvival and implantation.[2] Since the first live births resulting from FET were reported in 1984 and 1985, the techniques for cryopreservation have been extensively studied and modified in order to achieve the best results. This technology is now widely used in ART laboratories.

The typical cryopreservation process involves the following steps: (1) an initial exposure to cryoprotectants; (2) cooling to subzero temperatures in a controlled manner; (3) storage in liquid nitrogen; (4) thawing and removal of the cryoprotectants to return to a physiologic environment. The cells must maintain their structural integrity throughout the whole process. It is noted that the species, the embryo developmental stage, the type of cryoprotectant used, and the method of cryopreservation will all play important roles in affecting the cryosurvival rate. The most crucial principle is to reduce the damage caused by intracellular ice formation, which is usually achieved by dehydrating the cells before and during the cooling procedure.

KEY POINT

Many ethical and legal issues may arise from the cryopreservation of surplus embryos.

In addition to all the technical challenges, many logistical, legal, moral, and ethical problems may arise. Both partners must sign comprehensive consent forms that include the understanding of the risk involved in the procedure, how long the embryos are to be stored, legal ownership, and disposition, in case of a divorce or a separation, death of one partner, or loss of contact between the couple and the clinic, and so on.

Principles of Cryobiology

The main source of cell damage during cryopreservation is intracellular ice formation. This is usually prevented by dehydrating the cell with a nonpermeating substances, such as sucrose, followed by the addition of a permeating cryoprotectant. Other damage can be caused by high concentration of solute and osmotic shock during dehydration and rehydration process.[3–5]

INTRACELLULAR ICE FORMATION

Intracellular ice formation can mechanically damage oocytes and embryos by disrupting and displacing organelles, or slicing through membranes.

About 80% of the cell content is water. The water in the cell can remain unfrozen at −5 to −15°C, which is called supercooling, i.e., cooling well below the freezing point without ice formation. Addition of cryoprotectants helps to reduce the extracellular freezing point, which means the extracellular solution can be supercooled as well. When solutions supercool, the dehydration process is slowed down because membrane permeation highly depends on temperature.[6,7] Therefore, when the temperature drops to the freezing point, ice crystals form quickly in the extracellular solution and quickly penetrate the cell, which can cause large ice crystal formation inside the cell before the cell dehydrates enough.

The degree of this supercooling relies on several factors including the presence of ice nucleators. The nucleators are the molecules that mimic the molecular structure of ice, expediting the building of an ice lattice. The best nucleator of ice is ice itself. "Seeding" is a procedure to initiate extracellular ice formation before supercooling. In another words, the goal is to introduce extracellular ice formation at a higher subzero temperature point. The consequence is that extracellular ice forms slowly in the solution, which causes further increase in solute concentration of the extracellular solution producing an osmotic pressure difference between two sides of the cell membrane. This contributes to further intracellular dehydration as water leaves the cell to achieve equilibrium with the extracellular environment. In this process the risk for ice spreading into intracellular compartment is small because the cell has a marginally higher solute concentration, therefore a lower freezing point than the extracellular solution. The cytoplasm will not freeze because of the absence of the ice nucleators. By the time the cell is plunged into liquid nitrogen, there is virtually no, or very little, water left in the cell to form ice crystals that are detrimental to the cell viability.

The human oocyte and embryo have relatively small ratios of the surface area to the unit volume and hold a substantial amount of intracellular water. It is absolutely critical to cool at a lower rate when slow cooling method is used.

KEY POINT

The prevention of intracellular ice formation, by dehydration of the cell, is critical to survival during cryopreservation.

At temperatures below −120°C, little if any ice crystal formation or growth can occur. As soon as the temperature is raised above this point, as during the thaw, new ice crystals will form and both new and existing ice crystals will grow, which is defined as recrystallization. The thawing protocol must be designed, according to the specific freezing protocol, in order to avoid recrystallization during the thaw.

SOLUTE DAMAGE

The solute damage (toxicity) is less understood. High concentrations of solute are used to dehydrate the cell and to prevent intracellular ice formation. The problem is that many cells are sensitive to the high concentration of solutes during a relatively slow cooling process. This may cause cell death (e.g., shrink dramatically and cellular disruption). Another source of damage is the chemical toxicity of high concentrations of electrolytes.[8] Addition of permeating cryoprotectants, such as glycerol or ethylene glycol, reduces the relative concentration of electrolyte in the solution through their colligative action and can help cells to survive.

OSMOTIC TOLERANCE Volume excursions that occur with addition and removal of cryoprotectants can be detrimental, especially during the nonequilibrium cooling which often requires a higher concentration of cryoprotectants. The cryoprotectant concentration in solution causes cell to shrink (by adding the cryoprotectants) or swell (by removing the cryoprotectants), sometimes beyond the physical limits of the cell membrane.

CRYOPROTECTANTS The role of the cryoprotectant is to protect the cell from damage by ice and high concentrations of solutes. When cells are placed into a solution containing a cryoprotectant, intracellular water exits as a result of the higher extracellular concentration of cryoprotectant. This causes a cell to shrink until osmotic equilibrium is reached by the slower diffusion of the cryoprotectant into the cell. Once equilibrium is reached, the cell resumes a normal appearance. The rate of permeation of the cryoprotectant and water is dependent on temperature. For example, equilibrium is achieved faster at higher temperatures. But cells are more sensitive to solute toxicity at higher temperatures. Therefore, most processes of moving embryos through cryopreservation solutions are carried out at room temperature. It is necessary to use even lower temperatures if very high concentration of cryoprotectant solutions are used, e.g., in vitrification.

Cryoprotectant is able to slightly lower the freezing point of the solution by 2–3°C. Since the cryoprotectants are not part of the ice during extracellular ice crystal formation, their concentration in relation to the remaining nonfrozen fraction progressively increases as the temperature falls. The solutes become concentrated in the nonfrozen fraction and can reach toxic levels, which may, further, result in irreversible changes to important molecules, e.g., enzymes. Cryoprotectants can reduce this toxicity and serve as a buffer by replacing the water molecules around enzyme.

Most currently used cryoprotectants for human embryo cryopreservation usually include one or more of the following permeating compounds: dimethyl sulphoxide (DMSO), propanediol (propylene glycol, PG), polyethylene glycol (PEG), or glycerol. They have a molecular weight between 63 and 97, and are very water-soluble. Which one to use depends on the cell development stage or cryopreservation method, e.g., PG is commonly used for cleavage stage embryo freezing and glycerol is usually the cryoprotectant for blastocyst freezing. In order to achieve a better result of dehydrating and protect cells from osmotic shock, cryoprotectant additives are usually used. They are large molecules that do not penetrate cell membrane. Sucrose and ficoll are commonly used cryoprotectant additives, as are proteins and lipoproteins. Some other biological fluids such as egg yolk, milk, or serum also can be used as cryoprotectant additives. It has been established that at least one macromolecule in the freezing solution helps reduce the cell physical damage in particularly the zona pellucida; however, these macromolecules cannot be used alone. Buffer solution has to be used to maintain intracellular pH value. Either N-1-hydroxy ethylpiperazine-N'-1-ethanesulfonic acid (HEPES) buffered medium or Dulbecco's phosphate buffered saline (DPBS) can be used.

Generally speaking, extracellular solute concentration, constituents of permeating and nonpermeating solutes, and the rate of temperature changes are the important variables to control the cryoprotectant optimal effect.

KEY POINT

The selection of cryoprotectant is chosen based on the cell stage to be frozen and the specific protocol.

SEEDING

When slow cooling is used for oocytes or embryos, it is critical to prevent the rapid ice crystal formation during supercooling. An ice crystal is usually introduced in a controlled fashion (at temperature between −5 and −8°C) by touching the wall of the straw or vial with a cold object, e.g., forceps or cotton swabs dipped in liquid nitrogen. Typically, the first ice crystals are created relatively far away from the embryos. Once the ice formation has been initiated, the ice propagates itself from the starting point throughout the rest of the solution slowly, which furthers the dehydration process.

In summary, the goal of the freezing techniques is to use the cryoprotectants and control ice formation at critical temperatures. Cooling too quickly results in cells which cannot lose water fast enough to prevent intracellular ice formation. Cooling too slowly means that cells are exposed to high concentrations of salts and other solutes longer than necessary, thereby reducing the survival rate due to solute toxicity. Therefore, controlling the initial composition of the freezing media, controlling the rates of cooling and warming, and controlling the temperature at which the cells are plunged into liquid nitrogen are the ways to reduce the damage caused by intracellular ice formation and solute toxicity. The detailed optimal cooling rate has to be specific for each cell type. Even for a single cell type, there will be species differences, because the composition and permeability characteristics of the cell membrane are different and the surface-to-volume ratio is also different. In addition, both the temperature and the difference in osmotic pressure between the two sides of the membrane play important roles in setting an optimal cooling rate. Optimal cooling rate for human embryos is around 0.3–0.5°C/min. Different cooling mechanisms and their associated outcomes are listed in Table 15-1.

THAW

KEY POINT

Thaw rate is dependent on the freezing protocol and the cryoprotectants used.

A successful thaw must prevent recrystalization. Slow thaw or quick thaw methods are developed to achieve the same goal. Slow thaw protocols involve holding the straw in the air (room temperature) for 2 min or longer until all ice crystals are completely thawed. Quick thaw refers to plunging the straw into a 37°C water bath after only seconds at room temperature. Optimal warming rates depend on the cell type, the cryoprotectant used, and the amount of water remaining (which depends on the cooling procedure). From −196 to −120°C, if the straw is warmed up too quickly, the cell survival rate is reduced. This is possibly due to the brittleness of the straw contents at this temperature and to the fact that cells are prone to stress fractures. Two steps of thawing are usually performed: holding the straw in the air for seconds, to reduce the brittleness, then plunging the straw in water bath. The specific times depend on the freezing protocol previously used.

Materials and Methods

Cryopreservation of embryos requires a sophisticated laboratory arrangement. The cryopreservation itself is done in a programmable freezer. These units consist of not only the freezer unit and a source of liquid nitrogen, but also a computer which orchestrates

Table 15-1. **COOLING RATES VS. OUTCOME**

Type of Cooling	Cooling Rate (°C/min)	Definition	Description	Outcome
High rate cooling	10	Supercooling	Below nucleation temperature	Large ice crystal form Cell damage occurs No survival
Moderate rate cooling	2–10	Supercooling	Above nucleation temperature	Small ice crystal form, which may not be lethal, but may recrystallize on warming Cell damage occurs
Slow cooling	0.5	Equilibrium cooling	Extracellular pure water freezing Increasing the solution tonicity Decreasing the extracelullar chemicals Osmotic pressure drives water to leave the cell	Cell shrinks (decrease the amount of freezable water inside the cell) Intracellular chemicals decrease Cell may survive Disadvantage is the extended long exposure to high concentration of solute and cryoprotectants
Slow cooling	0.5	Nonequilibrium cooling	Cell dehydrates significantly The remaining cellular solution forms an amorphous glass-like solid undergoing vitrification (based on membrane integrity and initial cell division)	Efficient cell dehydration and shorter exposure to high concentration of solutes Disadvantage is the dramatic osmotic shock both during addition and removing of cryoprotectants
Ultrarapid cooling		Very rapid cooling	No dehydration High concentrations of cryoprotectants Rapid thaw in 37°C water bath	If no intracellular ice crystals, it is actually a vitrification procedure
Vitrification		Super-rapid cooling	High concentrations of cryoprotectants Very small volume	No intracellular ice crystals Cryoprotectant toxicity is the main concern. It

(*Continued*)

Table 15-1.   COOLING RATES VS. OUTCOME (CONTINUED)

TYPE OF COOLING	COOLING RATE (°C/MIN)	DEFINITION	DESCRIPTION	OUTCOME
			(<1 µL) results in both rapid and uniform heat exchange Solidify without the formation of ice crystals High rates of cooling prevent chilling damage	can be prevented at a lower temperature; however, lower temperature compromises the rate of diffusion of cryoprotectant across the cell membrane

the freezing process precisely for each stage of the cryopreservation process.

Embryos can be stored in liquid nitrogen (–196°C) without loss of viability for decades. There is virtually no movement of atoms and molecules at or below –196°C. Liquid nitrogen is potentially dangerous and must be handled with care.[5] Pure nitrogen gas can asphyxiate living organisms, therefore, tanks must be stored in a well-ventilated area. Oxygen concentration monitoring is also needed. Eye and hand protection must be worn to prevent frostbite. Liquid nitrogen spillage can damage a vinyl floor so covering the floor with metal sheets is recommended. Spills of liquid nitrogen can saturate a person's clothing, therefore, the affected clothing or shoes should be removed immediately to prevent cryoburn. A temperature monitoring system is required to make sure the liquid nitrogen in the storage tanks is sufficient. Since virus can be transmitted inside liquid nitrogen storage tanks,[9] infected specimens should be stored in specific identified tanks, or stored in the vapor phase of liquid nitrogen. However, the temperature in the vapor phase must be monitored carefully since a rise in temperature even as low as –130°C can compromise the frozen samples.

Plastic straws, plastic vials, or glass ampoules are used for holding the specimens. The size of the straw (0.25 mL versus 0.5 mL) may affect the cryopreservation outcome since differences may cause differences in heat transmission. Glass ampoules are no longer commonly used because they can be fragile or explode if not handled properly. Straws can be sealed by heat, polyvinal alcohol, or polyvinalpyrrolidone powder.[4]

Embryo Cryopreservation

IMPORTANCE OF EMBRYO STAGE

Embryos can be frozen at different developmental stages, i.e., 2 pronuclear stage (day 1 after fertilization), day 2, day 3, or at the blastocyst stage. It has been shown that the survival rate is better if the embryos are frozen at an earlier stage rather than a later stage, i.e., embryos frozen at 2 pronuclear stage tend to survive better than those frozen at a later stage. Numerous studies have confirmed that the embryo survival rate is similar regardless whether the embryos are generated from conventional IVF or intracytoplasmic sperm injection (ICSI), and it can reach an average of 80–90%.[10]

ZYGOTES (2 PRONUCLEAR)

Freezing at this stage has shown satisfactory results,[11] e.g., the survival rate after thaw for zygotes is consistently higher than that for embryos frozen at any other stages. One explanation is that the zygote lacks of a spindle. Technically, it is much easier to assess whether a zygote has survived the thaw, because it is a single cell, and less than 5% of the zygotes will survive the thaw and fail to cleave. It is important to freeze the zygotes before their pronuclei breakdown. Otherwise, freezing zygotes at the syngamy stage (when the male and female pronuclei have fused) will have a negative impact. Freezing the pronuclear stage embryos before syngamy has been suggested.[12]

The disadvantage of freezing at the zygote stage is a decrease in the number of fresh embryos for embryo selection. Furthermore, because morphologic parameters to aid in the selection of 2 pronuclear zygotes have not been optimized, zygotes with poor development potential are sometimes frozen leading to poor clinical outcome (Figs. 15-1 and 15-2).

EMBRYOS AT CLEAVAGE STAGE

Embryos can be frozen successfully at almost any cleavage stages, e.g., from 2-cell to 8-cell and at almost anytime. Also better embryo selection becomes possible because both morphology and growth

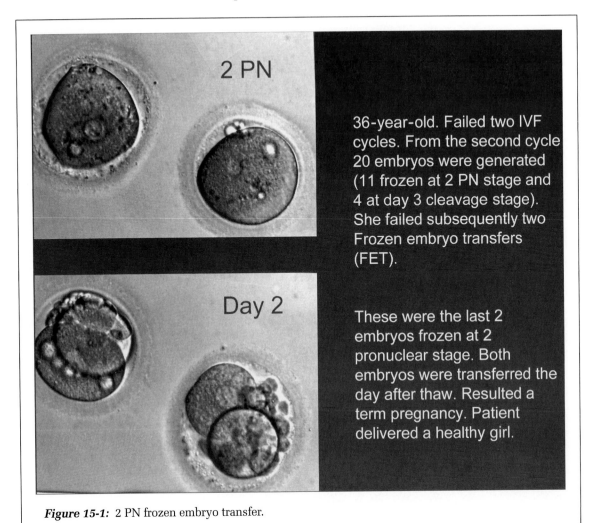

2 PN

36-year-old. Failed two IVF cycles. From the second cycle 20 embryos were generated (11 frozen at 2 PN stage and 4 at day 3 cleavage stage). She failed subsequently two Frozen embryo transfers (FET).

Day 2

These were the last 2 embryos frozen at 2 pronuclear stage. Both embryos were transferred the day after thaw. Resulted a term pregnancy. Patient delivered a healthy girl.

Figure 15-1: 2 PN frozen embryo transfer.

rate of the embryos are known. However, it is more difficult to evaluate whether an embryo has survived the thaw, because it has multiple cells, and not necessarily all the blastomeres will survive the freezing and thawing. Generally, an embryo demonstrating >50% survival of blastomeres after thaw is considered a survivor. It is observed that fully intact embryos demonstrate a higher implantation rate than partially intact ones. However, a live birth from FET when only one single blastomere survived the thaw has been reported.[13] Freezing and thawing protocols for cleavage stage embryo are similar to the ones for zygotes (Figs. 15-3 and 15-4).

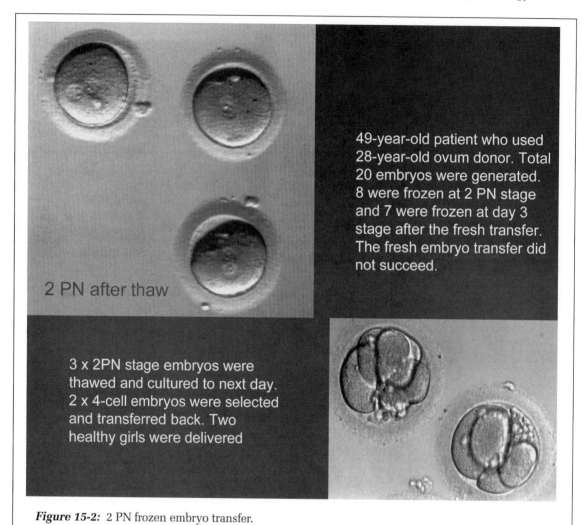

49-year-old patient who used 28-year-old ovum donor. Total 20 embryos were generated. 8 were frozen at 2 PN stage and 7 were frozen at day 3 stage after the fresh transfer. The fresh embryo transfer did not succeed.

2 PN after thaw

3 x 2PN stage embryos were thawed and cultured to next day. 2 x 4-cell embryos were selected and transferred back. Two healthy girls were delivered

Figure 15-2: 2 PN frozen embryo transfer.

BLASTOCYST

Blastocyst stage embryos are usually cryopreserved in glycerol-based solutions. It is yet to be established whether ethylene glycol would be more suitable than glycerol. Ethylene glycol has potential advantages over glycerol because it penetrates embryos significantly faster minimizing problems of osmotic shock. The physical properties of ethylene glycol are known to be different from propanediol, and it has been reported that embryos previously frozen in propanediol, having survived the thaw, could be killed when frozen in ethylene glycol.[5]

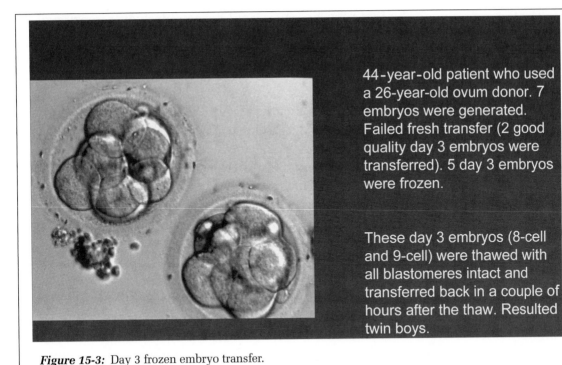

44-year-old patient who used a 26-year-old ovum donor. 7 embryos were generated. Failed fresh transfer (2 good quality day 3 embryos were transferred). 5 day 3 embryos were frozen.

These day 3 embryos (8-cell and 9-cell) were thawed with all blastomeres intact and transferred back in a couple of hours after the thaw. Resulted twin boys.

Figure 15-3: Day 3 frozen embryo transfer.

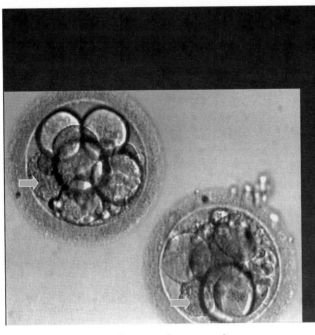

35-year-old. 6 embryos total. 2 embryos (9-cell grade 3 and 8-cell grade 2) were transferred 3 days after egg retrieval and resulted no pregnancy. 2 embryos were frozen after fresh transfer (8-cell grade 3 and 6-cell grade 3). 2 embryos with poor quality were discarded.

Both embryos were thawed with some blastomeres lysed. A singleton pregnancy was resulted from this FET.

Arrows indicate the lysed blasotmeres.

Figure 15-4: Day 3 frozen embryo transfer.

The first report of successful human blastocyst freezing dates back to 1985. A slow freezing protocol, with glycerol as the cryoprotectant, has been used to freeze blastocysts. However, the implantation rate of frozen blastocyst transfers is approximately half of that reported for the transfer of fresh blastocysts. By changing the starting temperature from room temperature to –6°C, the cooling rate of 2°C/min followed by 0.3°C/min to a cooling rate 0.5°C/min, and combining culture in hyaluronon-based media, a much higher implantation rate has recently been achieved.[14,15] Vitrification of the blastocyst has also been studied with post-thaw survival rates comparable to those for embryos frozen at cleavage stages. Vitrification uses very high concentrations of cryoprotectants such that, when cooled rapidly, the cell will be solidified in a glass state without the formation of ice crystals. Monosaccharides may be more effective than disaccharides when added to penetrating cryoprotectants, because they are less toxic to embryos and can form a stable glass at lower total solute concentrations. The success of vitrification procedures has been enhanced by techniques that substantially increase the cooling rate by vitrifying on electron microscope grids, thinly walled straws, and a nylon cryoloop. In the nylon cryoloop technique, the open system lacks any thermoinsulating layer. This, coupled with a small volume of <1 µL, results in both rapid and uniform heat exchange during cooling, which is very important in preventing chilling injury to sensitive cells (Fig. 15-5).[16]

Oocyte Cryopreservation

Before 1997, the only option for preserving female fertility after treatment for malignant disease was a full IVF treatment with cryopreservation of embryos (fertilized eggs) prior to the initiation of chemotherapy. This strategy raises the risk of creating embryos with higher chance of being orphaned. It is also only acceptable for women with a current partner. The young women who are often seeking fertility preservation may not be involved in a stable relationship at the time of their diagnosis. Oocyte cryopreservation has become very attractive, in theory, for those young or single women facing cancer treatments. It also offers an alternative for couples with religious or personal convictions that

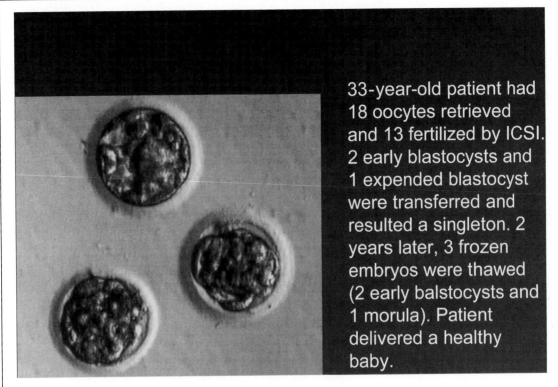

33-year-old patient had 18 oocytes retrieved and 13 fertilized by ICSI. 2 early blastocysts and 1 expended blastocyst were transferred and resulted a singleton. 2 years later, 3 frozen embryos were thawed (2 early balstocysts and 1 morula). Patient delivered a healthy baby.

Figure 15-5: Blastocyst cryopreservation.

prevent them from considering embryo cryopreservation. Furthermore, the demand for preserving fertility in the healthy young women who wish to delay reproductive process has also been growing.[17]

In mid-1980s, a few pregnancies after oocyte freeze-thaw and fertilization were reported. However, extremely low oocyte survival rates, and even lower fertilization and pregnancy rates, prevented the technique from being adopted clinically.

Human oocytes are particularly susceptible to freeze-thaw damage due to their size and complexity. (1) The meiotic spindle apparatus is highly temperature sensitive and depolymerizes with temperature reduction. Abnormal spindle organization after thawing may result in the presence of "stray" chromosomes in cytoplasm. (2) Premature cortical granule release with subsequent zona hardening and parthenogenetic activation. This zona hardening will also decrease the likelihood for fertilization with standard insemination techniques. (3) Oocytes are less permeable to cryoprotectants than zygotes so that they are far more likely to be damaged by osmotic shock than zygotes.

An alternative approach is the freezing of immature eggs containing a germinal vesicle (GV). Meiosis is arrested in prophase I of the dictyate stage, with the chromosomes located within a membrane bound nucleus or germinal vesicle, eliminating the risk of damaging the microtubules of the meiotic spindle. Nevertheless, there is still the risk of zona hardening and damage to the cytoskeleton, *plus* the challenges of *in vitro* maturation (IVM).

In mid-1990s, propanediol and sucrose were used to freeze human oocytes and achieve a recovery rate of 64%, with normal spindle and chromosome configuration after thawing. ICSI was used to overcome the zona hardening, and 50% fertilization with normal karyotypes was reported. In the late-1990s, more live births after oocyte cryopreservation were reported. Further investigation concluded that better survival rates occurred with cumulus enclosed, compared to denuded oocytes, and that increasing the concentration of nonpermeating sucrose further improved survival rates. Current data would support a 60% survival rate and 64% fertilization rate.[18] Listed in Table 15-2 are the most recent clinical outcomes for oocyte cryopreservation.

ICSI is recommended for insemination since the hardening of the zona pellucida after cryopreservation significantly decreases fertilization rate with standard insemination. The cumulus is removed after 1 h of culture. Survived oocytes are defined as intact zona pellucida and plasma membrane, clear periviteline space of normal size, no evidence of cytoplasmic leakage or oocyte shrinkage. ICSI is performed after 2–3 hours culture.

Although oocyte cryopreservation is a viable option in ART, the overall survival rate is about 60%, lower than the rates seen for human embryos which typically reach 85% or higher. The clinical pregnancy rate still remains low, such that only about 1–2% of frozen oocytes will result in a live birth. However, it is encouraging that, to date, all infants resulting from frozen oocytes are healthy (Fig. 15-6).

***Table 15-2.* RECENT PREGNANCY OUTCOME FROM
OOCYTE CRYOPRESERVATION**

AUTHOR	YEAR	CRYO METHOD	CRYO DETAIL	PREGNANCY
Porcu et al.[23]	1997	Slow freezing	12 oocytes frozen 4 survived thaw 2 fertilized by ICSI 1 cleaved to 4-cell	A healthy girl
Tucker et al.[24]	1998	Slow freezing	13 GV were frozen 3 survived thaw None of the MII did 2 fertilized by ICSI	A healthy girl
Antinori et al.[25]	1998	Slow freezing	MII were frozen 56% survival rate 75% cleaved after fertilization	2/37 ET were resulted pregnancies
Young et al.[26]	1998	Slow freezing	8 oocytes from donor were frozen 5 embryos transferred	Triplets Patient terminated pregnancy at 10 weeks
Porcu et al.[27]	1999	Slow freezing	1502 oocytes thawed 54% survived 58% fertilized 91% cleaved	9/112 cycle resulted pregnancy 11 healthy children
Cha et al.[28]	1999	Vitrification	MII oocytes 7 survived 6 fertilized 6 transferred	Singleton
Kuleshova et al.[29]	1999	Vitrification	Donor oocytes 40% ethylene glycol	A healthy pregnancy
Yoon et al.[30]	2000	Vitrification	MII oocytes	3/7 ET
Porcu et al.[31]	2001	Slow freezing		4 more healthy children

Ovarian Tissue Cryopreservation

Cryopreservation, and subsequent transplantation, of ovarian tissue are attractive strategies for fertility conservation for women or children who are faced with sterilizing chemotherapy, radiotherapy, or radical reproductive surgery. Oocyte freezing may not be the best approach for cancer patients because frequently they do not have enough time to complete a stimulated cycle before cancer

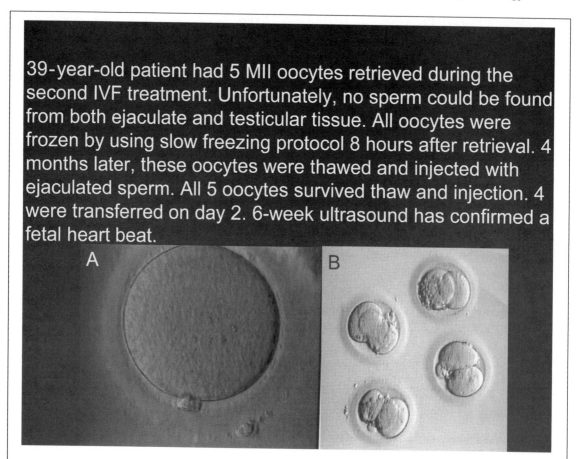

39-year-old patient had 5 MII oocytes retrieved during the second IVF treatment. Unfortunately, no sperm could be found from both ejaculate and testicular tissue. All oocytes were frozen by using slow freezing protocol 8 hours after retrieval. 4 months later, these oocytes were thawed and injected with ejaculated sperm. All 5 oocytes survived thaw and injection. 4 were transferred on day 2. 6-week ultrasound has confirmed a fetal heart beat.

Figure 15-6: Oocyte cryopreservation.

treatment. Also, given the limited number of oocytes that would be retrieved in a single cycle, and the still poor pregnancy rates with cryopreserved oocytes, preservation of fertility may be limited. Ovarian biopsy or oophorectomy can be carried out at any age and any stage of menstrual cycle. Small pieces such as 1 mm^3 of ovarian cortex contain large numbers of primordial follicles, which theoretically can either be later returned to the patient by grafting or cultured *in vitro* to generate oocytes for IVF. Oocytes in primordial follicles have very different properties compared to mature oocytes. They are very small, only about 1% of the size of a mature metaphase II (MII) oocyte. They are less differentiated with fewer organelles and no zona pellucida and no cortical granules. Lastly, they are arrested in prophase (lower risk of carrying cytogenetic errors).[4]

High rates of survival after freeze-thaw have been reported in mice, sheep, and human ovaries. When isolated primordial follicles are transferred in the mouse, or ovarian tissue slices are grafted into sheep, it is possible to obtain follicular survival with subsequent maturation, estrogen secretion, and restoration of fertility to the hosts. In 1999, University of Leeds reported the first study that human ovarian heterotopic autografting resulted in a survival rate of 27% and follicles were identified in all grafts.[4]

Current literature and research presentations suggest reasonable survival with freezing and thawing, but there is significant loss of viable tissue with the grafting procedure and reestablishment of vascularization. There are also questions about the safety of transferring tissue from a patient with active malignancy back into a patient with remission. Transmission of malignant cells from a transplanted ovary in an animal model has been documented.[19]

The other option is to perform *in vitro* maturation in the laboratory. However, the primordial follicle requires about 120 days for development in the human ovary. Recreating this process in the petri dish, while shortened, remains complex. There are very little animal data available for review. Prior to 2003, only one such birth had occurred. With aging, this animal appeared to have growth and neurologic health problems.[20]

The theory of how the cryopreserved ovarian tissue could be used after a successful recovery is shown in Fig. 15-7. While significant advances have been reported in this field, much more effort is needed to perfect this technology before it can be safely adopted clinically.

Risk of Cryopreservation

It is possible in theory to store oocytes or embryos at −196°C without loss of viability for decades. There is virtually no movement of atoms and molecules at −196°C. At approximately −130°C, atoms and molecules are able to move. Temperature of −90°C allows ice crystal formation. Therefore, short exposure to this temperature can cause lethal damage to embryos.[5]

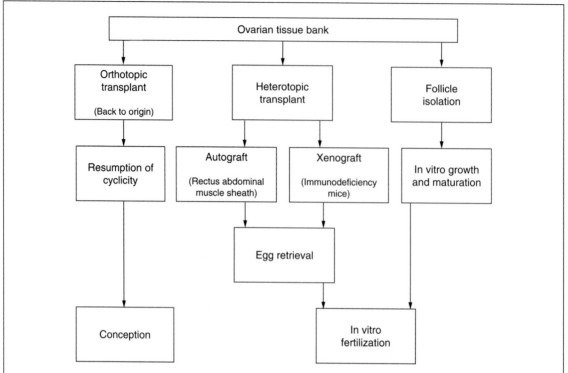

Figure 15-7: Theoretic options for the use of cryopreserved human ovarian tissue. (*Source*: Oktay K, et al. Cryopreservation of immature human oocytes and ovarian tissue: an emerging technology? Fertil Steril, Vol. 69, p. 5, 1998, with permission from The American Society for Reproductive Medicine.)

KEY POINT

The health of babies born from cryopreserved embryos appears to be no different from that seen in fresh ART cycles.

It has been demonstrated that the infectious agents such as viruses can be spread through liquid nitrogen. This is known to have caused hepatitis.[9] The risk can be significantly reduced if storing in liquid nitrogen vapor or −140 to −150°C biological freezers. But the effect on oocytes or embryos with long-term storage at those temperature conditions is clear. Embryos or eggs can be killed during cryopreservation process. Suboptimal cryopreservation can cause chromosomal anomalies, perturb the cell microtubules, cause parthenogenetic activation, and perturb fertilization process and cleavage. Fortunately, the clinical outcome from FET has been encouraging. A study from 283 babies resulting from cryopreserved embryos found no difference in the perinatal statistics and a statistically lower incidence of major congenital malformations as compared to a group of babies derived from fresh embryo transfer after IVF (1% versus 3%).[22]

REFERENCES

1 Tucker MJ, et al. *Cryopreservation of human embryos and oocytes. Curr Opin Obstet Gynecol* 7(3):188–192, 1995.

2 Trounson A, Jones G. *Freezing of embryos: early vs late stages. J Assist Reprod Genet* 10(3):179–181, 1993.

3 Johnson CA, Crister JK, Leibo SP, Toner M. *Embryo and Oocyte Cryopreservation: Fundamental Principles, Gamete Biology, and Developmental Strategies.* Seattle: American Society for Reproductive Medicine, Course 10, 2002.

4 Elder K, DB. *In Vitro Fertilization.* Cambridge, UK: Cambridge, 2000.

5 Trounson AO, GD. *Handbook of In Vitro Fertilization,* 2nd ed. Boca Raton, FL: CRC Press, 1999.

6 Paynter SJ, Fuller BJ, Shaw RW. *Temperature dependence of mature mouse oocyte membrane permeabilities in the presence of cryoprotectant. Cryobiology* 34(2):122–130, 1997.

7 Paynter SJ, et al. *Permeability characteristics of human oocytes in the presence of the cryoprotectant dimethylsulphoxide. Hum Reprod* 14(9):2338–2342, 1999.

8 Stachecki JJ, Cohen J, Willadsen S. *Detrimental effects of sodium during mouse oocyte cryopreservation. Biol Reprod* 59(2):395–400, 1998.

9 Tedder RS, et al. *Hepatitis B transmission from contaminated cryopreservation tank. Lancet* 346(8968):137–140, 1995.

10 Hu Y, et al. *A comparison of post-thaw results between cryopreserved embryos derived from intracytoplasmic sperm injection and those from conventional IVF. Fertil Steril* 72(6):1045–1048, 1999.

11 Veeck LL, et al. *Significantly enhanced pregnancy rates per cycle through cryopreservation and thaw of pronuclear stage oocytes. Fertil Steril* 59(6):1202–1207, 1993.

12 Ginsburg KA, et al. *Tetraploidy associated with human pronuclear embryo cryopreservation: a case report. J Assist Reprod Genet* 9(5):484–488, 1992.

13 Edgar DH, et al. *A quantitative analysis of the impact of cryopreservation on the implantation potential of human early cleavage stage embryos. Hum Reprod* 15(1):175–179, 2000.

14 Gardner DK, et al. *Changing the start temperature and cooling rate in a slow-freezing protocol increases human blastocyst viability. Fertil Steril* 79(2):407–410, 2003.

15 Lane M, et al. *Cryo-survival and development of bovine blastocysts are enhanced by culture with recombinant albumin and hyaluronan. Mol Reprod Dev* 64(1):70–78, 2003.

16 Lane M, Schoolcraft WB, Gardner DK. *Vitrification of mouse and human blastocysts using a novel cryoloop container-less technique.* Fertil Steril 72(6):1073–1078, 1999.

17 Oktay K, Kan MT, Rosenwaks Z. *Recent progress in oocyte and ovarian tissue cryopreservation and transplantation.* Curr Opin Obstet Gynecol 13(3):263–268, 2001.

18 Fabbri R, et al. *Human oocyte cryopreservation: new perspectives regarding oocyte survival.* Hum Reprod 16(3):411–416, 2001.

19 Shaw JM, et al. *Fresh and cryopreserved ovarian tissue samples from donors with lymphoma transmit the cancer to graft recipients.* Hum Reprod 11(8):1668–1673, 1996.

20 Eppig JJ, O'Brien MJ. *Comparison of preimplantation developmental competence after mouse oocyte growth and development in vitro and in vivo.* Theriogenology 49(2):415–422, 1998.

21 Oktay K, et al. *Cryopreservation of immature human oocytes and ovarian tissue: an emerging technology?* Fertil Steril 69(1):1–7, 1998.

22 Wada I, et al. *Birth characteristics and perinatal outcome of babies conceived from cryopreserved embryos.* Hum Reprod 9(3):543–546, 1994.

23 Porcu E, et al. *Birth of a healthy female after intracytoplasmic sperm injection of cryopreserved human oocytes.* Fertil Steril 68(4):724–726, 1997.

24 Tucker MJ, Wright G, Morton PC, Massey JB. *Birth after cryopreservation of immature oocytes with subsequent in vitro maturation.* Fertil Steril 70(3):578–579, 1998.

25 Antinori S, Dani G, Selman HA, et al. *Pregnancies after sperm injection into cryopreserved human oocytes.* In: *Proceedings of the 14th Annual Meeting of Eshre,* Göteborg, 1998.

26 Young E, et al. *Triplet pregnancy after intracytoplasmic sperm injection of cryopreserved oocytes: case report.* Fertil Steril 70(2):360–361, 1998.

27 Porcu E, Fabbri R, Ciotti PM, et al. *Cycles of human oocyte cryopreservation and intracytoplasmic sperm injection: results of 112 cycles.* Abstract, Fertility and Sterility, 1999.

28 Cha KY, Han SY, Chung HM, et al. *Pregnancy and Implantation from vitrified oocytes following in vitro fertilization (IVF) and in vitro culture (IVC).* Abstract Fertility and Sterility, 1999.

29 Kuleshova L, et al. *Birth following vitrification of a small number of human oocytes: case report.* Hum Reprod 14(12):3077–3079, 1999.

30 Yoon TK, et al. *Pregnancy and delivery of healthy infants developed from vitrified oocytes in a stimulated in vitro fertilization-embryo transfer program.* Fertil Steril 74(1):180–181, 2000.

31 Porcu E, Fabbri R, Ciotti P, et al. *Four healthy children from human oocytes and frozen human sperms.* Orlando: Abstract, Fertility and Sterility, 2001.

Oocyte Donation

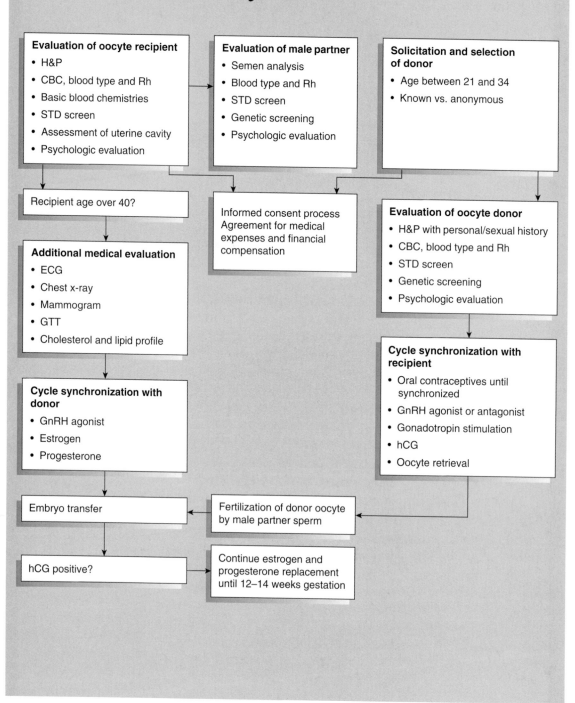

Evaluation of oocyte recipient
- H&P
- CBC, blood type and Rh
- Basic blood chemistries
- STD screen
- Assessment of uterine cavity
- Psychologic evaluation

Evaluation of male partner
- Semen analysis
- Blood type and Rh
- STD screen
- Genetic screening
- Psychologic evaluation

Solicitation and selection of donor
- Age between 21 and 34
- Known vs. anonymous

Recipient age over 40?

Informed consent process
Agreement for medical expenses and financial compensation

Evaluation of oocyte donor
- H&P with personal/sexual history
- CBC, blood type and Rh
- STD screen
- Genetic screening
- Psychologic evaluation

Additional medical evaluation
- ECG
- Chest x-ray
- Mammogram
- GTT
- Cholesterol and lipid profile

Cycle synchronization with recipient
- Oral contraceptives until synchronized
- GnRH agonist or antagonist
- Gonadotropin stimulation
- hCG
- Oocyte retrieval

Cycle synchronization with donor
- GnRH agonist
- Estrogen
- Progesterone

Embryo transfer

Fertilization of donor oocyte by male partner sperm

hCG positive?

Continue estrogen and progesterone replacement until 12–14 weeks gestation

16 Oocyte Donation

Jane I. Ruman
Mark V. Sauer

Introduction

Oocyte donation in humans began as a treatment for infertility in the early 1980s with the first reports of successful pregnancies and births following the transfer of donated embryos fertilized *in vitro* and *in vivo*.[1,2] Refinements in egg donation evolved rapidly, as improvements in endometrial stimulation of functionally agondal recipients, synchronization of donor-recipient cycles, and oocyte recovery techniques were introduced. Coupled with the sharply increasing efficiency and success of in vitro fertilization (IVF), a heightened demand for egg donation soon arose. Today oocyte donation affords women with ovarian failure, advanced reproductive age, heritable conditions, or recurrent implantation failure the ability to conceive. Over 6509 fresh donor oocyte cycles were performed in the United States in 1999, accounting for roughly 10% of all IVF cycles initiated that year.[3] This chapter reviews both the technical and clinical aspects of egg donation, including indications for treatment, recipient screening, recruitment and screening of donors, and synchronization of donor-recipient cycles. Ethical, psychosocial, and legal aspects of care are also referenced throughout the text; however, a detailed account of these issues is beyond the scope of this review.

Guiding Questions

- What is the likelihood for a successful pregnancy if a patient is to use her own oocytes compared with the use of donated oocytes?

- What aspects of the recipient's health and history need to be investigated prior to proceeding through a cycle?
- What makes for a "good" oocyte donor?

INDICATIONS FOR OOCYTE DONATION

Initially envisioned as an infertility therapy for young women with premature ovarian failure, oocyte and embryo donation are now commonly used to treat a broad array of conditions. Due to dismal success rates, conventional IVF (without donor oocytes) is not recommended for women above the age of 45. Therefore, patients older than 45 years desiring to bear a child should be triaged to oocyte donation. Although controversial, even younger patients who repeatedly fail to perform well with conventional IVF, may wish to consider egg donation, due to its high success rate. The majority of patients conceive following repetitive attempts at oocyte donation, reflecting the paramount biologic importance of genotype and age of the oocyte for the successful establishment of pregnancy (see Table 16-1).

Table 16-1. **GUIDING QUESTIONS TO DETERMINE IDEAL CANDIDATES FOR OOCYTE DONATION**

ASSESSMENT OF THE RECIPIENT	ASSESSMENT OF THE DONOR
Does the potential recipient have a history of gonadal dysgenesis or an inheritable disorder that would preclude her from using her own eggs for pregnancy?	Is the donor between the age of 20 and 35 and free of any inheritable conditions?
If the patient desiring pregnancy is over the age of 45, or has already undergone natural menopause, is she free of any major medical illness or condition that would jeopardize her or her fetus during pregnancy?	Is the donor physically healthy, and not at high risk for sexually transmitted infections or transmissible spongiform encephalopathies (TSEs)?
Does the potential recipient have indications of limited ovarian reserve or premature ovarian failure?	Is the donor psychologically stable and able to comply with the vigorous ongoing requirements of the egg donation cycle?
Does the potential recipient have a history of repeated IVF failure?	Is the donor willing and able to comply with strict contraceptive measures during and immediately following the cycle?
Are the recipient and her partner psychologically stable with a strong family support system?	Does the donor, if anonymous, possess phenotypic characteristics compatible with the recipient?

KEY POINT

Oocyte donation offers high success for women of advanced reproductive age and/or with elevations of FSH.

Patients with diminished ovarian reserve (FSH > 15 mIU/mL) should also be discouraged from undergoing IVF with their own eggs. The simplest and most common method to assess ovarian reserve is by basal (cycle days 2–3) serum follicle-stimulating hormone (FSH) and estradiol (E2) levels. Elevations of FSH above 15 mIU/mL and E2 above 75 pg/mL typically correlate with a poor follicular response to exogenous gonadotropin stimulation and extremely low pregnancy rates during conventional IVF.[5–8] The clinician must keep in mind, however, that while the positive predictive value of these tests is high, a normal result does not ensure success. Failure to produce multiple follicles and oocytes after repeated exposure to high gonadotropin doses (despite normal test results) is in effect functional evidence of poor ovarian reserve and may also indicate a need for donor eggs.

Use of donor oocytes in couples with heritable conditions has long been recommended as a means to avoid vertical transmission of disease to the offspring.[9] However, the need for donor eggs may be avoided if preimplantation genetic diagnosis by embryonic biopsy is available and able to detect the condition in question (see Chap. 17). Patients with balanced translocations in homologous chromosomes have little chance of bearing a fetus of normal chromosomal complement (either trisomic or monosomic pregnancies ensue), and egg donation is recommended. Egg donation may also be offered to older women who have experienced recurrent miscarriage, as pregnancy wastage in this age group reflects the poor quality of the resting pool of oocytes.[10] However, women with pregnancy loss due to a familial thrombophilia or antiphospholipid antibody syndrome require anticoagulant treatment regardless of the source of the oocyte, and should undergo egg donation only if other indications warrant its selection.

KEY POINT

Clinicians should consider oocyte donation in addressing the fertility needs of women with ovarian failure (premature or physiologic), advanced reproductive age, multiple prior IVF failures, and maternally transmitted heritable conditions.

Although in 1997, the Ethics Committee of the American Society for Reproductive Medicine (ASRM) published guidelines discouraging egg donation in women beyond the age of natural menopause,[11] studies have shown pregnancy outcomes in older recipients are favorable if women are appropriately screened and counseled.[12,13] There are no federal or state laws in the United States governing eligibility for egg donation, and the decision to treat lies with the individual practitioner. Age limits vary between programs, but most restrict egg donation to healthy recipients below 50 years of age (although successful pregnancy and delivery has been described in women in their midfifties and even early sixties). An ongoing concern is the financial and psychosocial welfare of children whose parents may become medically ill or even die while the children are young. Appropriate counseling and recipient screening (see below) will help minimize this risk.

Screening of Recipients

KEY POINT

Recipients over the age of 40 require a stringent medical evaluation that includes cardiovascular testing.

Thorough screening of prospective recipients is requisite to ascertain the physical and psychosocial well-being of the couple and future offspring. The clinician first needs to obtain a thorough preconceptual medical and reproductive history followed by a complete physical examination, including Papanicolaou testing and vaginal cultures (see Table 16-2). In addition to standard blood chemistry and infectious disease screening, recipients

Table 16-2. **SUGGESTED MEDICAL SCREENING OF OOCYTE RECIPIENT(S)**

Oocyte Recipient	Male Partner
Thorough medical history and physical examination	Blood Rh and type
CBC, blood Rh, and type	Hepatitis screen
Serum electrolytes, liver and kidney function	VDRL
Sensitive TSH	HIV-1, HTLV-1, HIV-2, HTLV-2
Rubella and hepatitis screen	Semen analysis and culture
Venereal disease research laboratory slide test (VDRL)	Appropriate genetic screening
HIV-1, HTLV-1, HIV-2, HTLV-2	
Urinalysis and culture	
Cervical cultures for gonorrhea and chlamydia	
Pap smear	
Transvaginal ultrasound	
Uterine cavity evaluation (sonohysterogram or hysterosalpingogram)	
Electrocardiogram[a]	
Chest x-ray[a]	
Mammogram[a]	
Glucose tolerance test[a]	
Cholesterol and lipid profile[a]	

[a]If over 40 years of age.

over the age of 40 should also have documentation of normal mammogram, chest x-ray, electrocardiogram, lipid panel, glucose tolerance test, and thyroid-stimulating hormone (TSH) level. Cardiovascular reserve may be better assessed by a treadmill stress test in recipients aged 50 and older. Based on the results of this preliminary screen, further investigation may be warranted. Historical or physical evidence of cardiopulmonary compromise, for example, would require additional workup or consultation with a cardiologist. If hypertension, diabetes, or other medical conditions are discovered, the clinician should also recommend consultation with a maternal-fetal-medicine specialist to better define risks and outcomes associated with pregnancy.

Evaluation of the uterine cavity is mandatory to rule out conditions known or thought to affect implantation and pregnancy. In oocyte donation, relatively few conditions of the fallopian tubes and pelvis are clinically significant. The presence of a significant hydrosalpinx (usually defined as a hydrosalpinx visible on transvaginal sonography) has been shown to be associated with lower pregnancy rates.[14] Salpingectomy should be offered to these patients in order to maximize the success of the upcoming embryo transfer. A sonohysterogram or hysterosalpingogram should be performed to confirm a normal uterine cavity. Hysteroscopic resection of significant endometrial polyps, submucosal myomas, or uterine septa is recommended prior to the egg donation cycle. Rarely, a patient may have a uterine cavity that cannot be accessed transcervically. A transtubal procedure may be required, and in these cases patency of a fallopian tube is mandatory. Endometriosis (even severe) does not affect pregnancy rates with oocyte donation, and additional treatment is indicated only if other symptoms coexist.[15,16]

The functional adequacy of the endometrium may be evaluated with a "mock cycle" and timed endometrial biopsy. The chances of discovering a significant abnormality (i.e., an inadequate response to hormonal priming and/or a luteal phase defect) is small, and in our center we omit this step except in patients at increased risk of a poor response. An increased risk of abnormality would include women who have received chemotherapy or pelvic radiation, have a history of severe intrauterine adhesive

KEY POINT

Optimizing the uterine cavity, by removing polyps and fibroids, is required prior to oocyte donation.

disease or significant prior uterine surgery, or have a history of multiple (>3) failed donor egg cycles.[17]

Screening for genetic disease is dictated by family history and ethnic background. For instance, Blacks and people of Mediterranean descent require tests of red cell indices and a hemoglobin electrophoresis to rule out sickle cell anemia, beta thalassemia, and hemoglobinopathies. Individuals with a normal hemoglobin electrophoresis at high risk for alpha-thalassemia (e.g., people of Southeast Asian ancestry) require DNA-based testing. All Whites should be screened for cystic fibrosis due to its high prevalence in the population. Ashkenazi Jews should additionally be screened for Tay-Sachs (recommended in French-Canadians as well), Gaucher, and Canavan diseases. Any family history significant for an inheritable condition (i.e., Fragile X syndrome, recurrent miscarriage due to parental balanced translocations) requires appropriate genetic screening. Referral to a genetic counselor is recommended in couples requiring more sophisticated testing to better define risk and obtain information regarding prenatal diagnosis.

KEY POINT

A complete evaluation prior to oocyte donation includes, not only history and physical examination with appropriate laboratory testing to exclude genetic and obstetrical risk, but also psychologic support.

Psychologic assessment of recipient couples is strongly recommended in addition to medical screening. For a woman requiring egg donation, the inability to bear a genetically related child may pose additional pressure to the preexisting stress of infertility. At stake are issues of self-esteem, guilt over the inability to provide the spouse a child, concerns surrounding disclosure to offspring, and worry over the impact on the personal relationship with the husband or family. The role of the clinician and/or psychologist caring for couples struggling with these issues is usually one of support and guidance. Most couples ultimately reconcile themselves to the fact that there is a loss of genetic lineage (with respect to the mother), as the desire to be a parent may be more important for positive parenting than a genetic link.[18] If social or psychologic concerns become evident, it is best to defer treatment until these issues are resolved.

Recruitment and Screening of Oocyte Donors

Most programs use either women known to the donor or recruited anonymously as a primary source of eggs. Anonymous donors are often solicited through advertisements, and matched according to phenotypic characteristics such as race, height, complexion, and other specifications requested by the recipient (e.g., educational background, religion, and so on). Known donors are typically close friends or family, including siblings, cousins, and even rarely children born from a previous marriage. Donors should be at least the age of their state's legal majority, preferably over the age of 21 and under the age of 35. Most IVF programs prefer anonymous donors under age 32, as pregnancy rates seem to be inversely related to the donor's age.[19,20] Recipients using known donors over age 35 should be informed of the increased risk of aneuploidy (in addition to a lower pregnancy rate) in the offspring, and be offered prenatal testing (amniocentesis) in the event of pregnancy.

Prior to initiating medical treatment, thorough informed consent must be completed. Donors should be given an overview of egg donation at the outset, as many may not be willing or able to commit the time required to complete a treatment cycle. A discussion of the risks involved may also dissuade potential donors from participating, and is best rendered early before time and money are spent on sophisticated laboratory screening tests. Risks to the donor have been shown to be minimal,[21] and are similar to those of women undergoing conventional IVF, which include the risk anesthesia, ovarian hyperstimulation syndrome (OHSS), postaspiration vaginal or intraabdominal bleeding, postaspiration urinary retention/bladder atony, and infection. Although few guidelines in the United States exist concerning the number of times an individual donor may participate, the ASRM suggests restricting donors to a maximum of six cycles to limit the cumulative risk.[22] No impairment of future fertility has been linked to egg donation, although the risks of controlled ovarian hyperstimulation with gonadotropins on future development of ovarian cancer remain unresolved.[23] It is recommended that physicians inform both recipients and donors prior to initiating a treatment cycle if the physician intends to divide the harvested oocytes amongst multiple patients. "Shared" donation is increasingly common due to the limited number of available oocyte donors. Financial responsibility for all medical expenses including those incurred after unexpected complications should be defined and agreed upon before treatment is begun. Most programs in the United States additionally compensate donors for the time, inconvenience, physical and emotional demands, and risk associated with egg donation. As there are no restrictions on payments to donors, reimbursement varies greatly with locale, depending on the supply and demand for suitable egg donors in that area. The amount of this monetary compensation should also be agreed upon prior to the start of ovarian stimulation.

Screening of donors should follow the guidelines recently published by the ASRM.[24] A thorough history and physical examination is mandatory. The donor should be screened for transmissible infectious diseases and inheritable genetic conditions (see Table 16-3). Unlike sperm donation, where a quarantine period for infectious diseases is mandatory, limitations in oocyte cryopreservation renders the quarantine of eggs infeasible. Therefore, a careful history of behavioral risk factors, including sexual history, contraception and drug use, body piercing or tattoos, and other factors known to be associated with transmittable diseases such as hepatitis and human immunodeficiency virus (HIV) is mandatory to minimize infectious risks to the recipient. A family history of or prior exposure to transmissible spongiform encephalopathy (TSE), such as Creutzfeldt-Jakob's disease, is also defined by the recent ASRM guidelines as a risk factor that excludes potential donors. As with recipient screening (see above), appropriate genetic testing depends largely on the ethnic background of the egg donor and recipient's male partner. Donors should be carefully questioned for any history

Table 16-3.	**SUGGESTED MEDICAL SCREENING OF OOCYTE DONORS**

Complete blood count with platelets
Blood type
Hepatitis screen
VDRL
HIV-1, HTLV-1, HIV-2, HTLV-2
Cervical cultures for gonorrhea and chlamydia
Pap smear
Transvaginal ultrasound of pelvis
Appropriate genetic tests

of heritable Mendelian disorders, whether dominant or recessive, and be tested accordingly. Donors should also be free of any serious malformations of multifactorial origin (e.g., spina bifida, cleft lip/palate, congenital heart defects, and so on) that may recur in future generations. Diseases such as diabetes, atherosclerosis, and some cancers (e.g., breast, ovarian, prostate, colon) have a familial tendency and may warrant exclusion from the program. The relative scarcity of donor eggs, however, may prompt some recipients to accept certain risks, particularly if the donor is an otherwise ideal candidate. Appropriate counseling and informed consent is mandatory in such instances.

A transvaginal ultrasound will ensure the pelvic viscera are free of pathology and the ovaries accessible for oocyte retrieval. Women with documented polycystic ovarian syndrome (PCOS) are excluded as potential donors due to their increased risk for severe OHSS, familial predisposition for androgen disorders, and higher miscarriage rates. Known donors with *polycystic appearing* ovaries should be counseled regarding the increased risk of OHSS, and should typically be started on lower doses of gonadotropins. Contraception is mandatory to ensure donors do not become pregnant during their participation in egg donation. Hormonal contraceptives, including Norplant, are contraindicated, although an intrauterine device may be left *in situ*. An inability to comply with an appropriate contraceptive method should result in exclusion of a prospective donor.

Psychologic counseling prior to participation is recommended for egg donors. The underlying motivation governing their participation, ability to handle stress, emotional stability, and coping skills should be ascertained. Donors that are known to the recipients merit special consideration. Occasionally nonanonymous donors feel obligated or even coerced to donate eggs to a close friend or relative. The impact of donation on the relationship between the donor and recipient, and issues of disclosure to resulting children should be explored. Grief or severe depression may occur in donors unable to successfully provide a child for a relative or friend.

Maintaining the anonymity of the donor is an important obligation. Most programs warrant that identity disclosure will not occur between recipients and donors unless required by court order. To date, this has never been necessary in the United States.

KEY POINT

Clinicians must ensure that egg donors are healthy and pose no infectious or genetic risk to the recipient or offspring. Oocyte donors, themselves, should undergo psychologic evaluation, not only to assure the ability to comply and handle the process of the procedure, but to assure a complete understanding of the process and free will in determination to move forward.

The Egg Donation Cycle

Egg donation begins with the synchronization of the menstrual cycles of the donor and recipient (Fig. 16-1). This is most easily accomplished by prescribing continuous oral contraceptives to the donor prior to synchronizing the start with the recipient. Gonadotropin-releasing hormone (GnRH) agonists or antagonists may be used to prevent a premature luteinizing hormone (LH) surge in both donor and recipient. Cycling recipients are usually given a GnRH agonist (for example, 1 mg leuprolide acetate daily until suppressed, then 0.5 mg daily thereafter) for pituitary receptor downregulation prior to commencing hormone replacement for endometrial preparation. Likewise, the cycling donor may be given either 2 weeks of GnRH agonist prior to initiation of gonadotropin stimulation of the ovary, or continue oral contraceptives until start of the stimulation during which time a GnRH antagonist is added to prevent a premature LH surge. Downregulation has been achieved and the synchronization may be completed once both donor and recipient attain serum estradiol levels below 30 pg/mL and the ovarian morphology viewed by transvaginal ultrasound is normal (without physiologic or pathologic cysts).

A minimum of 2 weeks of estrogen replacement in recipients is recommended before progesterone administration, although estrogenic priming for as little as 6 days has resulted in pregnancy.[25] Most practitioners begin estrogen treatment in recipients

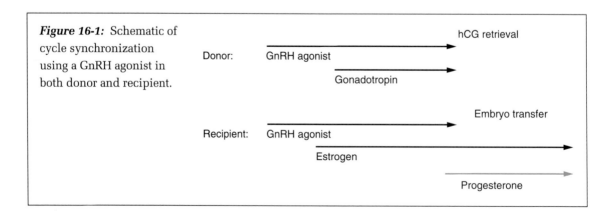

Figure 16-1: Schematic of cycle synchronization using a GnRH agonist in both donor and recipient.

a few days prior to gonadotropin therapy in the donor, since the stimulation period in the donor is usually shorter than the follicular phase of a normal menstrual cycle. The most common regimens use oral estradiol either in a constant dose (4–8 mg/day) or in a gradually increasing fashion. Alternatively, estrogen may be administered transdermally (0.2–0.4 mg/day). Since these estradiol preparations are relatively physiologic, and not contraceptive, failure to prescribe a GnRH agonist/antagonist may result in an undesired LH surge and a premature progesterone rise in up to 20% of recipient cycles. Monitoring of serum estradiol levels in recipients is unnecessary, as values vary widely depending on when the patient took her medications, her diet, and intestinal absorption. Furthermore, following the ingestion of oral estradiol, the weaker circulating metabolites of estradiol, including estrone, estrone sulfate, estriol, and estrone glucuronide are considerably elevated and also contribute to the physiologic stimulation of the endometrium. If necessary, estrogen replacement can be safely extended for several months prior to transfer to accommodate synchronization with the donor's cycle without decreasing treatment efficacy.

A more critical window exists for initiating and replacing progesterone in recipients. Evidence has shown the optimal time of transfer for 4–8-cell embryos is day 4–5 of progesterone therapy,[26] and for blastocysts day 7 of progesterone therapy.[27] Most programs add progesterone to the recipient's hormone replacement regimen the day prior to or the day of the donor's egg retrieval. Progesterone in oil is most commonly administered IM (100 mg in daily split doses) or transvaginally (Crinone 90 mg one to two times daily or micronized progesterone suppositories 400–600 mg daily). Vaginal progesterone results in an adequate, reliable endometrial response despite much lower serum concentrations of hormone (as compared with IM dosing).[28] Thus, measurement of serum progesterone levels following hormone administration to assess efficacy is also unnecessary. Transvaginal ultrasound monitoring of the endometrium during the treatment cycle is often suggested to assess the recipient's response to hormone replacement. Although thin linings (less than 6 mm) have been associated with decreased implantation rates, successful pregnancies have occurred in recipients with linings as thin as 4 mm.[29] Thus, an embryo transfer is still prudent despite sonographic evidence of a "thin" endometrium. Rarely, however, if the reason for poor development is discovered to be a result of noncompliance with the medication regimen, a delay in embryo transfer (i.e., freezing the embryos rather than transfer) or cycle cancellation is necessary.

KEY POINT

After synchronization of the donor-recipient cycle, recipients receive estradiol therapy for adequate endometrial priming (6–65 days), and progesterone replacement (beginning the day prior to or the day of egg retrieval) to maintain a receptive uterine lining until 12–14 weeks of gestation.

Following the donor's ovarian stimulation (usually after a minimum of 10 days of gonadotropin administration), human chorionic gonadotropin (hCG) is administered and egg retrieval is performed 34–36 h later. If the sperm to be used for fertilization is produced by the recipient's partner on the same day as retrieval, it is imperative that the anonymity of the donor is safeguarded (i.e., ensure there is no contact between the recipient couple and the donor). Recipients have been known to loiter in waiting rooms awaiting the departure of the donor postaspiration in an effort to "view" her. Mature donor oocytes are either inseminated in culture or undergo intracytoplasmic sperm injection (ICSI), as dictated by the quality of sperm and oocytes. Embryo transfer is performed 3–5 days after retrieval, depending on quality of embryo development. Both progesterone and estrogen replacement is continued by the recipient throughout the luteal phase. In the event of pregnancy, exogenous steroid therapy may be withdrawn after the luteo-placental transition (7–10 weeks gestation), although conventionally most programs discontinue hormone replacement at the end of the first trimester (12–14 weeks).

What's the Evidence?

Much of the data evaluating the use of oocyte donation to treat infertility in women with absent or diminished ovarian reserve consist of small series reports from various IVF centers, based on a relatively limited number of donor cycles.[12,13,29,31] However, more recent reviews of aggregated national cycles, such as that reported by the Society for Assisted Reproductive Technology/Center for Disease Control (SART) dataset of donor egg cycles performed in the United States between 1996 and 1998,[30] provide comparative data by which to assess relative efficacy. Reviewing 17,339 recipient cycles, success rates remained relatively constant (a delivery rate of roughly 40%) among recipients aged 25–49 years. Beyond age 50 rates were noted to decline to about 30%. The study also concluded that once a woman became pregnant through the use of donor eggs, she had greater than an 80% chance of successful delivery.[30]

Outcomes of Oocyte Donation

Success rates following egg donation are among the highest experienced using any assisted reproductive technique. Implantation and pregnancy rates in women undergoing egg donation are comparable or even higher than those of young women undergoing conventional IVF using their own oocytes.[12,31] Despite the recent tallied results from SART, many programs have repeatedly demonstrated that recipient age does not adversely impact the success of egg donation,[12,13,29] implicating the oocyte as the primary determinant of reproductive senescence (Table 16-4). Success rates are relatively constant regardless of the indication for treatment, although patients with Turner's syndrome may have a higher incidence of early pregnancy failure.[32]

Table 16-4. **RESULTS OF THE TRANSFER OF FERTILIZED DONOR OVA**

	≥40 YEARS WITH DONOR IVF	<40 YEARS WITH DONOR IVF	≥40 YEARS WITH STANDARD IVF
No. of recipients	65	35	57
No. of recipient cycles	93	46	79
No. of oocytes per recipient	15.2 ± 9.0	15.3 ± 6.8	6.7 ± 4.1^a
No of transfer cycles	86	43	70
No. of embryos transferred per cycle, mean ± SD	4.4 ± 1.0	4.7 ± 0.7	2.9 ± 1.2^a
Implantation rate per transferred embryo, %	19.7	15.9	4.8^a
Ratio of clinical pregnancies per transfer attempt (%)	34/86 (34.5)	14/43 (32.6)	8/70 (11.4)
Ratio of ongoing pregnancies or deliveries per transfer (%)	29/86 (33.7)	13/43 (30.2)	6/70 (8.6)

[a] $P < 0.05$ comparing women 40 years of age and above undergoing standard IVF with either group undergoing oocyte donation.

The number of embryos transferred during an egg donation cycle varies, but is generally limited to three in recipients with good embryo quality. Transferring two embryos of high quality from donors under age 35 may avoid higher-order multiple gestations while preserving success rates. One program reports a lower multiple gestation rate with a comparable success rate following transfer of two versus three day 3 (6–10 cell) embryos.[33] Other programs have chosen to preferentially transfer only blastocysts, resulting in a 12.6% increase in clinical pregnancy rates coupled with a greater than sixfold decrease in the incidence of high-order multiple gestations after adoption of blastocyst culture and transfer.[27]

Obstetric outcomes following egg donation generally parallel those of conventional IVF. When comparing singleton pregnancies, the incidence of perinatal complications (IUGR, low birth weight, prematurity, congenital malformation) are similar.[34,35] However, the enhanced implantation and pregnancy rates noted in recipients of oocyte donation lead to high multiple gestation rates, which increases maternal and neonatal morbidity. In addition, egg donation pregnancies have been associated with a higher incidence of pregnancy-induced hypertension (PIH), controlling for recipient age and multiple gestations.[34–36] In women older than 55, the incidence of both PIH and glucose intolerance was found to be markedly increased compared to recipients in

Table 16-5.   **MEDICAL CONDITIONS ENCOUNTERED AT HIGHER FREQUENCY IN RECIPIENTS OF ADVANCED MATERNAL AGE AND THOSE WITH TURNER'S SYNDROME**

Advanced Maternal Age	*Turner's Syndrome*
Glucose intolerance/diabetes mellitus	Glucose intolerance/diabetes mellitus
Hypertension	Hypertension
Cardiac disease	Autoimmune thyroiditis
Renal/liver abnormalities	Aortic coarctation
Thyroid disease	Ventricular septal defect
Malignancy	Horseshoe kidney
	Unilateral renal agenesis

the 50–54 years age group.[13] All recipients should be monitored closely during their pregnancies for development of these conditions. Exaggerated cesarean section rates (30–60%) have also been consistently noted within this patient population.[34,35] Older recipients and women with Turner's syndrome merit special attention, as they are more likely to have coexistent medical conditions (Table 16-5). Postnatal growth and development of children born to egg donor recipients has been only sporadically studied, but appears no different than the general population.[37]

Discussion of Cases

CASE 1

You are asked to evaluate a 49-year-old, recently married Black woman for oocyte donation. The patient has two healthy children, aged 17 and 23, from a previous marriage. She is married to a 39-year-old Black male who brings documentation of a normal semen analysis performed 1 year ago. The patient states she is "perimenopausal," with menses occurring irregularly every 30–60 days. The couple would like to have an anonymous donor, also of Black descent.

What would be the next step in her evaluation?

Both the patient and her husband require appropriate medical screening (see Table 16-2). As the patient is over 40, in addition to the standard medical screen, an electrocardiogram, chest x-ray, mammogram, glucose tolerance test, and lipid profile are needed. Cardiopulmonary reserve should be assessed by a treadmill stress test. Both individuals require testing (SS prep or hemoglobin electrophoresis) to rule out sickle cell anemia and other hemoglobinopathies. Further genetic screening should be dictated by any family history of inherited diseases. The patient should have a sonohysterogram to assess her uterine cavity and basal day 3 serum FSH and E2 levels drawn. A second semen analysis should be performed using your own andrology facility, to confirm the results from the other institution. Finally, the couple should have an appropriate psychologic and social assessment by a qualified individual (i.e., psychologist, psychiatrist, social worker) prior to initiation of the cycle.

The patient's medical and genetic screens are largely unremarkable. Her FSH level is 22 mIU/mL and E2 level 45 mIU/mL. Sonohysterogram reveals a small 1 cm polyp at the fundus of the uterus, but no other abnormalities. All other screening tests are within normal limits. The husband's semen analysis is confirmed as normal. The husband is found to be positive for sickle cell trait (Hgb AS), but has no family history of sickle cell disease.

How would you manage these findings?

The patient requires a hysteroscopic resection of the endometrial polyp to ensure it is not malignant. Also, implantation success may be compromised if inadvertent evulsion of the polyp occurs at the time of embryo transfer which may create bleeding. The patient may proceed with the egg donation cycle 1 month after the procedure, if no complications are encountered. The detection of sickle cell trait in her partner requires that the donor also be screened for any hemoglobinopathies. If present, the donor should be excluded from consideration. The informed consent process should be completed in its entirety before the cycle is begun. Once the donor has been selected and appropriately screened (see Table 16-3), the recipient should begin GnRH agonist therapy on either day 2 or 21 of her cycle to synchronize her to the donor's cycle. Once both the donor and the recipient are suppressed, the recipient begins her estrogen replacement as per the standard protocol (see above).

Case 2

A 32-year-old White married woman with primary infertility and secondary amenorrhea presents for evaluation for IVF. Her partner is a healthy White male with normal semen analysis. Her reproductive history reveals menarche at age 14, with irregular menses for several years, followed by cessation of menses at age 18. On physical examination, the patient is found to be 4 ft and 11 in. tall, average weight, and has normal pubertal development—normal pubic hair distribution, normal vagina and cervix, and small, but normal breast development. The ovaries are difficult to visualize on transvaginal ultrasound and appear to be devoid of antral follicles. Serum blood tests reveal an FSH of 88 mIU/mL, LH of 65 mIU/mL, and E2 <20 pg/mL.

What further tests would you recommend?

Spontaneous puberty and menstruation has been reported in up to 5% of women with Turner's syndrome, usually in women with a mosaic complement, such as 45X/46XX. This patient presents with hypergonadotropic hypogonadism and some of the physical stigmata of Turner's syndrome. A karyotype is mandatory. In addition, a sensitive TSH, fasting glucose, autoimmune antibody screen, complete blood count (CBC), and serum electrolytes including calcium and phosphorus are warranted to exclude other endocrine gland autoimmune disorders. Cardiac and renal imaging is imperative to rule out other known associated defects (Table 16-5). A bone density evaluation is also helpful to determine if osteopenia or osteoporosis is present.

The patient's karyotype returns 45X/46XX, and she has normal serum TSH and electrolyte levels. No cardiac or renal defects were found. She still desires pregnancy and requests oocyte donation.

How do you counsel this patient?

The patient has gonadal dysgenesis and premature ovarian failure. Although patients with Turner's syndrome may have a slightly higher incidence of early pregnancy loss, prognosis is still favorable using donor oocytes. However, maternal fatalities secondary to cardiovascular abnormalities (i.e., aortic aneurysm dissection and rupture) have occurred during pregnancy in these patients. In addition, she will be at higher risk for glucose intolerance and hypertension during her pregnancy. A cardiology consult and electrocardiogram are prerequisite prior to initiating the cycle. The patient should be monitored very closely by her cardiologist throughout the pregnancy with serial echocardiograms. Both the patient and her partner should undergo standard medical and genetic screening (including tests for cystic fibrosis) prior to cycle start.

How would you manage this patient's treatment cycle?

In patients with hypergonadotropic hypogonadism, GnRH agonist treatment prior to hormone replacement is unnecessary, as the patient is already "suppressed." Thus, cycle synchronization merely requires the patient's donor be adequately downregulated with either GnRH agonist or oral contraceptives, prior to starting estrogen in the recipient. The remainder of the patient's egg donation cycle (including dosages of estrogen and progesterone) would be similar to the standard protocol described earlier. Sonographic imaging of the endometrium after 2 weeks of hormonal priming may be useful to ensure adequate response. Once pregnant, the patient should remain on progesterone and estrogen until the 12th week of gestation. As mentioned above, she will require close cardiac and obstetrical monitoring throughout her pregnancy. Postdelivery, the patient should be counseled to begin hormone replacement therapy with calcium supplementation to prevent further bone loss and osteoporosis.

REFERENCES

1 Trounsen A, Leeton J, Besanko M, et al. Pregnancy established in an infertile patient after transfer of a donated embryo fertilized in vitro. *Br Med J Clin Res ed* 286:835–838, 1983.

2 Lutjen P, Trounson A, Leeton J, Findlay J, Wood C, Renou P. The establishment and maintenance of pregnancy using in vitro fertilization and embryo donation in a patient with primary ovarian failure. *Nature* 307:174–175, 1984.

3 Society for Assisted Reproductive Technology and the American Society for Reproductive Medicine. Assisted reproductive technology in the United States: 1999 results generated from the American Society for Reproductive Medicine, Society for Assisted Reproductive Technology Registry. *Fertil Steril* 78:918–931, 2002.

4 Bustillo M, Buster JE, Cohen SW, et al. Nonsurgical ovum transfer as a treatment in infertile women. Preliminary experience. *JAMA* 251:1171–1173, 1984.

5 Muasher SJ, Oehninger S, Simonetti S, et al. The value of basal and/or stimulated serum gonadotropin levels in prediction of stimulation response and in vitro fertilization outcome. *Fertil Steril* 50:298–307, 1988.

6 Scott RT, Toner JP, Muasher SJ, et al. Follicle-stimulating hormone levels on cycle day 3 are predictive of in vitro fertilization outcome. *Fertil Steril* 51:651–654, 1989.

7 Licciardi FL, Liu HC, Rosenwaks Z. Day 3 estradiol serum concentrations as prognosticators of ovarian stimulation response and pregnancy outcome in patients undergoing in vitro fertilization. *Fertil Steril* 64:991–994, 1995.

8 Smotrich DB, Widra EA, Gindoff PR, et al. Prognostic value of day 3 estradiol on in vitro fertilization outcome. *Fertil Steril* 64:1136–1140, 1995.

9 Levran D, Ben-Shlomo I, Dor J, et al. Aging of endometrium and oocytes: observations on conception and abortion rates in an egg donation model. *Fertil Steril* 56(6):1091–1094, 1991.

10 Van Voorhis BJ, Williamson RA, Gerard JL, et al. Use of oocytes from anonymous, matched, fertile donors for prevention of heritable genetic diseases. *J Med Gen* 29:398–399, 1992.

11 Ethics Committee of the American Society for Reproductive Medicine. Ethical considerations of assisted reproductive technologies. *Fertil Steril* 67(Suppl 1):1S–9S, 1997.

12 Sauer MV, Paulson RJ, Lobo RA. Reversing the natural decline in human fertility: an extended clinical trial of oocyte donation to women of advanced reproductive age. *JAMA* 268:1275–1279, 1992.

13 Paulson RJ, Boostanfar R, Saadat P, et al. Pregnancy in the sixth decade of life obstetric outcomes in women of advanced reproductive age. *JAMA* 288:2320–2323, 2002.

14 Cohen MA, Lindheim SR, Sauer MV. Hydrosalpinges adversely affect implantation in donor oocyte cycles. *Hum Reprod* 14:1087–1089, 1999.

15 Bustillo M, Krysa LW, Coulam CB. Uterine receptivity in an oocyte donation programme. *Hum Reprod* 10:442–445, 1995.

16 Diaz I, Navarro J, Blasco L, et al. Impact of stage III-IV endometriosis on recipients of sibling oocytes: matched case-control study. *Fertil Steril* 74:31–34, 2000.

17 Li TC, Dockery P, Ramsewak SS, et al. The variation of endometrial response to a standard hormone replacement therapy in women with premature ovarian failure. An ultrasonographic and histological study. *Br J Obstet Gynecol* 98:656–661, 1991.

18 Golombok S, Cook R, Bish A, Murray C. Families created by the new reproductive technologies: quality of parenting and social and emotional development of the children. *Child Dev* 66:285–298, 1995.

19 Faber BM, Mercan R, Hamacher P, Muasher SJ, Toner JP. The impact of an egg donor's age and her prior fertility on recipient pregnancy outcome. *Fertil Steril* 68:370–372, 1997.

20 Cohen MA, Lindheim SR, Sauer MV. Donor age is paramount to success in oocyte donation. *Hum Reprod* 14:2755–2758, 1999.

21 Sauer MV. Defining the incidence of serious complications experienced by oocyte donors: a review of 1000 cases. *Am J Obstet Gynecol* 184(3):277–278, 2001.

22 Committee Opinion, American Society for Repoductive Medicine. *Repetitive Oocyte Donation* 1–4, 2000.

23 Konishi I, Kuroda H, Mandai M. Gonadotropins and development of ovarian cancer. *Oncology* 57(Suppl 2):45–48, 1999.

24 The American Society for Reproductive Medicine. Guidelines for oocyte donation. *Fertil Steril* 77(Suppl 5):S6–S8, 2002.

25 Navot D, Anderson TL, Droesch K, Scott RT, Kreiner D, Rosenwaks Z. Hormonal manipulation of endometrial maturation. *J Clin Endocrinol Metab* 68:801–807, 1989.

26 Prapas Y, Prapas N, Jones EE, et al. The window for embryo transfer in oocyte donation cycles depends on the duration of progesterone therapy. *Hum Reprod* 13:720–723, 1998.

27 Schoolcraft WB, Gardner DK. Blastocyst culture and transfer increases the efficiency of oocyte donation. *Fertil Steril* 74;482–486, 2000.

28 Franchin R, De Ziegler D, Bergeron C, et al. Transvaginal administration of Progesterone. *Obstet Gynecol* 90:396–401, 1997.

29 Noyes N, Hampton BS, Berkeley A, et al. Factors useful in predicting the success of oocyte donation: a 3-year retrospective analysis. *Fertil Steril* 76(1):92–97, 2001.

30 Toner JP, Grainger DA, Frazier LM, et al. Clinical outcomes among recipients of donated eggs: an analysis of the U.S. national experience, 1996–1998. *Fertil Steril* 78:1038–1045, 2002.

31 Paulson RJ, Hatch IE, Lobo RA, Sauer MV. Cumulative conception and live birth rates after oocyte donation: implications regarding endometrial receptivity. *Hum Reprod* 12:835–839, 1997.

32 Press F, Shapiro HM, Cowell CA, Oliver GD. Outcome of ovum donation in Turner's syndrome patients. *Fertil Steril* 64:995–998, 1995.

33 Licciardi F, Berkeley AS, Krey L. A two-versus three-embryo transfer: the oocyte donation model. *Fertil Steril* 73:510–513, 2001.

34 Abdalla HI, Billett A, Kan AK, et al. Obstetric outcome in 232 ovum donation pregnancies. *Br J Obstet Gynecol* 105:332–337, 1998.

35 Soderstrom-Anttila V, Tiitinen A, Foudila T, Hovatta O. Obstetric and perinatal outcome after oocyte donation: comparison with in-vitro fertilization pregnancies. *Hum Reprod* 13:483–490, 1998.

36 Salha O, Sharma V, Dada T, et al. The influence of donated gametes on the incidence of hypertensive disorders of pregnancy. *Hum Reprod* 14:2268–2273, 1999.

37 Soderstrom-Anttila V, Sajaniemi N, Tiitinen A, Hovatta O. Health and development of children born after oocyte donation compared with that of those born after in-vitro fertilization, and parents' attitudes regarding secrecy. *Hum Reprod* 13:2009–2015, 1998.

17 New Technologies in Assisted Reproduction

David Keefe

Introduction

Since the advent of *in vitro* fertilization (IVF) more than 25 years ago, great progress has been made in the application of assisted reproductive technology (ART) to the treatment of tubal, male, and anovulatory forms of infertility. The diagnosis of egg infertility, however, remains crude, and its treatment, short of egg donation, inefficient[1] controlled ovarian hyperstimulation (COH), combined with intrauterine insemination (IUI), IVF with transfer of multiple embryos, or egg donation[2-4] remain the mainstays in the treatment of egg infertility, but result only in modest pregnancy rates in the case of the former, or loss of the woman's genetic legacy in the case of the latter. Not only are the benefits of COH slim, but also when it does work, it carries a risk of multiple gestations.[5] New approaches to predict egg and embryo developmental potential are needed, not only to stave the epidemic of multiple gestations, but also to help women decide whether to pursue treatments which depend on their own eggs, or to seek alternatives, such as egg donation or adoption, which improve their chances of having a baby, but provide genetically unrelated offspring.

Egg infertility presents a significant diagnostic challenge to clinicians, because its onset is so variable and difficult to predict.[6] Ovarian reserve testing with day 3 follicle-stimulating hormone (FSH), estradiol, and inhibin B levels, and the clomiphene citrate challenge test provide only insensitive assays for egg infertility.[7-11]

405

Not only is egg infertility the most refractory form of infertility to treat but also it is becoming more prevalent, as women increasingly delay attempts at childbearing and are exposed to tobacco smoke and environmental toxicants.

Egg infertility has become more prevalent, but reproductive senescence itself is not a new phenomenon. Ample evidence suggests that reproductive senescence in women is an evolutionarily conserved biological process, which no longer provides adaptive advantage.[12] Until safe and effective contraceptive technology and obstetrical care became available, women risked conceiving involuntarily, though pregnancy carried significant risks to themselves and to their offspring. Moreover, perinatal death of older women was especially disruptive to traditional societies, because in most such cultures, women carried inordinate responsibility for the reproductive success of kin. Reproductive senescence provided a kind of natural contraception, and thus served to control population size, at the same time preserving strategically important members of traditional societies. Of course, in the modern era of effective contraceptive technology and obstetrical care, the adaptive value of reproductive senescence is outweighed by the detrimental effects of aging on the reproductive potential of those who have delayed attempts at childbearing.

Even during the peak years of women's fertility (early twenties), reproductive efficiency is low. In fact, reproductive wastage is a universal characteristic not only of human reproduction, but also throughout the animal kingdom, with all forms of life devoting enormous energies toward production of germ cells far in excess of the number that eventually develop into a new adult capable of repeating the life cycle. Female fetuses contain millions of oocytes, but by midgestation oogonial proliferation ceases, and oocytes and follicles immediately begin to die.[13,14] By birth, the cohort of follicles will have been reduced to hundreds of thousands. The majority of oocytes never ovulate, but rather undergo atresia. Because these prenatal events play such a large role in the determination of the number of oocytes within the adult ovary, paradoxically understanding these early stages of oogenesis should provide key insights into reproductive senescence.

Explosive growth in the fields of molecular, cellular, and developmental biology has provided new methods to study individual cells, including eggs and embryos, often without disturbing them.

At the same time, ART provides unprecedented access to human eggs and embryos for translational research providing new approaches to the diagnosis of egg infertility. Fluorescence *in situ* hybridization (FISH), polymerase chain reaction (PCR), and related technologies have demonstrated a prominent role for aneuploidy detection in eggs and embryos. Recent developments in light microscopy and single cell physiology also promise to help assess the viability of living eggs and embryos in the IVF laboratory. Finally, the emerging field of genomics, especially expression profiling through microarray, holds great promise to unlock the mysteries of egg and embryo senescence.

Aneuploidy Detection in Eggs and Embryos

The most striking effect on egg function in women is the logarithmic increase in the rate of aneuploidy with age, resulting in follicular atresia, cell cycle arrest, and apoptosis in preimplantation embryos, failure of implantation, and/or spontaneous abortion, and in some cases, birth of aneuploid offspring. The marked age-related increase in aneuploidy in second trimester amniocenteses and births represents only the tip of the iceberg. Multiprobe fluorescent hybridization (FISH) currently allows detection of up to eight pairs of chromosomes in chromosome spreads generated from individual blastomeres biopsied from living human embryos and/or polar bodies. Multiprobe FISH focuses on detection of the chromosome pairs most affected by age-related nondisjunction, chromosomes 13, 14, 15, 16, 18, 21, 22, X, and Y.[15] Aneuploidy screening by multiprobe FISH of these chromosomes before embryo transfer has improved outcome for women who have failed multiple cycles of IVF, and reduced the rate of miscarriage following IVF. Preimplantation genetic diagnosis (PGD) also helps couples deal with the complex choice between donor egg versus IVF with the woman's own eggs.

FISH has been employed to diagnose aneuploidy in the polar body[16–20] and in blastomeres biopsied from cleavage stage embryos.[21,22] The applicability of FISH for PGD of aneuploidy is currently constrained by the number of chromosomes which can be distinguished in a single cell, because of the overlapping emission spectra of available fluorophores. Other chromosomes have been studied, and some evidence suggests that nondisjunction of chromosomes 1 and 17 can occur in preimplantation human embryos, but rarely is found in spontaneous abortions, presumably because they seldom implant or they die shortly after implantation.[23] Because of the significant level of mosaicism in cleavage stages human embryos[22] and the diversity of chromosomes involved in nondisjunction, attempts have been made to increase the number of chromosomes analyzed by multiple (up to three) rounds of FISH on the same chromosome spread, enabling PGD of aneuploidy for up to 13 chromosomes (13, 16, 18, 21, and 22; X, Y, 15, 17; and 2, 3, 4, and 11).[24]

A number of alternative approaches have been developed in research settings to scan the entire complement of chromosomes from individual cells, and these technologies are just beginning to find their application in PGD of aneuploidy in individual eggs and embryos. Spectral karyotyping (SKY) employs a combinatorial approach to label all chromosomes from a single cell. After labeling a set of chromosomes with all available fluorophores, SKY then labels additional chromosomes by combining multiple fluorophores and digitally assigning a unique pseudocolor to identify the additionally labeled chromosomes.[25]

Comparative genomic hybridization employs the PCR to amplify sequences from the entire genome in order to detect all chromosomes from a single cell. The prolonged time and technical challenge required to complete these techniques have limited their widespread application to ART, but a recent approach circumvents these problems by performing complete genomic hybridization (CGH) on polar body chromosomes, thus providing up to 6 days to complete the analysis of the full complement of chromosomes before embryo transfer.[26]

In general, the more chromosomes analyzed, the higher the rate of aneuploidy detected in oocytes and cleavage stage embryos. When chromosome pairs are studied in oocytes or embryos from older women, the vast majority are found to be aneuploid. Moreover, PGD of aneuploidy facilitates single embryo transfer with pregnancy rates of up to 35% in women over the age of 40.[27]

Gene expression profiling by microarray now is feasible, even on a single blastomere or oocyte. The small copy number of RNAs within an individual cell requires amplification by T7 or by CGH before performing the microarray, but this has been carried out

KEY POINT

New technologies will allow evaluation of the entire genome to exclude embryos affected by aneuploidy from embryo transfer.

successfully in mammalian embryos.[28,29] Microarray technology can also be used to scan the entire genome of a single cell for numerical, insertional, or deletional abnormalities.[30]

CAUSES OF AGE-RELATED ANEUPLOIDY

Our group has focused on attempts to understand the mechanisms underlying age-related aneuploidy, in the hope that it will open up new avenues to the diagnosis of egg infertility in women. Since multiple chromosomes are predisposed to nondisjunction, and since nondisjunction can arise throughout development, identifying markers of susceptibility to aneuploidy might better predict outcome. Up to 80% of aneuploidies found in embryos and fetuses have their origin in the oocyte,[31] and 80% of aneuploidies of oocyte origin arise during metaphase I (MI), so studying the germinal vesicle (GV) to MI transition should facilitate the study of aneuploidy as it occurs *in vitro*. We have employed two strategies—imaging the meiotic spindle with a novel, digital, orientation-independent polarized light microscope, called the polscope, and measuring telomere length—to diagnose egg infertility.

Spindle Imaging by Polarized Light Microscopy

Evidence suggests that the physical state of the spindle reflects its function, and that increased maternal age, the single most important predictor of female fertility, is associated with disruption of spindle architecture.[32] Conventional methods of spindle imaging (e.g., fluorescence labeling techniques), however, are invasive, and thus not compatible with clinical use. A new, orientation-independent polarized light microscope, the polscope, reveals the spindle's architecture noninvasively.[33] Instead of using exogenous dyes or exposing the spindle to damaging levels of light, the polscope generates contrast to image spindles based on a fundamental optical property of the spindle's molecular structure, called birefringence.

Why Focus on the Condition of the Oocyte as a Way to Improve IVF Success Rates?

Evaluation of oocyte quality has been difficult in humans. Attempts to estimate oocyte developmental potential demonstrate a number of morphologic features, such as darkness, granularity, vacuoles, fragmentation, and irregularity[34] are associated with poor developmental potential. However, standard imaging techniques used in the IVF laboratory do not provide a sensitive method of diagnosing egg infertility. Moreover, the pathobiological basis of these morphologic markers remains unclear.

IVF offers a unique opportunity to study the role of the meiotic spindle in human egg developmental potential. Eggs are ovulated at the metaphase II (MII) stage of development when chromosomes are poised on the metaphase plate, tethered by microtubules that are inherently unstable, with more birefringent than other structures in the oocyte. In patients who undergo immature oocyte retrieval and *in vitro* maturation (IVM),[35] the MI spindle also is available for imaging. Unfortunately, imaging methods currently used in the IVF laboratory, i.e., Hoffman, Nomarski or bright field microscopy, cannot image clearly the meiotic spindle.[33]

KEY POINT

Alterations in the meiotic spindle may be important in the increased risk for aneuploidy seen with aging.

A previous study by Battaglia et al.[32] compared spindles of eggs from two groups of women, aged 20–25 and 40–45, imaged by immunofluorescence labeling, and found that meiotic spindles from older women exhibited significantly more abnormalities in chromosome placement and structure. Seventy-nine percent of oocytes from the older group exhibited abnormal spindle structure, including abnormal tubulin placement and displacement of one or more chromosomes from the metaphase plate. In the younger group, only 17% exhibited such abnormalities. Spindles in the younger group appeared well ordered, and held chromosomes aligned on the metaphase plate. These data suggest that the architecture of meiotic spindles is altered in older women, possibly explaining their higher prevalence of aneuploidy.

While intriguing, these results originated from experiments that destroyed eggs by fixing and staining them, then illuminating them with intense, high frequency light. Moreover, because it employed invasive imaging, it could not link spindle architecture to developmental outcome of individual eggs.

Imaging Spindles Noninvasively With the Polscope

Oocytes, like most living cells, are almost entirely translucent when viewed with a standard optical microscope. The meiotic spindle is not too small to be imaged by conventional light microscopy, but rather lacks contrast, making it necessary to employ methods to enhance contrast of the spindle against the translucent cytoplasm. Nomarksi (also called differential interference contrast or DIC), Hoffman, and phase contrast microscopy use optical interference effects to create contrast. While noninvasive, they cannot image spindles.[33] Other imaging methods mark spindles with exogenous, absorptive colored stains or fluorescent labels. While producing the high level of contrast needed to image the spindle within the oocyte, these latter methods kill the egg or disrupt its function, and therefore, provide limited value for clinical and/or developmental studies.

Birefringence is an optical property that derives from the molecular order inherent to such macromolecules as membranes, microtubules, microfilaments, and other cytoskeletal components.[36,33] Polarized light microscopy has the unique potential to visualize and measure birefringent structures, such as spindles, dynamically and nondestructively, in living cells. However, the low sensitivity of conventional polarized light microscopes make them marginally suitable for application to mammalian experimental and clinical embryology.[33] Polarized light microscopy introduces contrast based on retardance, which arises when the optical paths between two orthogonal, polarized light beams are differentially slowed as they pass through highly ordered molecules within the specimen, such as microtubules. Birefringent objects present differences in the paths encountered by polarized light beams as they traverse the specimen. Compared to nonbiological materials, the birefringence of biological samples is weak, with only a few nanometers of retardance, so the low level of birefringence in biological specimens requires the use of manually adjusted compensators and rotating stages, a complicated procedure,[36,33] which is prohibitively slow and cumbersome for clinical applications. Moreover, quantification of retardance levels, necessary to compare spindles between eggs, is complicated when using conventional, plane polarized light microscopes, because the observed image originates from both the inherent birefringence of the specimen and the settings of the manually adjusted compensator and analyzer.

The polscope uses digital image processing to enhance sensitivity, and nearly circularly polarized light, combined with electrooptical hardware, to achieve orientation-independence, so even low levels of retardance of mammalian spindles can be measured without confounding orientation dependence.[33] CCD technology, liquid-crystal compensator optics, and computer algorithms are used to quantify birefringence magnitude (i.e., retardance) and orientation (called azimuth) at every image point in the field of view. The polscope's orientation-independence enables quantification of retardance magnitude and azimuth of spindle fibers within microtubules, because differences in these parameters results from the tissue itself rather than settings of the compensators and stages.

To produce a retardance image, the polscope generates four intensity images (which are in perfect register because there are no moving parts) at four liquid-crystal compensator settings. This gives four numbers at each pixel of the 480×640 pixel image. These four values are used in a ratio-metric calculation to determine the sample's retardance and azimuth at each pixel. An additional four images, without the sample in the optical field, are taken to serve as a background correction. Quantification of the specimen's retardance is carried out by grayscale thresholding. With this strategy, the polscope can measure retardances of as little as 0.05 nm or 0.03 degrees of phase change (which corresponds to 10^{-4} wavelengths of light). In comparison, conventional polarized light techniques have a retardance sensitivity limit of 5–10 nm, barely enough to image the meiotic spindle of mammalian oocytes, which has a retardance of approximately 3 nm in mouse oocytes. Moreover, since it illuminates specimens with the same intensity of light as used for Nomarski DIC, and since Nomarski DIC also employs polarized light, the polscope should be nontoxic to oocytes. Indeed, we have demonstrated no detrimental effects on mouse or human oocytes or on mouse embryo developmental potential following exposure to the polscope.[37]

In collaboration with Dr. Oldenbourg of the Marine Biological Laboratory at Woods Hole, Massachusetts (MBL), the polscope was adapted for use in mammalian embryology.[38] First, we optimized the optical path of the polscope for imaging with an inverted microscope. Next, we observed a number of unique features of oocyte morphology, including a laminar structure of the zona pellucida, as well as the meiotic spindle[39,40] of mouse and hamster oocytes with our polscope at the Women and Infants Laboratory for Reproductive Medicine at the Woods Hole Marine

Biological Laboratory. After establishing the safety of polscope imaging in animals, we installed polscopes at our IVF centers, at Women and Infants Hospital in Providence, RI and at Tufts-New England Medical Center in Boston, to study human eggs and embryos.

Hoffman or Nomarski DIC microscopy reveals the position of the polar body, but not the meiotic spindle. Since clinical embryologists use the polar body to orient the injection site during intracytoplasmic sperm injection (ICSI), we examined whether the location of the polar body could predict the position of the spindle. We found discordance between the location of the spindle and the polar body in eggs from hamster, mouse, cow, and humans.[38,41] To perform these experiments, oocytes were adjusted until the first polar body and spindle appeared in the same optical plane. Polscope images were saved and the angle formed between these two structures was calculated by Metamorph (Universal Imaging, Chester, PA). Using the polscope, we found that the polar body does not predict accurately the location of the meiotic spindle in mouse, hamster, or human eggs. In only 5 of 18 hamster eggs did the polar body accurately predict the placement of the meiotic spindle. For approximately 30% of the eggs, if the polar body had been used to direct ICSI the needle would have approached the meiotic spindle. The risk of injury to spindle or chromosomes during needle insertion must be small, because the needle itself is so small relative to the egg, but injury would be more likely to occur when the oocyte's cytoplasm is aspirated just before the sperm is injected. The lack of close relationship between the spindle and the polar body in MII oocytes raises the question of whether oocytes should be oriented on the holding pipette based on the location of the spindle rather than of the polar body. It also introduces the question of whether egg infertility could result from abnormalities in the establishment of normal polarity during oogenesis.

The Zona Pellucida has a Multilaminar Structure

Since the zona pellucida is comprised of three related filamentous glycoproteins (ZP1, ZP2, and ZP3), we hypothesized that it would exhibit a high level of birefringence. The impairment of hatching identified in embryos after *in vitro* culture also begged the question of whether the artificial conditions associated with IVF might change the biophysical properties of zona proteins, and thus alter the retardance and/or azimuth of specific zona layers. When imaged under Hoffman or Nomarski DIC optics, the zona pellucida appears as a uniform, thick layer. However, when imaged with the polscope, the zona exhibits a multilaminar structure, with three layers differing in their degree of retardance and orientation.[39] Moreover, when comparing embryos cultured *in vitro* or *in vivo*, the polscope revealed that *in vitro* cultured embryos exhibited impaired thinning of the inner layer of the zona. Culturing embryos appears to disrupt the normal process of zona thinning by selectively affecting the inner layer of the zona, visible only with the polscope.[40]

The Polscope Does not Disrupt Preimplantation Mouse Embryo Development

Since the polscope uses light of approximately the same intensity as Nomarski DIC and Hoffman optics (unpublished observation), and since Nomarski DIC uses polarized light, yet exerts no significant detrimental effects on embryo development, we hypothesized the polscope would be safe for embryos. To test this hypothesis, the implantation rate of mouse embryos following imaging with the polscope was compared to control embryos not imaged with the polscope, after transfer into the uterus of pseudopregnant young recipients. Results confirmed that the light exposure levels encountered during polscope operation have no apparent affect on blastocyst rate, cell number, or pregnancy rates after transfer.[38]

Spindle Observation in Living Human Eggs with Polarized Microscope

Spindles imaged by immunofluorescence of human eggs appear to be smaller than spindles from mouse eggs, so we needed to determine whether the polscope could image spindles in human oocytes. We examined human eggs aspirated from stimulated ovaries of consenting patients undergoing oocyte retrieval for ICSI. Five hundred and thirty-three oocytes from 51 cycles were examined by the polscope. Spindles were imaged in 61.4% of oocytes.[37] Interestingly, after ICSI, more oocytes with spindles fertilized and developed normally than oocytes lacking spindles.[37]

We also needed to confirm that the polscope was safe for human eggs, so we conducted an observational study comparing development of *in vitro* embryos, which either had or had not been imaged with the polscope at the egg stage of development.[37,42] The average age was 33.3 ± 3.9 for patients whose oocytes were exposed to the polscope and 34.7 ± 3.7 for the patients whose oocytes were not exposed to the polscope. Three hundred and thirty-seven oocytes from 35 cycles were examined with the polscope, and spindles were imaged in 59.3% of oocytes. The fertilization rate of imaged eggs was 62.3%, the same as that (64.0%) of eggs (433 from 52 cycles) not exposed to the polscope. The rate of viable embryos (57.1%) from eggs that had been exposed to the polscope did not differ statistically from that of oocytes not exposed (59.6%). These results indicate that exposure of human oocyte to polscope for spindle imaging is not detrimental to human eggs.

Comparison of Polscope and Confocal Microscope Images of Spindles from Oocytes

The polscope measures spindle retardance while immunocyto-chemistry directly images immunolabeled microtubules, so we needed to compare spindles imaged by both methods. Two sources of oocytes were used: unfertilized oocytes from mice and spare human eggs from women undergoing ICSI. While immunocyto-chemistry provided greater detail of spindle microtubules, excellent overlap could be seen when the same mouse eggs were imaged with the polscope before fixation and immunostaining.[38] Imaging spare human eggs, on day 1 after ICSI, spindles could be imaged in 73% oocytes with the polscope.[37] Interestingly, spindles from aged eggs were shorter (8.08 ± 0.84 μm) than from fresh eggs (11.2 ± 3.4 μm). Spindle structure obtained with the polscope was comparable to that imaged by confocal microscopy. Of the 27% oocytes on day 1, and all oocytes from days 2 to 4, in which no birefringent spindles could be imaged by the polscope, confocal immunostaining also failed to demonstrate meiotic spindles, suggesting that the sensitivities of these two methods to image the spindle were comparable. Indeed, eggs lacking spindle birefringence exhibited only disassembled microtubules and dispersed chromosomes on confocal immunostaining.

Culture of immature human oocytes yielded MI and MII stage oocytes, in which spindles could readily be observed with the polscope. When oocytes with birefringent spindles were fixed and examined by confocal microscopy, 75% of oocytes at MI and 71% of oocytes at MII had typical metaphase spindles. Most oocytes (75%) with birefringent spindles had normal chromosome configuration, confirmed by a series of confocal microscopic images. However, all oocytes without a birefringent spindle and 25% of oocytes with a birefringent spindle exhibited abnormal chromosomal configurations. Thus, the polscope provides nearly the same information about spindle structure, though less sensitive than confocal immunostaining, to detect chromosome misalignment.

Spindle Microtubules can be Quantified by Retardance Measurements

Because of its orientation-independence, the polscope provides quantitative information about spindle structure. Conversely, quantification of spindle structure following fixation and immunostaining is problematic because of the confounding effects of fixation and fluorescence quenching. We employed the quantitative features of the polscope to image mouse spindles during activation and demonstrated increased assembly of microtubules in the spindle's midpiece, suggesting that the spindle's microtubules may be pushing as well as pulling chromosomes during anaphase.[38]

We also demonstrated the feasibility of studying spindle kinetics. Since polscope imaging is noninvasive, we performed time-lapse pole imaging of activated mouse oocytes. We even succeeded in performing time-lapse polscope imaging of meiotic spindles in karyoplasts generated either by enucleation[38] or centrifugation.

During egg aging *in vitro*, meiotic spindle structure may deteriorate. We measured retardance in human spindles and found large differences in retardance among eggs as a function of *in vitro* aging. Aged eggs had smaller spindles with less birefringence compared to freshly aspirated eggs.[42] The level of spindle birefringence thus may prove useful to monitor egg quality or cytoplasmic maturation before "rescue ICSI." These results indicate that spindle retardance can be qualified in living human eggs, and that retardance may be an important parameter for evaluation of egg quality and to predict cytoplasmic maturation.

Thermodynamic Regulation of Spindle Assembly

Mammalian spindles are remarkably temperature-sensitive. Previous studies had demonstrated profound effects of even transient cooling on spindle assembly, so we studied the temperature sensitivity of human meiotic spindles, and demonstrated that reassembly following significant cooling on rewarming is only partial.[42] Moreover, conventional heating plates employed in most IVF laboratories only poorly maintain thermal stability of eggs, while they are being imaged and injected. A system which maintained rigorous thermal control during ICSI, by thermostaining both the petri dish and the microscope's objective, nearly doubled the development of embryos to morula and blastocyst stages following the ICSI procedure.[43]

Prediction of Aneuploidy by Polscope Imaging of the Meiotic Spindle

KEY POINT

Animal models support the key role of the spindle for chromosomal arrangement and the negative impact of aging.

Abnormal spindle structure has been indirectly implicated in the generation of aneuploidy by the association of advanced maternal age and structurally abnormal spindles,[32] and by the obviously important role of the meiotic spindle in partitioning chromosomes during meiotic maturation and fertilization. An association between chromosome misalignment and spindle abnormalities also has been observed in immunostained spindles.[32] We demonstrated that noninvasive imaging of the MI spindle in human eggs provides an excellent predictor of chromosome misalignment.[44] We also demonstrated abnormal spindle birefringence in eggs from the senescence accelerated mouse (SAM), a naturally occurring strain of mouse which exhibits precocious reproductive senescence compared to wild-type strains. Although the retardance of chromosomes is much less than that of microtubules, we were able to image chromosomes noninvasively in SAM eggs and by doing so, demonstrated higher rates of chromosome misassembly in eggs from SAM compared to eggs from wild-type strains.[45]

Mechanisms Underlying Aging-Related Spindle Disruption

How aging disrupts spindles from older females remains unclear. We have hypothesized that the effects of reproductive aging on egg function are mediated by telomere shortening in eggs ovulated late in the life of the female. Telomeres are TTAGGG repeats which cap and protect the ends of all chromosomes. Telomere shortening occurs with each cell cycle, and unless telomeres are restored, results in cell cycle arrest and apoptosis, a process called crises. Telomerase activity is almost nonexistent during late oogenesis,[46] so telomere length provides a bottleneck during early development. Eggs ovulating late in the life of a female exited late from the production line during fetal oogenesis,[47,48] and therefore must have traversed more cell cycles, so unless telomerase is an unusually efficient enzyme, late ovulating eggs would be expected to start life with shorter telomeres than eggs ovulated early in the life of the female, which exited early from oogenesis and therefore traversed fewer cell cycles. Moreover, during early meiosis telomeres establish the homology search necessary for chiasmata formation, and during the prolonged interval between early into prophase and completion of meiotic maturation, telomeres anchor the oocytes' chromosomes in the nuclear membrane.[49–53] Here telomeres are susceptible to chronic attack by reactive oxygen species, the inevitable by-products of cellular metabolism, which promote aging in virtually every type of cell. Using quantitive digital fluorescence microscopy (Q-FISH) to measure telomere length,[54] we demonstrated that reactive oxygen species can further shorten telomeres and induce chromosome abnormalities[55] in mouse zygotes. Moreover, mice genetically engineered to have short telomeres exhibited abnormalities in the structure of their meiotic spindles, but only when telomere length reached a critical length.[56] Eggs with short telomeres also gave rise to embryos which exhibited cell cycle arrest and apoptosis,[57] a phenotype remarkably similar to that of embryos from older women.[1,34] Thus, it is likely that chromosomal structure itself, rather than cytoplasmic factors predisposes to spindle dysfunction, and ultimately to nondisjunction.

Egg Reconstitution Techniques for the Treatment of Infertility

Numerous studies have demonstrated the efficacy of egg donation for the treatment of egg infertility, but couples faced with egg infertility almost invariably resist the most effective therapy available to them—egg donation. Faced with the logistic, ethical, and financial limitations of egg donation, most hope and pray for some way to transmit the woman's genetic legacy. One strategy that has been proposed to combine the benefits from donor eggs, yet still transmit the genetic legacy of the infertile woman, is oocyte reconstitution. Developments in egg and embryo biotechnology over the past 25 years now make it technically feasible to reconstitute human eggs and embryos from nuclei, cytoplasm, or cytoplasmic organelles originating from different eggs from the same individual, from polar bodies from the same egg, or from eggs from different individuals.[58] Although technically feasible, currently inadequate evidence supports the efficacy of oocyte reconstitution procedures in the treatment of human infertility. Moreover, no long-term studies support the safety to offspring conceived following these procedures. Indeed, studies from a number of animal models suggest significant potential for generation of abnormalities in offspring arising from oocyte reconstitution. Since the cytoplasm contains mitochondrial DNA (mtDNA), oocyte reconstitution manipulates the germ line genome and therefore contravenes the existing voluntary moratorium on germ line gene therapy.[59] Finally, since cytoplasm mediates most of the protective effects of apoptosis to prevent transmission of defective germ cells across generations, and chromosome structure may play as important a role in mediating age-related egg dysfunction as cytoplasm, by replacing senescent cytoplasm while leaving senescent chromosomes, oocyte reconstitution may disarm this important protective mechanism.

Oocyte reconstitution techniques employ various strategies to manipulate the oocyte's cytoplasm, while preserving the nuclear genome. Nuclear transfer involves the transfer of the nucleus from a somatic cell,[60,61] polar body,[62] or other oocyte into an enucleated donor oocyte or zygote.[62-65] Cytoplasmic transfer involves transfer of cytoplasm from a donor oocyte or zygote into a recipient oocyte or zygote.[66] Mitochondrial transfer involves the infusion of mitochondria fractionated from another source, either somatic or germ cells, into an oocyte or zygote.[67]

Nuclear transfer can be performed at the prophase[64,65,68] or metaphase stages[69] of meiotic maturation, procedures called germinal vesicle and spindle transfer, respectively. Nuclear transfer can also be performed at the zygote stage, called pronuclear transfer, or at later stages of development.[63,70,71] Nuclear transfer involves an enucleation step, typically employing pretreatment with cytoskeletal toxins to free the nucleus from surrounding cytoplasm, followed by mechanical enucleation. Centrifugation of oocytes also has been employed to separate nucleus and cytoplasm.[38] Additional interventions are required to fuse the nuclear material (called karyoplast) and the cytoplasm (called cytoplast). The most commonly used methods to reconstitute the karyoplast and cytoplast are electrofusion, which jolts the cell constituents with a brief pulse of high voltage electricity, or chemical fusion mediated by inactivated Sendai virus.[72–76] Technically it is difficult to transfer pure nuclear material, since the karyoplast invariably also carries varying amounts of cytoplasmic material, including mitochondria.

Cytoplasmic transfusion uses a micropipette to deliver small quantities of cyptoplasm into the oocyte, typically at the time of ICSI. Most published protocols recommend transfer of no more than 3% of cell volume to reduce risk to the recipient cell from the procedure.[77] Thus, in contrast to nuclear transfer, cytoplasmic transfer typically exchanges only a minuscule proportion of the oocyte's cytoplasm. Transfusion of mitochondria fractionated from other cells types, or from other oocytes also has been successfully carried out.[67] Although debate exists as to the survival of mitochondria injected into oocytes and zygotes,[78–80] sensitive molecular methods, such as PCR, demonstrate survival of injected mitochondria at least to the blastocyst stage in a mouse model.[67]

When oocyte reconstitution techniques have been used to study nuclear-cytoplasmic interactions during development, most studies conclude that cytoplasm exerts powerful control over meiotic maturation of the egg and subsequent development of the preimplantation embryo.[81] Testimony to the powerful effects of egg cytoplasm on the birth is the first mammal by somatic cell cloning from fusion of a somatic cell with an enucleated egg.[60] Considered one of the most important breakthroughs in developmental biology and medicine, this basic application of the nuclear transfer method underscored the ability of oocyte cytoplasm to alter nuclear function, even to the extent of completely reprogramming it.[76,82] Other important roles of cytoplasm include regulation of cell cycle,[81] commitment of the cell to apoptosis,[83,84] transmission of mitochondrial genome,[85] and regulation of metabolism.

Oocyte reconstitution procedures also have been proposed as medical therapies, including cell replacement therapy of degenerative diseases,[86–88] gene therapy to prevent transmission of mitochondrial diseases,[62,85] treatment of idiopathic cytoplasmic dysfunction during infertility,[62] haploidization of somatic cells to produce gametes for agonadal women, and prevention of aneuploidy.[62,64] A major rational for application of oocyte reconstitution procedures to reproductive medicine is that egg infertility is an important cause of idiopathic infertility, since egg donation achieves excellent pregnancy rates for such patients. However, egg donation, like adoption, requires significant modification of the personal goals of the infertile couple, and the pace of achieving this emotional shift varies among couples. Furthermore, critical shortages of egg donors limit the availability of this procedure, so alternative treatments for egg infertility are urgently needed. If egg viability could be enhanced by reconstitution of oocytes from the infertile woman's nucleus and cytoplasm from a healthy donor's eggs, the prospective mother could transmit her genetic legacy and the donor would provide only that part of the egg which does not carry her nuclear genome. It is important to note that nuclear or cytoplasmic transfer used this way would not be expected to confer fertility to menopausal women, since most menopausal women have no oocytes at all.

For menopausal women, some investigators have proposed transfer of nuclei from somatic cells into immature, enucleated donor oocytes in an attempt to generate gametes by artificial haploidization. However, cells are committed to the germ line only very early during development and germ line commitment involves formation of chiasmata and other molecular and cytogenetic machinery for recombination.[89] Indeed, normal execution of the critical steps of early meiosis, i.e., pairing of homologous chromosomes, cohesion between sister centromeres, and monopolar attachment during meiosis I, depend more on features of the chromosomes, egg telomere length, and the action of molecules, such as cohesions and monopolin, than on cytoplasmic or spindle-based factors.[90] Thus, this strategy is destined to fail unless the somatic cell is used to generate a clone, which then is allowed to develop until the stage of germ line commitment, a strategy which currently is considered ethically unacceptable.[59,90–92]

The major hope for application of nuclear transfer to the treatment of human infertility has been to prevent aneuploidy. Most aneuploidy arises at anaphase I,[90,91] so it has been hypothesized that transfer of the nucleus from the prophase stage oocyte, called

KEY POINT

Oocyte reconstitution procedures are not likely to improve outcome in older women as chromosomal damage is likely to have occurred long before the point of in vitro intervention.

germinal vesicle transfer, into a more favorable cytoplasmic environment provided by an enucleated egg from a young donor, might correct factors responsible for aneuploidy. However, the most widely accepted theory of aneuploidy in humans postulates that, while aneuploidy first appears at anaphase I, its origin actually was much earlier during oogenesis, during fetal life, when chiasmata between sister chromosomes were established.[90] The "Production Line" theory suggests that eggs ovulated late in life themselves were born predisposed to aneuploidy because they had fewer chiasmata.[92] Thus, later manipulation of their cytoplasmic environment by nuclear or cytoplasmic transfer would be unlikely to alter their cytogenetic configuration. Indeed, since apoptosis may prevent transmission of defective oocytes to succeeding generations, and since cytoplasm mediates apoptosis, replenishing older eggs with cytoplasm from younger eggs may in fact disarm this important mechanism to prevent transmission of aneuploidy to succeeding generations.[84]

The biologic rationale for clinical application of cytoplasmic and mitochondrial transfer is that abnormalities of some constituents of cytoplasm, such as cell cycle regulatory molecules[81] or mitochondria,[93–96] might contribute to oocyte dysfunction and replacement of such a defective constituent by transfer of healthy cytoplasm or mitochondria may overcome this problem. However, these procedures exchange such small quantities of cytoplasm relative to the large amount of cytoplasm which remains in the oocyte, they are unlikely to impact egg or embryo function. For example, mutations in mtDNA have been reported in human eggs from infertile women, but the proportion of total mtDNA they represent is so small that the mutations themselves are unlikely to affect abnormal embryo development. Published reports indicate no more than 0.1% of mtDNA are affected by individual mtDNA mutations.[94] Although numerous mutations have been reported in human oocytes,[93–96] human oocytes contain hundreds of thousands of mtDNA molecules and mitochondria, so infusion of a few mitochondria or trace amounts of mtDNA into oocytes during cytoplasmic or mitochondrial transfer are unlikely to produce significant physiologic effects. Indeed, the low oxygen consumption and the lack of cristae in mitochondria from oocytes and embryos demonstrate relative quiescence of this organelle until the morula stage of preimplantation development, further suggesting that transfer of trace numbers of mitochondria into oocytes from infertile women are unlikely to affect early preimplantation embryo development.[97]

Inadequate clinical evidence supports the clinical efficacy of these experimental procedures. Nuclear transfer, performed at the germinal vesicle or metaphase I stages, is hindered by the poor development *in vitro* even of unoperated immature oocytes.[98] Indeed, no deliveries following this procedure have been reported in women. A handful of pregnancies have been reported following cytoplasmic transfer,[66] but the lack of untreated controls and the favorable profile of treated patients (age less than 40, excellent ovarian reserve) make it impossible to know to what extent the cytoplasmic transfer procedure actually may have influenced outcome. No pregnancies have been reported following mitochondrial transfer.

While the rationale for clinical application of nuclear and cytoplasmic transfer rests in translation of findings from animal studies to humans, these same animal studies also demonstrate substantial risks to offspring born after these procedures. Risks to offspring born after nuclear transfer include large body size, idiopathic sudden death, pulmonary dysfunction, imprinting metabolic and placental abnormalities.[99,100] These abnormalities are thought to arise from the detrimental effects of mitochondrial heteroplasmy[101–104] and prolonged culture *in vitro*.[105] mtDNA is the most rapidly evolving functional component of the genome, so considerable mtDNA heteroplasmy exists even within species.[85] While heteroplasmy also arises in nature, naturally occurring heteroplasmy has survived a number of stringent bottlenecks during development. The effects of experimentally produced heteroplasmy in humans are unknown, although abnormal nuclear-mitochondrial interactions have been shown to underlie some mtDNA diseases, which may exhibit a phenotype only late in life. Moreover, since mtDNA molecules harboring some deletions preferentially replicate over wild-type mtDNA molecules, aging promotes further deletions and some abnormal mtDNA molecules invariably are transferred with the karyoplast, offspring conceived after nuclear transfer theoretically could go on to develop premature senescence.

Prolonged culture, required after germinal vesicle or spindle transfer, may also induce abnormalities in genomic imprinting,[105] a condition associated with a number of human genetic diseases, including Prader-Willi's and Angelmann's syndromes,[106] as well as pregnancy-induced hypertension.[107] Other potential risks of oocyte reconstitution include abrogation of the protective effects of apoptosis during preimplantation embryo development. During normal oogenesis and preimplantation embryo development, apoptosis blocks further development of aneuploid offspring. Cytoplasm is a critical regulator of this process, so transfer of an aneuploid nucleus into normal cytoplasm might allow continued development of an aneuploid offspring that otherwise would have been sentenced to death.[83,84] Perhaps most troubling is that many of these problems, especially imprinting and mitochondrial abnormalities, may not be expected to appear until late in the life of affected offspring.

Current evidence suggests that clinical application of oocyte reconstitution procedures to the treatment of human infertility should be discouraged until studies establish the safety and efficacy of these procedures in a number of animal models, including some long-lived animals. If studies are to be pursued in humans, they should be performed only under the auspices of human investigational review board (IRB) approval. Since many local IRBs may not include experts with sufficient background in this rapidly evolving field, guidelines for consideration of IRB approval of projects involving clinical application of oocyte reconstitution are provided below.

Guidelines for Responsible Research on the Application of New Technologies for Treatment of Human Infertility

Advances in cellular and molecular biology of early development have created unprecedented opportunities to unlock the mysteries of the beginning of human life, and also to relieve the suffering associated with human infertility by developing new diagnostic and treatment approaches to egg infertility. However, because of the refractory nature of their problem, couples suffering from egg infertility are among the most vulnerable encountered by the clinician. While clinical studies in this area clearly are needed, investigators must provide informed consent, which discusses not only the theoretical benefit of the proposed research procedures, but also the theoretical risks to offspring. In the case of oocyte reconstitution, risks include large offspring, sudden death, placental and pulmonary abnormalities, and abnormalities in mitochondrial function and imprinting, as well as premature senescence in offspring. The availability of effective alternatives, including continued treatment with own gametes, egg donation, and adoption should be broached. Psychologic counseling should be available for all subjects, and should focus on interpreting resistance to pursuing currently available alternatives and on grieving loss of the ability to transmit the woman's own genetic material to her offspring. Any studies of oocyte reconstitution for the treatment of human infertility should include testing of all resulting conceptions for aneuploidy, as well as mtDNA heteroplasmy,[108] and should include prolonged follow-up of any offspring born after such treatment.

Summary

Egg infertility remains the greatest challenge facing ART. As women continue to delay attempts at childbearing the magnitude of this problem will only increase. Attempts to overcome relative egg infertility by controlled ovarian stimulation, followed by IUI or IVF, have contributed to an epidemic, of multiple gestations, that has become a major public health concern. The pathophysiology of egg infertility centers on nondisjunction resulting in aneuploidy. For now, cytogenetic analyses of polar bodies and/or cleavage stage embryos provide the most powerful predictor of aneuploidy-related egg infertility.

The clinical use of cytogenetic analysis, however, is limited by the difficulty of imaging more than a handful of the diverse chromosomes predisposed for nondisjunctures in the human egg. A number of alternative approaches have been developed to be able to identify all (SKY, CGH) or a large subset of chromosomes. Other approaches aim to identify and diagnose the underlying etiology of germ line genomic instability, including noninvasive imaging of the spindle apparatus with polscope and measurement of telomeres by Q-FISH.

For the foreseeable future, the treatment options for egg infertility will be limited to egg donation for severe cases, and to identifications of the most viable among a cohort of superovulated eggs for milder cases. Oocyte reconstitution not only lacks evidence of clinical efficacy, but also lacks biological credibility, with growing evidence to support the primacy of chromosomes themselves in the regulation of meiosis.

REFERENCES

1 Ezra Y, Laufer SA. Defective oocytes in a new subgroup of unexplained infertility. *Fertil Steril* 58:24–27, 1992.

2 Lutjen PJ, Leeton JF, Findlay JK. Oocyte and embryo donation in IVF programmes. *Clin Obstet Gynaecol* 12(4):799–813, 1985.

3 Navot D, et al. Poor oocyte quality rather than implantation failure as a cause of age-related decline in female fertility. *Lancet* 337(8754):1375–1377, 1991.

4 Sauer MV, Paulson RJ. Oocyte and embryo donation. *Curr Opin Obstet Gynecol* 7(3):193–198, 1995.

5 Callahan TL, et al. The economic impact of multiple-gestation pregnancies and the contribution of assisted-reproduction techniques to their incidence. *N Engl J Med* 331:244–249, 1994.

6 Abdalla HI, et al. Age, pregnancy and miscarriage: uterine versus ovarian factors. *Hum Reprod* 8(9):1512–1517, 1993.

7 Toner JP, et al. Basal follicle-stimulating hormone level is a better predictor of in vitro fertilization performance than age. *Fertil Steril* 55(4):784–791, 1991.

8 Corson SL, et al. Inhibin-B as a test of ovarian reserve for infertile women. *Hum Reprod* 14:2818–2821, 1999.

9 Gulekli B, et al. Accuracy of ovarian reserve tests. *Hum Reprod* 14(11):2822–2826, 1999.

10 Hall JE, Welt CK, Cramer DW. Inhibin A and inhibin B reflect ovarian function in assisted reproduction but are less useful at predicting outcome. *Hum Reprod* 14(2):409–415, 1999.

11 Sharara FI, Scott RT Jr, Seifer DB. The detection of diminished ovarian reserve in infertile women. *Am J Obstet Gynecol* 179(3 Pt 1): 804–812, 1998.

12 Keefe DL. Reproductive aging is an evolutionarily programmed strategy that no longer provides adaptive value. *Fertil Steril* 70(2): 204–206, 1998.

13 Baker TG. A quantitative and cytological study of germ cells in human ovaries. *Proc Roy Soc B* 158:417–433, 1963.

14 Baker TG, Sum OW. Development of the ovary and oogenesis. *Clin Obstet Gynecol* 3:3–26, 1976.

15 Gianaroli L, et al. Preimplantation diagnosis for aneuploidies in patients undergoing in vitro fertilization with a poor prognosis: identification of the categories for which it should be proposed. *Fertil Steril* 72(5):837–844, 1999.

16 Verlinsky Y, et al. Polar body diagnosis of common aneuploidies by FISH. *J Assist Reprod Genet* 13(2):157–162, 1996.

17 Verlinsky Y, et al. Prepregnancy genetic testing for age-related aneuploidies by polar body analysis. *Genet Test* 1(4):231–235, 1997.

18 Verlinsky Y, et al. Preimplantation diagnosis of common aneuploidies by the first- and second-polar body FISH analysis. *J Assist Reprod Genet* 15(5):285–289, 1998.

19 Verlinsky Y, et al. Prevention of age-related aneuploidies by polar body testing of oocytes. *J Assist Reprod Genet* 16(4):165–169, 1999.

20 Verlinsky Y, Evsikov S. Karyotyping of human oocytes by chromosomal analysis of the second polar bodies. *Mol Hum Reprod* 5(2):89–95, 1999.

21 Marquez C, et al. Chromosome abnormalities in 1255 cleavage-stage human embryos. *Reprod Biomed Online* 1(1):17–26, 2000.

22 Munne S, et al. Chromosome mosaicism in cleavage-stage human embryos: evidence of a maternal age effect. *Reprod Biomed Online* 4(3):223–232, 2002.

23 Bahce M, Cohen J, Munne S. Preimplantation genetic diagnosis of aneuploidy: were we looking at the wrong chromosomes? *J Assist Reprod Genet* 16(4):176–181, 1999.

24 Abdelhadi I, et al. Preimplantation genetic diagnosis of numerical abnormalities for 13 chromosomes. *Reprod Biomed Online* 6(2):226–231, 2003.

25 Sandalinas M, Marquez C, Munne S. Spectral karyotyping of fresh, non-inseminated oocytes. *Mol Hum Reprod* 8(6):580–585, 2002.

26 Wells D, et al. First clinical application of comparative genomic hybridization and polar body testing for preimplantation genetic diagnosis of aneuploidy. *Fertil Steril* 78(3):543, 2002.

27 Obasaju M, et al. Pregnancies from single normal embryo transfer in women older than 40 years. *Reprod Biomed Online* 2(2):98–101, 2001.

28 Schultz RM. Gene expression in mouse embryos: use of mRNA differential display. In: Richter JD (ed.), *Advances in Molecular Biology*. New York, NY: Oxford University Press, 1999, pp. 149–156.

29 Tanaka TS, et al. Genome-wide expression profiling of mid-gestation placenta and embryo using a 15,000 mouse developmental cDNA microarray. *Proc Natl Acad Sci USA* 97(16):9127–9132, 2000.

30 Weier HG, et al. Towards a full karyotype screening of interphase cells: "FISH and chip technology." *Mol Cell Endocrinol* 183(Suppl 1): S41–S45, 2001.

31 Hassold T, Hunt P. To err (meiotically) is human: the genesis of human aneuploidy. *Nat Rev Genet* 2(4):280–291, 2001.

32 Battaglia DE, et al. Influence of maternal age on meiotic spindle assembly in oocytes from naturally cycling women. *Hum Reprod* 11(10):2217–2222, 1996.

33 Oldenbourg R. Polarized light microscopy of spindles. *Methods Cell Biol* 61:175–208, 1999.

34 Bolton VN, et al. Development of spare human preimplantation embryos in vitro: an analysis of the correlations among gross morphology, cleavage rates, and development to the blastocyst. *J In Vitro Fert Embryo Transf* 6:30–35, 1989.

35 Cha KY, Chian RC. Maturation in vitro of immature human oocytes for clinical use. *Hum Reprod Update* 4:103–120, 1998.

36 Sato H, Ellis GW, Inoue S. Microtubular origin of mitotic spindle for birefringence. *J Cell Biol* 67:501–517, 1975.

37 Wang WH, et al. The spindle observation and its relationship with fertilization after intracytoplasmic sperm injection in living human oocytes. *Fertil Steril* 75(2):348–353, 2001.

38 Liu L, et al. A reliable, noninvasive technique for spindle imaging and enucleation of mammalian oocytes. *Nat Biotechnol* 18(2):223–225, 2000.

39 Keefe DL, et al. Polarized light microscopy and digital image processing identify a multilaminar structure of the hamster zona pellucida. *Hum Reprod* 12:1250–1252, 1997.

40 Silva CP, et al. Effect of in vitro culture of mammalian embryos on the architecture of the zona pellucida. *Biol Bull* 193(2):235–236, 1997.

41 Silva CP, et al. The first polar body does not predict accurately the location of the metaphase II meiotic spindle in mammalian oocytes. *Fertil Steril* 71:719–721, 1999.

42 Wang WH, et al. Developmental ability of human oocytes with or without birefringent spindles imaged by Polscope before insemination. *Hum Reprod* 16(7):1464–1468, 2001.

43 Wang WH, et al. Rigorous thermal control during intracytoplasmic sperm injection stabilizes the meiotic spindle and improves fertilization and pregnancy rates. *Fertil Steril* 77:1274–1277, 2002.

44 Wang WH, Keefe DL. Prediction of chromosome misalignment among in vitro matured human oocytes by spindle imaging with the Polscope. *Fertil Steril* 78(5):1077–1081, 2002.

45 Liu L, Keefe DL. Aging-associated aberration in meiosis of oocytes from senescence-accelerated mouse (SAM). *Hum Reprod* 17:2678–2685, 2002.

46 Wright DL, et al. Characterization of telomerase activity in the human oocyte and preimplantation embryo. *Mol Hum Reprod* 7(10):947–955, 2001.

47 Henderson SA, Edwards RG. Chiasma frequency and maternal age in mammals. *Nature* 217(136):22–28, 1968.

48 Polani PE, Crolla JA. A test of the production line hypothesis of mammalian oogenesis. *Hum Genet* 88(1):64–70, 1991.

49 Bass HW, et al. Telomeres cluster de novo before the initiation of synapsis: a three-dimensional spatial analysis of telomere positions before and during meiotic prophase. *J Cell Biol* 137(1):5–18, 1997.

50 Bass HW, et al. Evidence for the coincident initiation of homolog pairing and synapsis during the telomere-clustering (bouquet) stage of meiotic prophase. *J Cell Sci* 113(Pt 6):1033–1042, 2000.

51 de Lange T. Ending up with the right partner. *Nature* 392(6678): 753–754, 1998.

52 Scherthan H, et al. Mammalian meiotic telomeres: protein composition and redistribution in relation to nuclear pores. *Mol Biol Cell* 11(12):4189–4203, 2000.

53 Scherthan H, et al. Centromere and telomere movements during early meiotic prophase of mouse and man are associated with the onset of chromosome pairing. *J Cell Biol* 134(5):1109–1125, 1996.

54 Poon SS, et al. Telomere length measurements using digital fluorescence microscopy. *Cytometry* 36:267–278, 1999.

55 Liu L, et al. Mitochondrial dysfunction leads to telomere attrition and genomic instability. *Aging Cell* 1:40–46, 2002.

56 Liu L, Blasco MA, Keefe DL. Requirement of functional telomeres for metaphase chromosome alignments and integrity of meiotic spindles. *EMBO Rep* 3:230–234, 2002.

57 Liu L, et al. An essential role for functional telomeres in mouse germ cells during fertilization and early development. *Dev Biol* 249:74–84, 2002.

58 Foote RH. In: Wolf DP, Zelinski-Wooten (eds.), *Contemporary Endocrinology: Assisted Fertilization and Nuclear Transfer in Mammals.* Totowa, NJ: Humana Press, 2001, pp. 3–20.

59 Gene therapy and the germline. *Nat Med* 5(3):245, 1999.

60 Wilmut I, et al. Viable offspring derived from fetal and adult mammalian cells. *Nature* 385(6619):810–813, 1997.

61 Willadsen SM. Nuclear transplantation in sheep embryos. *Nature* 320(6057):63–65, 1986.

62 Wolfe DP. Cloning and nuclear transfer in humans. Contemporary Endocrinology: Assisted fertilization and nuclear transfer in mammals 285–297, 2001.

63 McGrath J, Solter D. Nuclear transplantation in the mouse embryo by microsurgery and cell fusion. *Science* 220(4603):1300–1302, 1983.

64 Zhang J, et al. In vitro maturation of human preovulatory oocytes reconstructed by germinal vesicle transfer. *Fertil Steril* 71(4):726–731, 1999.

65 Takeuchi T, et al. A reliable technique of nuclear transplantation for immature mammalian oocytes. *Hum Reprod* 14(5):1312–1317, 1999.

66 Cohen J, et al. Birth of an infant after transfer of anucleate donor oocyte cytoplasm into recipient eggs. *Lancet* 350:186–187, 1997.

67 Rinaudo P, et al. Microinjection of mitochondria into zygotes creates a model for studying the inheritance of mitochondrial DNA during preimplantation development. *Fertil Steril* 71:912–918, 1999.

68 Takeuchi T, et al. Preliminary findings in germinal vesicle transplantation of immature human oocytes. *Hum Reprod* 16(4):730–736, 2001.

69 Tatham BG, Dowsing AT, Trounson AO. Enucleation by centrifugation of in vitro-matured bovine oocytes for use in nuclear transfer. *Biol Reprod* 53:1088–1094, 1995.

70 McGrath J, Solter D. Nuclear transplantation in mouse embryos. *J Exp Zool* 228(2):355–362, 1983.

71 McGrath J, Solter D. Nucleocytoplasmic interactions in the mouse embryo. *J Embryol Exp Morphol* 97(Suppl):277–289, 1986.

72 Collas P, Robl JM. Factors affecting the efficiency of nuclear transplantation in the rabbit embryo. *Biol Reprod* 43(5):877–884, 1990.

73 Kubiak JZ, Tarkowski AK. Electrofusion of mouse blastomeres. *Exp Cell Res* 157(2):561–566, 1985.

74 Saltman D, et al. Telomeric structure in cells with chromosome end associations. *Chromosoma* 102(2):121–128, 1993.

75 Prather RS, et al. Nuclear transplantation in the bovine embryo: Assessment of donor nuclei and recipient oocyte. *Biol Reprod* 37:859–866, 1987.

76 Collas P, Robl JM. Relationship between nuclear remodeling and development in nuclear transplant rabbit embryos. *Biol Reprod* 45:455–465, 1991.

77 Mehlmann LM, Kline D. Regulation of intracellular calcium in the mouse egg: calcium release in response to sperm or inositol trisphosphate is enhanced after meiotic maturation. *Biol Reprod* 51(6):1088–1098, 1994.

78 Sutovsky P, Navara CS, Schatten G. Fate of the sperm mitochondria, and the incorporation, conversion, and disassembly of the sperm tail structures during bovine fertilization. *Biol Reprod* 55(6):1195–1205, 1996.

79 Ebert KM, et al. Mouse zygotes injected with mitochondria develop normally but the exogenous mitochondria are not detectable in the progeny. *Mol Reprod Dev* 1(3):156–163, 1989.

80 Cummins JM, Wakayama T, Yanagimachi R. Fate of microinjected sperm components in the mouse oocyte and embryo. *Zygote* 5(4):301–308, 1997.

81 Smith GD. In: Wolf DP, Zelinski-Wooten (eds.), *Control of Oocyte Nuclear and Cytoplasmic Maturation. Contemporary Endocrinology: Assisted Fertilization and Nuclear Transfer in Mammals.* Totowa, NJ: Humana Press, 2001, pp. 53–65.

82 Liu L, et al. Nuclear remodeling and early development in cryopreserved, procine primordial germ cells following nuclear transfer into in vitro-matured oocytes. *Int J Dev Biol* 39:639–644, 1995.

83 Liu L, Trimarchi JR, Keefe DL. Involvement of mitochondria in oxidative stress-induced cell death in mouse zygotes. *Biol Reprod* 62(6):1745–1753, 2000.

84 Liu L, Keefe DL. Cytoplasm mediates both development and oxidation-induced apoptotic cell death in mouse zygotes. *Biol Reprod* 62(6):1828–1834, 2000.

85 Wallace DC. Report of the committee on human mitochondrial DNA. *Cytogenet Cell Genet* 55(1–4):395–405, 1990.

86 Lanza RP, et al. The ethical validity of using nuclear transfer in human transplantation. *JAMA* 284:3175–3179, 2000.

87 Juengst E, Fossel M. The ethics of embryonic stem cells-now and forever, cells without end. *JAMA* 284:3180–3184, 2000.

88 Lanza RP, Cibelli JB, West MD. Prospects for the use of nuclear transfer in human transplantation. *Nat Biotech* 17:1171–1174, 1999.

89 Cowan CR, Carlton PM, Cande WZ. The polar arrangement of telomeres in interphase and meiosis. rabl organization and the bouquet. *Plant Physiol* 125(2):532–538, 2001.

90 Hassold T, Chiu D. Maternal age-specific rates of numerical chromosome abnormalities with special reference to trisomy. *Hum Genet* 70(1):11–17, 1985.

91 Pellestor F. Frequency and distribution of aneuploidy in human female gametes. *Hum Genet* 86(3):283–288, 1991.

92 Medicine ASFR. *Human Cloning Through Nuclear Transplantation*, 1997.

93 Keefe DL, et al. Mitochondrial deoxyribonucleic acid deletions in oocytes and reproductive aging in women. *Fertil Steril* 64(3):577–583, 1995.

94 Chen X, et al. Rearranged mitochondrial genomes are present in human oocytes. *Am J Hum Genet* 57(2):239–247, 1995.

95 Reynier P, et al. Long PCR analysis of human gamete mtDNA suggests defective mitochondrial maintenance in spermatozoa and supports the bottleneck theory for oocytes. *Biochem Biophys Res Commun* 252(2):373–377, 1998.

96 Barritt JA, et al. Mitochondrial DNA rearrangements in the human oocyte and embryo. *Mol Hum Reprod* 5:927–933, 1999.

97 Trimarchi JR, et al. Oxidative phosphorylation-dependent and -independent oxygen consumption by individual preimplantation mouse embryos. *Biol Reprod* 62:1866–1874, 2000.

98 Nagy ZP, et al. Pregnancy and birth after intracytoplasmic sperm injection of in vitro matured germinal-vesicle stage oocytes: case report. *Fertil Steril* 65(5):1047–1050, 1996.

99 Gartner K, et al. High variability of body sizes within nucleus-transfer-clones of calves: artifacts or a biological feature? *Reprod Com Anim*, 33:67–75, 1998.

100 Japan studies elevated cloning deaths. *Nat Biotech* 16:992, 1998.

101 Takeda K, et al. Dominant distribution of mitochondrial DNA from recipient oocytes in bovine embryos and offspring after nuclear transfer. *J Reprod Fertil* 116:253–259, 1999.

102 Meirelles FV, Smith LC. Mitochondrial genotype segregation during preimplantation development in mouse heteroplasmic embryos. *Genetics* 148(2):877–883, 1998.

103 Steinborn R, et al. Mitochondrial DNA heteroplasmy in cloned cattle produced by fetal and adult cell cloning. *Nat Genet* 25(3):255–257, 2000.

104 Hiendleder S, et al. Transmitochondrial differences and varying levels of heteroplasmy in nuclear transfer cloned cattle. *Mol Reprod Dev* 54(1):24–31, 1999.

105 Doherty AS, et al. Differential effects of culture on imprinted H19 expression in the preimplantation mouse embryo. *Biol Reprod* 62(6):1526–1535, 2000.

106 Reik W, Walter J. Evolution of imprinting mechanisms: the battle of the sexes begins in the zygote. *Nat Genet* 27(3):255–256, 2001.

107 Dekker GA, Sibai BM. Etiology and pathogenesis of preeclampsia: current concepts. *Am J Obstet Gynecol* 179(5):1359–1375, 1998.

108 Ruitenbeek W, et al. The use of chorionic villin in prenatal diagnosis of mitochondriopathies. *J Inherit Metab Dis* 15:303–306, 1992.

Genetics and Infertility

Renee A. Reijo Pera

Introduction

KEY POINT

The genetics of human reproduction are complex and likely involve several hundred to several thousand genes.

Although infertility is a common health problem and has been recorded in the earliest documents of humankind, the study of the genetic basis of infertility is in its early stages. In contrast, basic research has dissected the genetics of reproduction in model organisms such as the fruitfly, *Drosophila melanogaster* and the common mouse, *Mus musculus*, and demonstrated that reproduction is genetically complex and may require as many as several hundred to several thousand genes for the formation of a functional germ cell, a sperm or an egg.[1-4] When we consider reproduction in men and women, it is undoubtedly as complex genetically as that of model organisms, and yet just a handful of genes have been linked to human infertility. Here, the genetic basis of infertility is discussed, as it relates to formation and differentiation of mature germ cells that are capable of forming a viable embryo. In discussing each of these topics, current genetic knowledge is reviewed. Then, genetic assays that are likely to be developed in the future and find their way into infertility management are outlined. The genetics of causes of infertility other than defective germ cell development, that are linked to reproductive tract or hormonal dysfunction such as polycystic ovarian syndrome (PCOS) or endometriosis, are discussed elsewhere (see Chaps. 1–4).

The Development of Human Germ Cells from Blastocyst to Maturation

Human reproduction entails complex processes that are just beginning to be outlined at the genetic level (Fig. 18-1). Conception

435

Figure 18-1: An outline of the development of the human germ cell lineage from the formation of the blastocyst (on day 5 of embryo development) to the formation of primoridal germ cells (PGCs) that migrate from the embryo into the extraembryonic membranes to the differentiation of mature germ cells (the sperm and oocytes).

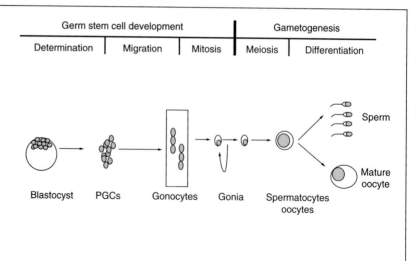

KEY POINT

The cells that ultimately give rise to mature sperm and oocytes have identical prenatal development up to meiosis. Genes required for early oocyte development may also be required for early germ cell development in males.

begins with fusion of the egg and sperm to form the first cell.[5] For the first 2 days of life, the embryo is transcriptionally silent; very few or no new RNAs are made and instead, development relies solely on RNAs that have been produced from the genetic information of the mother, in the oocyte. Shortly thereafter, the nascent genome, which contains the unique combination of female and male information each embryo inherits, is reprogrammed by destruction of maternal oocyte-specific transcripts and activation of the embryonic genetic programs.[6] During the next few days, continued growth within the zona pellucida produces the blastocyst, which is composed of a few hundred embryonic cells. Those on the outer surface, termed trophoblasts, will become the placenta, whereas, the inner cell mass will give rise to the embryo proper.[5] During implantation, the trophoblasts attach the blastocyst to the uterus, which is receptive during a brief window in time. Then, during subsequent development, a small group of cells is set aside or allocated to form the germ cell lineage (the primordial germ cells [PGCs]) that ultimately gives rise to eggs or sperm. At this time, the PGCs are identical in male and female embryos. They leave the embryo and reside in the placenta for several weeks before they migrate back into the embryo, and find their way to the newly formed testis or ovary. Following an initial period of expansion to form several million immature gonocytes, the germ cells assume sex-specific properties for the first time. The female germ cells enter meiosis; male germ cells go into a quiescent period that lasts until puberty, when meiosis resumes. Coincident with meiotic cell cycle entry, male and female germ cells undergo complex morphologic changes to assume the familiar structure of an egg or sperm. To begin to understand these processes and how genetic mutations or polymorphisms may lead to defective germ cell development in infertile men and women, the genes that function in these processes must be identified and characterized.

Genetics of Early and Premature Menopause

OOCYTE RESERVES AND MENOPAUSE

The "biological clock" is a reality for women and is a product of the unique biology of germ cell formation and maintenance and hormonal regulation of gametogenesis. Early in development of the mammalian female, a defined number of cells are set aside and destined to become germline stem cells.[7] The stem cells are first positioned outside of the fetus but later migrate to the undifferentiated gonad where they continue to divide. In the human female embryo, between the weeks of 12 and 18, the germ cells terminally differentiate; they enter meiosis and differentiate into immature oocytes. Thus, in the female, all germline stem cells have differentiated prior to birth.[5] In the woman, the germ cells may remain quiescent, may be recruited for further development and ovulation, or may apoptose. Over time, the population of oocytes will be depleted through recruitment and apoptosis until less than a 1000 oocytes exist and menopause ensues.[8] Conflict exists as to whether the depletion of oocytes triggers menopause or is a result of hormonal changes which precipitate the close of the reproductive era for each woman. Molecular analysis of genes which may be associated with variation in age of onset of menopause holds promise of addressing this conflict.

PREMATURE AND EARLY MENOPAUSE ARE GENETICALLY DETERMINED

The age of onset of menopause has not changed in recent history. Approximately 90% of women experience menopause in their early 50s. The other 10% of women experience menopause prior to 46 (early menopause) with 1% of women experiencing menopause at an age less than 40 (premature menopause).[9,10] A number of studies, based on different methods of population sampling, have demonstrated that age of onset of menopause may be largely dictated by genetics.[8,11–16] In 1995, Cramer et al. demonstrated that family history is a predictor of early menopause in a case-control study designed to examine inheritance of menopausal age. These authors found that risk for early menopause was greatest with a family history in a sister or in cases in which multiple relatives were affected. In fact, 37.5% of premature ovarian cases reported a family history of premature ovarian failure (POF) and the overall risk for POF—if a mother or sister had experienced POF—was more than six times greater than if no family history was observed. Thus, the overall odds ratio (OR) of early menopause with a reported family history was 6.1 with a confidence interval (CI) of 3.9–9.4. The findings of Cramer et al. were confirmed in additional case-control studies,[12,14] in twin studies,[13,17] and in sib-pair analysis.[17] Furthermore, Tibiletti et al. demonstrated that premature menopause or ovarian failure (<40 years of age) and early menopause (<45 years of age, in their study) demonstrated the same genetic pattern of inheritance.[15]

KEY POINT

Abundant evidence links early and premature menopause to genetics.

Given the data that oocyte depletion in humans and model organisms can trigger early menopause, several studies have sought to identify genes that trigger early menopause and are presumably required for the formation and maintenance of oocyte populations in women. To date, however, the genetic causes of early oocyte depletion and early menopause are poorly understood, though it is likely that genes on both the X chromosome and autosomes may be major determinants.

THE X CHROMOSOME HAS LONG BEEN CONSIDERED THE "POF" OR "PREMATURE OVARIAN FAILURE" CHROMOSOME

Premature ovarian failure has frequently been linked to X chromosome abnormalities including monosomy of the X chromosome and X chromosome deletions that map to the long arm, Xq (X-linked inheritance of POF; MIM 311360). Deletions of the X chromosome define two POF loci, Xq26-q28 (POF1) and Xq13.3-q22 (POF2), respectively.[18] Based on numerous studies, over the last 25 years, it has been proposed that these loci contain genes required for oocyte development and maintenance and that their loss of function is linked to oocyte depletion and early age of onset of menopause. However, the region of the X chromosome implicated in ovarian failure constitutes roughly one-half of the long arm of the X chromosome and so it has been difficult to obtain definitive proof that a particular gene is implicated in ovarian failure. Moreover, competing hypotheses exist as to how deletions of the X chromosome result in oocyte depletion.

Recently, a number of X/autosomal translocations, that map to the Xq critical region associated with premature ovarian failure, were molecularly mapped in hopes of identifying the genes that might constitute candidates for ovarian failure.[19] The authors found that translocations and deletions of the X chromosome in women with premature or early menopause can fall within genes but also surprisingly, can clearly map outside of any X chromosome genes.[19] Thus, these authors suggested that there are two alternatives to consider in exploring how X chromosome deletions may cause ovarian failure. In the first alternative, X chromosome deletions may simply be structural chromosome abnormalities that interfere with X-Y pairing during meiosis. In that case, no particular gene is required on the X chromosome for maintenance of the oocyte reserve. Instead, perhaps in response to poor meiotic pairing, oocytes are triggered to enter apoptosis. The second alternative is that the expression of a specific gene or genes is disrupted. In this case, structural genes required for oocyte maintenance have been disrupted and ovarian depletion and menopause ensue.

Two recent studies implicate the *DIA* (*Diaphonous*) and *XPNPEP2* genes in the ovarian depletion and failure associated with POF1 and POF2 loci, respectively. In the first study, Bione et al. found that the *DIA* gene was associated with the POF1 locus.[20] Essentially, these authors mapped the *DIA* gene to Xq22 (POF1) and demonstrated that it is disrupted in a family with POF. This gene is notable in that it is a homolog of *diaphanous* in flies where its disruption leads to loss of germ cells and sterility in both males and females.[21,22] The *diaphanous* gene encodes four transcripts, three are ubiquitously expressed and the fourth is testis specific.[20] With the observation of a disruption that occurs within the gene, and considering the phenotype in flies, the authors suggest that *DIA* is an excellent candidate for a gene that maps to the X chromosome and may be required for normal ovarian function.

In a similar manner, the breakpoints of nine women with translocations of the X chromosome and ovarian failure were molecularly examined.[23] The authors reported that in one patient, the breakpoint of the X chromosome interrupted the open reading frame (ORF) of a gene termed *XPNPEP2*, a ubiquitously expressed enzyme that is a member of the aminopeptidase P gene family. Again, these authors suggest the possibility that this gene is a candidate for a second ovarian failure gene. However, it is important to recognize that definitive evidence of a role for either of these genes in ovarian failure has not yet been reported.

***FMR1* PREMUTATION AND OVARIAN FAILURE**   The *fragile-X mental retardation-1* (FMR1) gene was discovered in a search for genes that cause fragile X syndrome, a syndrome characterized by moderate-to-severe mental retardation and the presence of a fragile site on the X chromosome at Xq28.[24] The gene encodes an RNA-binding protein that contains a triplet repeat, CCG, within the coding sequence; expansion of the number of CCG repeats is associated with fragile X syndrome.[24] In addition, premutations in the *FMR1* gene also exist; rather than a completely expanded number of CCG repeats, some women may be carriers of an *FMR1* allele that is intermediate between normal and that associated with fragile X syndrome. In these women, the manifestation of increased CCG repeat length is termed a premutation; the consequences to reproductive health are of interest.[25] Although the *FMR1* gene maps outside the POF loci, there is substantial evidence to suggest that premutations are implicated in ovarian failure.[26] Several notable reports have recently affirmed this link. In one report, 75 fragile X families were screened for female carriers, and then assessed for age at menopause.[27] In this study, it was noted that 30 families had a history of premature ovarian failure.[27] Moreover, when they further screened 89 families without a history of fragile X, there were 108 subjects who experienced POF, of which 6.5% had a fragile X premutation. This is a 70-fold increase in prevalence of the *FMR1* premutation over the background prevalence in Italy.[27] Similar results have been reported in a second study.[28] These authors found that 6% of 106 women with POF carried an *FMR1* premutation, again approximately 70-fold above population estimates. Moreover, results such as these are not specific to a single population; they have been confirmed in women of diverse backgrounds.[29] Finally, evidence from model organisms, especially the mouse, indicates that there is enhanced expression of the murine *FMR1* gene during germ cell proliferation in both males and females, suggesting that there may be a direct role in allocation of the oocyte population.[30] To date, however, an association of an expansion of the CCG repeats in *FMR1* with reduced oocyte reserves or a lower antral follicle count have not been demonstrated, though this might be the expected prelude to premature ovarian failure in *FMR1* carriers if the effect on age at menopause is a direct result of an oocyte-specific function.

AUTOSOMAL GENES ARE ALSO LIKELY TO DETERMINE OOCYTE DEPLETION AND AGE OF ONSET OF MENOPAUSE

The clearest correlation of premature ovarian failure and oocyte depletion with an autosomal locus is observed in patients affected with blepharophimosis-pstosis-epidanthus-inversus (BPES).[31–35] Patients afflicted with BPES, a complex eyelid malformation accompanied by premature ovarian failure, demonstrate a spectrum of mutations in a putative transcription factor, *FOXL2*, a member of the forkhead family of genes that encode DNA binding proteins.[31] *FOXL2* is expressed predominantly in follicular cells.[36] Several studies have sought to associate mutations or polymorphisms in the *FOXL2* gene with ovarian failure in the absence of associated defects in eyelid formation. In several studies, mutations of the *FOXL2* have not been observed in isolated cases of premature ovarian failure or early menopause.[37] However, in one study, two variants were observed.[38] One variant was observed in a single woman and resulted in the removal of 10 of 12 alanines at a stretch. The other was also observed in a single woman and predicts a change of a tyrosine to an asparagine at amino acid 258. Neither variant was observed in 200 women with normal age of onset of menopause.

Other autosomal genes that may contribute to determination of the age of onset of menopause include the follicle-stimulating hormone (FSH), leuteinizing hormone (LH), FSH receptor, KIT, and ataxia-telangiectasia (ATM) genes.[39] In addition, autosomal genes such as phosphomannomutase 2 (PMM2) gene, the galactose-1-phosphate uridyltransferase (GALT) gene, and the autoimmune regulator (AIRE) gene, responsible for polyendocrinopathy-candidiasis-ectodermal dystrophy, have been identified in patients with POF in association with other somatic abnormalities.[39] Taken together, however, all of these genes likely account for a small portion of premature or early menopause. In fact, in a recent study of the KIT gene, no polymorphisms were observed in 40 women with severe ovarian failure with onset between the ages of 14 and 40.[40] Thus, to date, these genes have not explained the large variation in age of onset of menopause that likely reflects the variation in initial oocyte pool and rate of depletion from woman to woman in the general population.

A PROMISING CANDIDATE GENE: THE *DAZL* GENE AND OVARIAN FAILURE

Some genes, such as the human *DAZL* (*Deleted in AZoospermia-Like*) gene are excellent candidate genes for linkage to ovarian failure and early menopause. This conclusion is based on several lines of evidence discussed below.

First, the *DAZL* genes are highly conserved through evolution with homologs already identified in flies and worms, fish, salamanders, frogs, mice, rats, old and new world primates, and humans.[41–52] In all cases, where relevant functional studies have been done, the genes are shown to function exclusively in germ cell development with loss of function causing loss of germ cells. Evidence for a special role in females has been demonstrated in worms, frogs, and mice. In *Caenorhabditis elegans*, disruption of the *DAZL* homolog, *ceDaz*, leads to female infertility characterized by arrest in meiosis I and subsequent apoptosis of oogenic cells.[47] In frogs, reduction in the activity of *XDazl* in the oocyte results in a reduction in the number of germ cells formed in progeny and their ability to develop and migrate to the gonad.[45] In the mouse, disruption of the single-copy *Dazl* homolog causes infertility in both sexes.[53] In the female, loss of oocytes occurs prenatally; ovarian steroidogenic function is maintained though gonadotropin secretion is altered.[54] The role of the *DAZL* gene in women is likely similar to that observed in model organisms but has yet to be explored.

Second, the human *DAZL* gene is expressed only in oocytes and precursor germ cells in humans as in mice.[53,55–57] In both organisms, expression ensues prenatally in the earliest identifiable germ cells and continues throughout the reproductive life of the female. In both species, DAZL protein is abundant in the cytoplasm of the oocytes in developing follicles in the fetus and adult. The similarity of the distribution of human DAZL1 protein and mouse Dazl1 protein implies that mutations that cause loss of function of the *DAZL1* genes in women would mirror loss of function mutations in mice and likely cause oocyte depletion resulting either in primary amennorhea, perhaps due to prenatal loss of the entire oocyte population, or premature ovarian failure or menopause, due to depletion of a smaller than average oocyte reserve. Thus, whether a woman presents with primary amennorhea or premature ovarian failure could reflect whether one or both copies of the *DAZL1* genes are deleted or mutated and the severity of mutations in the gene. For example, a stop codon introduced before the functional domain, that is required for RNA binding, is translated would likely cause a more severe phenotype than an amino acid substitution near the carboxyl terminus of the protein.

KEY POINT

Genes that map to autosomes (chromosomes other than the X and Y) are also likely to determine age at menopause.

Third, the human *DAZL* gene is variable. We expect that variation in age of onset of menopause reflects, in many cases, variation in the formation and maintenance of the oocyte population. If a gene is to contribute to the variability of age of onset of menopause in women, that gene must demonstrate variation in sequence. Variants of the *DAZL* gene, and other genes of interest, have been identified and deposited in the LocusLink database (http://www.ncbi.nlm.nih.gov/LocusLink/).

THE FUTURE: THE CASE FOR GENETIC CASE-CONTROL STUDIES

The case-control study has been the workhorse of the epidemiologic community for decades. Essentially, in a case-control study, one collects information, whether it be physical parameters, behavioral characteristics, or genetic information, on a population of affected individuals (cases) and a population of individuals who closely match (controls) in ethnicity, education, age, environmental exposures, diet, and other parameters deemed to be appropriate to the particular study.[58] Case-control studies have flourished in large part due to the ease of data collection; a set of cases and controls is easier to assemble than families, twins, or siblings for example. Case-control studies can, however, suffer from hidden confounding factors. For example, a particular nucleotide sequence may be associated much more frequently with ethnicity than the genetic characteristic under investigation. This is a more significant problem when a disease or disorder is strongly associated with a particular ethnic group to such a degree that case ascertainment is almost certain to involve over-sampling a subdivision of an ethnic group in which the disorder is most common. This can be especially confounding when ethnicity is masked by subsequent mixing of populations. Further problems with the case-control design in genetics may also be introduced when genetic outliers exist in individuals among the cases and controls due to different disease-inducing mutational spectra. In addition, usefulness of case-control studies may be limited when we consider that the power of a study to detect associations between a particular polymorphism and a disorder is severely reduced by diversity in mutational spectra. Moreover, the case-control study can suffer additional loss of power if pleotrophic polymorphisms occur and the ability to assess physiologic significance is restricted. In the face of these limitations, however, recent publications have lauded the design as one with a great future for the genetic studies on complex disorders.[58–61] As the availability of high throughput genotyping and polymorphic markers increases, undoubtedly the case-control study will become increasingly valuable.

Genetic case-control studies of the onset of menopause are warranted now, especially given the observation that familial history is a predictor of early menopause, an observation verified in studies with several design protocols, as noted above. Moreover, promising genes, such as *DAZL*, and numerous others that affect oocyte development specifically in other mammals, continue to be identified. Studies aimed at probing the role of gene sequence variants in well-defined genes in a case-control study population are likely to demonstrate the gene-based foundations for the heritability of early menopause and ultimately allow the examination of the role of specific mutations in altering protein function and outcomes of fertility such as oocyte number and age at menopause (Fig. 18-2).

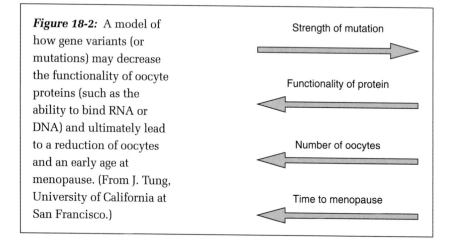

Figure 18-2: A model of how gene variants (or mutations) may decrease the functionality of oocyte proteins (such as the ability to bind RNA or DNA) and ultimately lead to a reduction of oocytes and an early age at menopause. (From J. Tung, University of California at San Francisco.)

Strength of mutation

Functionality of protein

Number of oocytes

Time to menopause

Genetics of Azoospermia and Oligospermia in Men

THE GENESIS OF Y CHROMOSOME ANALYSIS IN INFERTILE MEN

The role of the Y chromosome in sperm production in men was first illustrated in 1976 in the classic work of Tiepolo and Zuffardi.[62] These authors reported the karotype analysis of 1170 subfertile and infertile men; they demonstrated that six azoospermic men had deletions of the long arm of the Y chromosome. In two cases, they further showed that the deletions were *de novo*, i.e., the fathers of these men did not have deletions, as expected, if the deletions had caused azoospermia. Based on these findings, the hypothesis that a fertility gene(s) was present on the Y chromosome, and that in its absence men were infertile, was introduced. However, the identity of the Y chromosome genes that might be the key to sperm production was not to be known for nearly two decades.

The history of mapping deletions that cause infertility in men has been reviewed extensively.[63,64] Early karyotype analysis gave way to Southern blot analysis and finally to analysis of multiple markers or landmarks across the Y chromosome via polymerase chain reaction (PCR). These developments opened the door to rapid and reliable genetic analysis of infertile men and led to the identification of three genetic regions on the Y chromosome whose deletion results in infertility.[65] These regions have been termed the Azoospermia factor (AZF)-a, -b, and -c regions and encompass several gene families, a few of which are described below (Fig. 18-3).

KEY POINT

The Y chromosome harbors at least three distinct regions implicated in male infertility.

THE *AZFa* REGION AND THE *USP9Y*, *DBY*, AND *UTY* GENES

Complete deletions of the *AZFa* region are most frequently associated with severe spermatogenic failure or Sertoli cell only (SCO) syndrome.[65–68] *AZFa* deletions are relatively rare occurring in less than 1% of azoospermic men.[65] In spite of the rarity of the deletions, this region has the clearest association of infertility with specific genes. This is in large part to the fact that the *AZFa* region of the Y-chromosome long arm was the first region to be completely sequenced and spans approximately 1 Mb (megabase or 1 million basepairs) of sequence. The completed sequence revealed that *AZFa* contained just three genes, *USP9Y*, *DBY*, and *UTY*, all of which have X chromosome relatives or homologs. Both the X and Y chromosome copies of these genes

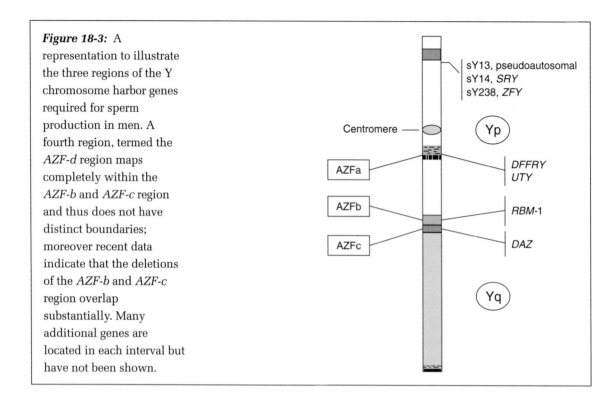

Figure 18-3: A representation to illustrate the three regions of the Y chromosome harbor genes required for sperm production in men. A fourth region, termed the *AZF-d* region maps completely within the *AZF-b* and *AZF-c* region and thus does not have distinct boundaries; moreover recent data indicate that the deletions of the *AZF-b* and *AZF-c* region overlap substantially. Many additional genes are located in each interval but have not been shown.

KEY POINT

The AZFa region of the Y chromosome contains two candidate fertility factors, USP9Y and DBY, that both likely function to insure male fertility.

are expressed ubiquitously throughout the body in men and women.

The loss of function of one or both of the *USP9Y* and *DBY* genes that map to the *AZFa* region is the cause of spermatogenic failure in men harboring deletions. Besides substantial deletion evidence, mutations within the *USP9Y* gene in infertile men definitively demonstrate its role in infertility in men.[67] The *DBY* gene has also been linked to infertility by deletion analysis, as well, and appears to cause more severe spermatogenic failure, frequently resulting in testis completely devoid of spermatogenic cells.[68]

THE *AZFb* REGION AND THE *RBM* GENES   The *RBM* genes, *RBM1* and *RBM2*, are present on the Y chromosome in approximately 15–30 copies that are dispersed along the short and long arms.[69] It is probable that the *RBM1* genes are required for normal fertility in men. However, to overcome ambiguity of multiple copies of the gene, the use of both PCR and Southern blotting is preferable to ascertain *RBM1* deletions with certainty.[65]

The use of multiple detection methods has demonstrated that deletions of the AZFb region encompass at least one copy of the RBM1 gene. This gene encodes an RNA-binding protein that is only distantly related to other RNA-binding proteins on the Y chromosome. The gene that maps to the *AZFb* region is translated and produces a protein that localizes to the nucleus of all spermatogenic cell types.[70]

THE *DAZ* GENES AND THE *AZFc* REGION

ANALYSIS OF PHENOTYPES ASSOCIATED WITH Y CHROMOSOME DELETIONS OF THE AZFc GENE CLUSTER Deletions of the *AZFc* region of the Y chromosome, that encompass the *DAZ* genes, are the most common deletions. Interestingly, early studies demonstrated that there was no apparent correlation between the extent of the deletion in an azoospermic man and the severity of the phenotype. Some men with no germ cells had equivalent deletions to those who had meiotic arrest.[71] And in fact, further analysis indicated that the *AZFc* region is not absolutely required to complete spermatogenesis and led to the demonstration that oligospermia is also associated with *AZFc* deletions.[72] AZFc deletions occur in approximately 10–15% of azoospermic men and 5% of oligospermic men.[65,71,73]

THE *DAZ* GENES HAVE HOMOLOGS IN DIVERSE ORGANISMS: LOSS OF FUNCTION CAUSES INFERTILITY

Sequencing of a *DAZ* cDNA revealed that the predicted protein contains a single RNA-binding domain and a series of repeated 24 amino acid motifs called *DAZ* repeats.[71] There are four copies of *DAZ* arranged in two head to head clusters on the Y chromosome, all deleted in infertile men containing *DAZ*-region deletions.[74,75] In addition, there are more divergent members of the *DAZ* gene family, called *DAZL* on chromosome 3 (see discussion of *DAZL* in oocytes above) and *BOULE* on chromosome 2 (Fig. 18-4).[57,74] The *DAZ* genes arose from the autosomal *DAZL* gene during primate evolution; *DAZL* arose via duplication of *BOULE* at the time of divergence of invertebrates and vertebrates. As discussed above, homologs of *DAZ* and *DAZL* have been identified in diverse organisms and in all cases, they are required for germ cell development.

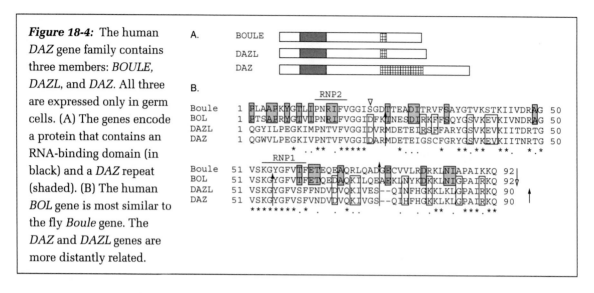

Figure 18-4: The human *DAZ* gene family contains three members: *BOULE, DAZL,* and *DAZ*. All three are expressed only in germ cells. (A) The genes encode a protein that contains an RNA-binding domain (in black) and a *DAZ* repeat (shaded). (B) The human *BOL* gene is most similar to the fly *Boule* gene. The *DAZ* and *DAZL* genes are more distantly related.

A number of studies have reported the localization of the DAZ proteins during the progression from fetal gonocytes to spermatogonia to spermatocytes to spermatids.[76] The proteins exist throughout male germ cell development and are dynamic in their subcellular localization. In the prenatal male gonocytes, the DAZ proteins are present in both the nucleus and the cytoplasm. In spermatogonia, DAZ and DAZL were most abundant in the nucleus, but could also be detected in the cytoplasm. In contrast, in spermatocytes, the proteins appear to be entirely restricted to the cytoplasm. Finally, as the spermatogenic cells mature into round spermatids and begin to elongate, the proteins become concentrated within the shrinking cytoplasmic volume. Thus, the DAZ proteins appear to be predominantly nuclear in spermatogonia, but at meiosis the proteins become concentrated in the cytoplasm, where they persist in differentiating spermatids. This expression pattern suggests that the proteins may begin to function early in spermatogenesis, a finding that fits well with previous evidence that men who are deleted for the Y-borne *DAZ* gene cluster are infertile because of a problem in the generation or maintenance of spermatogonial stem cell populations (an *early* function) and not a defect in the differentiation pathway of spermatogenesis itself (a *late* function). Thus, infertility in DAZ-deleted men may have its origins long before puberty, and perhaps even during fetal development.

THE SEQUENCE OF
THE Y CHROMOSOME
IS COMPLETE

Recently, the complete sequence of the Y chromosome has been determined.[77] In contrast to common belief, the Y chromosome is not gene poor and instead codes for 156 transcription units, including 78 proteins that fall into 27 distinct families. The role of these genes, individually and collectively, in determining male fertility and infertility is the subject of considerable research. In the future, we should see that much smaller deletions and mutations than are currently associated with male infertility will be identified; the result will be that the Y chromosome will be linked to an even greater number of genetic cases of male infertility. In addition, we may find that not only low or absent spermatogenic activity will be associated with Y chromosome abnormalities, but other traits such as poor motility or abnormal morphology will also display linkage to the Y chromosome.

KEY POINT

The human Y chromosome contains many genes; the functions of most are completely unexplored.

SHOULD Y
CHROMOSOME
ANALYSIS AND
GENETIC COUNSELING
BE OFFERED TO
INFERTILE MEN?

Although thus far there have been no health risks or diseases linked with Y chromosome microdeletions other than infertility, the practice of testing for Y chromosome deletions is gaining ground.[73,78] This is in part a reflection of the desires of the infertile couple to understand the etiology of their infertility. It is also due to the observation that the field of infertility genetics is still in its infancy and somatic defects that are associated with individuals who possess deletions may appear as further research is completed. Finally, it has been noted that one cannot predict whether the son of a man who carries a deletion will be oligospermic or completely sterile. Because of these observations, perhaps, the safest assumption may be to genetically test men who present with a high likelihood of harboring Y chromosome deletions (Fig. 18-5).

The population of infertile men who warrant Y chromosome testing presently is not yet precisely defined. Moreover, in the future, as our ability to detect genetic variants and smaller gene-specific deletions of the Y chromosome is enhanced, it is likely that the population of men who warrant testing will increase. Nonetheless, from what is presently known, it can be comfortably recommended that the following groups of men be offered Y chromosome analysis: (1) men with idiopathic (unexplained) oligospermia who have sperm concentrations less than 10 million sperm/mL and who are considering the use of *in vitro* fertilization (IVF) and intracytoplasmic sperm injection (ICSI), (2) men with

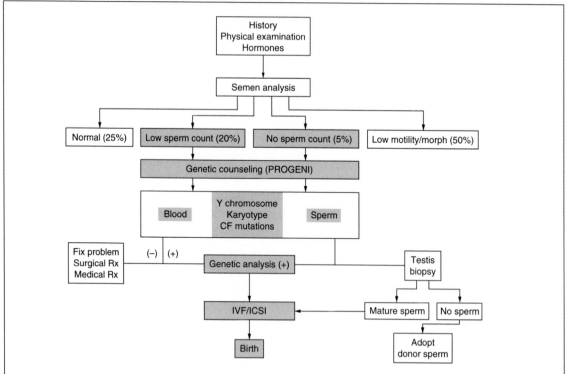

Figure 18-5: The role of genetic testing, in particular as related to the above discussion of the Y chromosome, in evaluation of male infertility. (From Dr. Paul J. Turek, University of California at San Francisco.)

oligospermia (<10 million sperm/mL) and a defined anatomic problem (e.g., varicocele) and who are considering IVF and ICSI, and (3) men with nonobstructive azoospermia who are to undergo testis sperm extraction in association with IVF and ICSI. In all cases, where genetic testing is performed, thorough and informed genetic counseling is essential, preferably by a trained genetic counselor, to take advantage of special expertise in the identification of trends in family pedigree and in the recognition of more subtle phenotypic patterns with which these patients may present.[79]

Research on the genetics of male reproductive failure holds immense clinical importance, given that 50% of male infertility remains unexplained.[80] Psychologically, it may comfort those afflicted to know the cause of their infertility. Moreover, the existence of a causal relationship between genetics and spermatogenic failure may also encourage the use of more rationale treatment regimens, and decrease unnecessary and empirical approaches to the problem.

DNA Repair and Recombination: Increased Frequency of Mutations in DNA from Men with Meiotic Arrest

Although Y chromosome deletions may occur in 10–15% of infertile men characterized by severe spermatogenic defects, as many as 85% of men do not have deletions. The infertility in these men may result from defects in crucial events in germ cell development related to the function of Y chromosome gene deletions or mutations still to be identified. Alternatively, the cause of infertility in these men may be due to mutations or polymorphisms in genes that are homologous to those that are required to efficiently complete meiosis in other organisms. Some of these genes may encode proteins that tightly regulate the recombination of genetic material and the repair of DNA should mutations occur during replication.

Genetic Evidence That Infertility in Men may be Caused by Defective DNA Repair and/or Recombination

Nearly half of infertility in men is linked to faulty gametogenesis characterized as nonobstructed azoospermia or oligospermia.[81] These disorders could result from defects in crucial events in germ cell development. Recently, many genes required to complete meiosis in other organisms have been identified.[82] Some of these genes encode proteins that tightly regulate the recombination of genetic material and the repair of DNA should mutations occur during replication. In diverse organisms from yeast to mice, mutations in genes required for DNA repair lead to infertility characterized by arrest in meiosis I at a meiotic checkpoint.[82–86]

Evidence that infertility in humans associated with maturation arrest of germ cells may be genetic has been documented in several studies. The first evidence was presented in the 1970s when Chaganti and German reported a family in which human male infertility appeared to be genetically determined.[87,88] In this family, three of eight brothers in one generation were azoospermic or oligospermic and four of six brothers in the subsequent generation were infertile. Histologic examination of biopsies of two of the infertile men indicated complete meiotic arrest in one man and nearly complete arrest in the other. Based on these observations, the authors suggested that infertility in this family might be due to mutations in genes that regulate meiotic progression. In another report, Pearson et al. observed a reduced ability to repair induced DNA damage in lymphocytes of an azoospermic man who presented with desynaptic germ cells that progressed no further than meiosis.[89] This report is the only association of somatic defects in DNA repair and infertility in men. Finally, in a third study, a polymorphic chromosomal marker was sequenced from testis and blood DNA obtained from both infertile men with meiotic arrest and infertile men with normal spermatogenesis who were obstructed.[90] The authors noted that the infertile testis DNA had significantly increased numbers of mutations in the markers than did the blood DNA from the same man or blood and testis DNA from men with normal biopsies. These results merit follow-up in order to determine whether defective DNA repair is a primary cause of infertility, to identify the genes defective in infertile men, and to determine if these defects impact the outcomes of assisted reproductive techniques (ART). Taken together, these observations suggest the possibility that human meiotic arrest could be genetic and possibly linked to mutations in genes required for the repair of DNA.

Finally, several different assays have increased in usage in recent times including aneuploidy detection via fluorescence *in situ* hybridization (FISH; Fig. 18-6), detection of mutations via inverse restriction site mutation (iRSM) assay, sperm chromatin structure assay (SCSA), and the DNA comet assay. Numerous individual studies have documented defects in DNA repair and DNA integrity in small populations of infertile men. Moreover, a single study has documented multiple genetic lesions, in oligospermic men, that indicate elevated aneuploidy as well as elevated disturbances in sperm chromatin and sperm DNA strand breakage.[91] Taken together these results indicate what has been suspected, that is, oligospermia and azoospermia likely are largely genetic pathologies and long-term studies are required to follow-up the use of assisted reproductive techniques with sperm obtained from severely affected men.

KEY POINT

The causes of male infertility are likely to extend beyond the Y chromosome to defective DNA repair and recombination.

Preimplantation Genetic Diagnosis

In recent years, the methodology that underlies preimplantation genetic diagnosis has advanced as progress on sequencing of the human genome and mapping genes for disease loci has accelerated.[92]

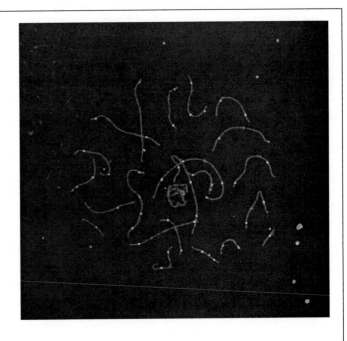

Figure 18-6: Fluorescence *in situ* hybridization (FISH) analysis of a human spermatogenic cell. The chromosomes are in meiosis as indicated by the presence of synaptonemal complex protein 3 (SCP3) along their length and foci of Mut-L Homolog 1 (MLH1) staining of recombination nodules (generally 1 per chromosome arm). The centromere is identified by use of CREST antibodies. (From J. Gonsalves, University of California at San Francisco.)

KEY POINT

The tools of human genetics are rapidly acquired for clinical analysis such as that of preimplantation genetic analysis.

The current diagnostic methods include methodologies to detect structural chromosomal abnormalities and aneuploidies and methodology to assess single gene defects. Commonly used chromosome-based assays include classical karyotypic analysis and FISH to detect aneuploidies and translocations. Single gene defects such as mutations in the cystic fibrosis transporter (CFTR) are generally detected in multiplex PCR with informative markers that indicate small nucleotide changes and/or deletions and insertions. In all cases, the analysis of parental samples to detect mutations and rearrangements, along with a single embryonic cell, is advantageous. Future advances are aimed at increasing the number of genes that can be assayed via novel strategies such as multiplexed genotyping with sequence-tagged molecular inversion probes,[93] DNA sequence arrays,[94] and comparative genomic hybridization to detect genome-wide insertions and deletions at the subchromosome level.[95] Currently, the ability to use techniques such as these to detect potential abnormalities exceeds the ability to predict the outcomes of the embryo diagnosed.

Future Assays: Imprinting Assays and Genome-Wide Genetic Screens of Infertile Couples and in Embryos

MOLECULAR GENETIC ANALYSIS OF IMPRINTING IN THE ASSISTED REPRODUCTIVE CLINIC

Genomic imprinting was first demonstrated in the 1980s in mammals when it was shown that both a paternal and a maternal set of chromosomes were required to give rise to a mature animal. In humans, it is estimated that approximately 100 genes may be imprinted or require both a paternal and maternal copy for normal development to occur. Recent studies that report an increased incidence of imprinted birth defects in children conceived via ART are cause for disquieting reflection by ART professionals and by current and future parents seeking reproductive assistance.[96,97]

Understanding imprinting is directly relevant to understanding human birth defects and reproductive health. Several studies have recently documented defects in imprinting associated with the use of ART. In one study, the incidence of Beckwith-Wiedemann's syndrome, a disorder of imprinting, was increased in children conceived via ART (4% incidence) relative to the general population (1.2% incidence).[96] In a second study, two children conceived via ICSI developed Angelman's syndrome, another disorder of imprinting; moreover, molecular analysis indicated that the imprinting in both patients was sporadic, suggesting the possibility that ICSI may interfere with establishment of the maternal imprint in the oocyte or embryo.[97] There are two critical periods for imprinting in mammalian development, one during sex-specific gametogenesis (development of sperm and eggs) and the second during preimplantation embryogenesis.[98] Thus, in some respects, imprinting defects might be expected in assisted reproduction given that the process is central to gametogenesis and early embryonic development and that the major reason to attempt assisted reproduction is faulty gametogenesis. In any case, it is abundantly clear that although we are amassing a tremendous amount of knowledge regarding imprinted gene expression and genome reprogramming in mice, we know virtually nothing of imprinting in humans apart from investigations into a few specific imprint-related diseases.[98] We do not know how frequently imprinting of multiple genes is defective in the gametes of couples who report for ART and we know even less of defective reprogramming in early preimplantation embryos obtained via ART.

IMPRINTING ASSAYS Loci that are imprinted generally demonstrate differential methylation and differential expression from maternal and paternal chromosomes. There are several assays by which defective genomic imprinting can be assessed including (1) direct assessment of expression of imprinted genes in oocytes, sperm samples, or embryos derived from ART via microarrays and (2) the single nucleotide primer extension (SNuPE) assay to assess imprinting in the male and female germline and embryos from the ART clinic. Well-established assays for the genes *NNAT, MEG1, PEG1, DLK1, H19, SLC22A1L, INSL, IGF2R, NECDIN, NESP, CDKN1C, IGF2, US1F1-RS1, SGCE,* and *PEG3* have been reported.[99]

THE FUTURE OF GENOME-WIDE ANALYSIS OF INFERTILITY

The future discovery of novel genes required for human reproduction entails the identification of genetic variants that are enriched among subclasses of infertile men and women. Historically, infertility was linked to environmental or behavioral factors. It is increasingly clear that genetics is a major determinant of infertility in both the male and female partners.[100–103] Frequently, the causes are unexplained defects in gametogenesis manifested as low or no production of normal sperm or eggs. Alternatively, poor-quality gametes are produced. When defects in gametogenesis are absent, problems that negatively affect post-fertilization development, implantation, placentation, and uterine receptivity are frequently suspected. In nearly all cases, regardless of the diagnosis, the molecular causes of infertility are unknown. As approximately 10–15% of couples worldwide are infertile, there is ready access to reproductive information and DNA samples from affected human populations. Surprisingly, however, the collection of samples from infertile patients along with clinical data in the form of strict phenotypic analyses has been attempted, on a small-scale, by only a few laboratories. These banks, which typically contain only a few hundred samples, are not large enough to perform the types of genetic screening analyses that will be possible in the near future. Therefore, establishment of large cohorts of affected and unaffected individuals is necessary. A number of different population structures, with individual advantages and disadvantages for genetic studies, will constitute the optimum human resource bank. These populations include case-control, sibling and twin pairs, related individuals, multigenerational families, and isolated population cohorts (such as the populations of Finland or Iceland).[104–107]

DEVELOPMENT OF THE APPROPRIATE TOOLS FOR GENOME-WIDE SCREENS

As the cohorts of infertile men and women are assembled, we must develop the best approaches for identifying genetic determinants of infertility. In recent years, a theory termed the "common variant/common disease" hypothesis has gained favor.[104,108] Simply stated, this theory suggests that common variants (e.g., SNPs [single nucleotide polymorphisms], genomic insertions/deletions, or chromosomal haplotypes) likely account for the common diseases and/or phenotypic traits that define the human population. This hypothesis, which is intuitively appealing, has been substantiated by considerable evidence, including metaanalysis of multiple genetic association studies.[109] In considering the inheritance of human reproductive characteristics, it is clear that fertility and infertility must be linked either to common variants that determine these common phenotypes or to unique associations with hundreds of different reproductive genes scattered throughout the population. Traditionally, linkage analysis has been the workhorse of human genetics, but the complex nature of infertility indicates that studies of association, linkage disequilibrium, and haplotype analysis are likely to be fruitful.[58,108,110–112] In this regard, the latter approach is especially intriguing. As SNP analysis of the human genome progresses, it is now clear that many genetic haplotypes (groups of SNPs that travel together on a chromosomal segment) exist in humans. Furthermore, these haplotypes exhibit limited diversity, such that a small number of variants characterize the vast majority of the human population.[113–115] To date, the role of the human sex chromosomes (the X and Y) in controlling the ability of humans to reproduce has been the primary focus.[23,79,116,117] As a result, the functions of the other chromosomal variants in reproduction await exploration and eventual introduction into clinical practice.

REFERENCES

1 Castrillon DH, Gonczy P, Alexander S, et al. Toward a molecular genetic analysis of spermatogenesis in *Drosophila melanogaster*: characterization of male-sterile mutants generated by single P element mutagenesis. *Genetics* 135:489, 1993.

2 Bellotto M, Bopp D, Senti KA, et al. Maternal-effect loci involved in *Drosophila* oogenesis and embryogenesis: P element-induced mutations on the third chromosome. *Int J Dev Biol* 46:149, 2002.

3 Mohr SE, Boswell RE. Genetic analysis of *Drosophila melanogaster* polytene chromosome region 44D-45F: loci required for viability and fertility. *Genetics* 160:1503, 2002.

4 Swan A, Hijal S, Hilfiker A, et al. Identification of new X-chromosomal genes required for Drosophila oogenesis and novel roles for fs(1)Yb, brainiac and dunce. *Genome Res* 11:67, 2001.

5 Moore KL, Persaud TVN. Human reproduction. *Before We are Born*, 5th ed. Philadelphia, PA: W.B. Saunders, 1998, p. 13.

6 Schultz RM. The molecular foundations of the maternal to zygotic transition in the preimplantation embryo. *Hum Reprod Update* 8:323, 2002.

7 Tam PPL, Zhou SX. The allocation of epiblast cells to ectoderman and germline lineages is influenced by the position of the cells in the gastrulating mouse embryo. *Dev Biol* 178:124, 1996.

8 Wise PM, Krajnak KM, Kashon ML. Menopause: the aging of multiple pacemakers. *Science* 273:67, 1996.

9 Coulam CB, Adamson SC, Annegers JF. Incidence of premature ovarian failure. *Obstet Gynecol* 67:604, 1980.

10 Conway GS. Premature ovarian failure. *Br Med Bull* 56:643, 2000.

11 Cramer DW, Xu H, Harlow BL. Family history as a predictor of early menopause. *Fertil Steril* 64:740, 1995.

12 Vegetti W, Tibiletti MG, Testa G, et al. Inheritance in idiopathic premature ovarian failure: analysis of 71 cases. *Hum Reprod* 13:1796, 1998.

13 Snieder H, MacGregor AJ, Spector TD. Genes control the cessation of a woman's reproductive life: a twin study of hysterectomy and age at menopause. *J Clin Endocrinol Metab* 83:1875, 1998.

14 Testa G, Chiaffarino F, Vegetti W, et al. Case-control study on risk factors for premature ovarian failure. *Gynecol Obstet Invest* 51:40, 2001.

15 Tibiletti MG, Testa G, Vegetti W, et al. The idiopathic forms of premature menopause and early menopause show the same genetic pattern. *Hum Reprod* 14:2731, 1999.

16 Vegetti W, Marozzi A, Manfredini E, et al. Premature ovarian failure. *Mol Cell Endocrinol* 161:53, 2000.

17 de Bruin JP, Bovenhuis H, van Noord PAH, et al. The role of genetic factors in age at natural menopause. *Hum Reprod* 16:2014, 2001.

18　Powell CM, Taggart RT, Drumheller TC, et al. Molecular and cytogenetic studies of an X; autosome translocation in a patient with premature ovarian failure and review of the literature. *Am J Med Genet* 52:19, 1994.

19　Mumm S, Herrera L, Waeltz PW, et al. X/autosomal translocations in the Xq critical region associated with premature ovarian failure fall within and outside genes. *Genomics* 76:30, 2001.

20　Bione S, Sala C, Manzini C, et al. A human homologue of the *Drosophila melanogaster* diaphanous gene is disrupted in a patient with premature ovarian failure: evidence for conserved function in oogenesis and implications for human sterility. *Am J Hum Genet* 62:533, 1998.

21　Castrillon DH *Diaphanous* is required for cytokinesis in *Drosophila* and shares domains of similarity with the products of the limb deformity gene. *Development* 120:3367, 1994.

22　Afshar K, Stuart B, Wasserman SA. Functional analysis of the *Drosophila* diaphanous FH protein in early embryonic development. *Development* 127:1887, 2000.

23　Prueitt RL, Ross JL, Zinn AR. Physical mapping of nine Xq translocation breakpoints and identification of XPNPEP2 as a premature ovarian failure candidate gene. *Cytogenet Cell Genet* 89:44, 2000.

24　Kremer EJ, Pritchard M, Lynch M, et al. Mapping of DNA instability at the fragile X to a trinucleotide repeat sequence p(CCG)n. *Science* 252:1711, 1991.

25　Murray A. Premature ovarian failure and the FMR1 gene. *Semin Reprod Med* 18:59, 2000.

26　Sherman SL. Premature ovarian failure in the fragile X syndrome. *Am J Med Genet* 97:189, 2000.

27　Uzielli ML, Guarducci S, Lapi E, et al. Premature ovarian failure (POF) and fragile X premutation females: from POF to fragile X carrier identification, from fragile X carrier diagnosis to POF association data. *Am J Med Genet* 84:300, 1999.

28　Marozzi A, Vegetti W, Manfredini E, et al. Association between idiopathic premature ovarian failure and fragile X premutation. *Hum Reprod* 15:197, 2000.

29　Allingham-Hawkins DJ, Babul-Hirji R, Chitayat D, et al. Fragile X premutation is a significant risk factor for premature ovarian failure: the International Collaborative POF in Fragile X study–preliminary data. *Am J Med Genet* 83:322, 1999.

30　Bachner D, Manca A, Steinbach P, et al. Enhanced expression of the murine *Fmr1* gene during germ cell proliferation suggests a special function in both the male and the female gonad. *Hum Mol Genet* 2:2043, 1993.

31 de Baere E, Dixon MJ, Small KW, et al. Spectrum of *FOXL2* gene mutations in blepharophimosis-ptosis-epicanthus inversus (BPES) families demonstrates a genotype-phenotype correlation. *Hum Mol Genet* 10:1591, 2001.

32 Crisponi L, Deiana M, Loi A, et al. The putative forkhead transcription factor *FOXL2* is mutated in blepharophimosis/ptosis/epicanthus inversus syndrome. *Nat Genet* 27:159, 2001.

33 Fraser IS, Shearman RP, Smith A, et al. An association among blepharophimosis, resistant ovary syndrome, and true premature menopause. *Fertil Steril* 50:747, 1988.

34 Panidis D, Rousso D, Vavilis D, et al. Familial blepharophimosis with ovarian dysfunction. *Hum Reprod* 9:2034, 1994.

35 Smith A, Fraser IS, Shearman RP, et al. Blepharophimosis plus ovarian failure: a likely candidate for a contiguous gene syndrome. *J Med Genet* 26:434, 1989.

36 Loffler KA, Zarkower D, Koopman P. Etiology of ovarian failure in blepharophimosis ptosis epicanthus inversus syndrome: FOXL2 is a conserved, early-acting gene in vertebrate ovarian development. *Endocrinology* 144:3237, 2003.

37 Baere ED, Lemercier B, Christin-Maitre S, et al. FOXL2 mutation screening in a large panel of POF patients and XX males. *J Med Genet* 39:e43, 2002.

38 Harris SE, Chand AL, Winship IM, et al. Identification of novel mutations in FOXL2 associated with premature ovarian failure. *Mol Hum Reprod* 8:729, 2002.

39 Laml T, Preyer O, Umek W, et al. Genetic disorders in premature ovarian failure. *Hum Reprod Update* 8:483, 2002.

40 Shibanuma K, Tong ZB, Vanderhoof VH, et al. Investigation of KIT gene mutations in women with 46,XX spontaneous premature ovarian failure. *BMC Womens Health* 1:8, 2002.

41 Chai NN, Phillips A, Fernandez A, et al. A putative human male infertility gene *DAZLA*: genomic structure and methylation status. *Mol Hum Reprod* 3:705, 1997.

42 Cooke HJ, Lee M, Kerr S, et al. A murine homologue of the human DAZ gene is autosomal and expressed only in male and female gonads. *Hum Mol Genet* 5:513, 1996.

43 Cheng MH, Maines JZ, Wasserman SA. Biphasic subcellular localization of the DAZL-related protein Boule in *Drosophila* spermatogenesis. *Dev Biol* 204:567, 1998.

44 Houston DW, Zhang J, Maines JZ, et al. A *Xenopus DAZ-like* gene encodes an RNA component of germ plasm and is a functional homologue of *Drosophila boule. Development* 125:171, 1998.

45 Houston DW, King ML. A critical role for *Xdazl*, a germ plasm-localized RNA, in the differentiation of primordial germ cells in *Xenopus. Development* 127:447, 2000.

46 Johnson AD BR, Drum M, Masi T. Expression of axolotl *dazl* RNA, a marker of germ plasm: widespread maternal RNA and onset of expression in germ cells approaching the gonad. *Dev Biol* 234:402, 2001.

47 Karashima T, Sugimoto A, Yamamoto M. *Caenorhabditis elegans* homologue of the human azoospermia factor *DAZ* is required for oogenesis but not for spermatogenesis. *Development* 127:1069, 2000.

48 Maegawa S, Yasuda K, Inoue K. Maternal mRNA localization of zebrafish *DAZ-like* gene. *Mech Dev* 81:223, 1999.

49 Maiwald R, Luche RM, Epstein CJ. Isolation of a mouse homolog of the human *DAZ (Deleted in AZoospermia)* gene. *Mamm Genome* 7:628, 1996.

50 Mita K, Yamashita M. Expression of *Xenopus* Daz-like protein during gametogenesis and embryogenesis. *Mech Dev* 94:251, 2000.

51 Shan Z, Hirschmann P, Seebacher T, et al. A *SPGY* copy homologous to the mouse gene *Dazla* and the *Drosophila* gene *boule* is autosomal and expressed only in the human male gonad. *Hum Mol Genet* 5:2005, 1996.

52 Yen PH, Chai NN, Salido EC. The human autosomal gene *DAZLA*: testis specificity and a candidate for male infertility. *Hum Mol Genet* 5:2013, 1996.

53 Ruggiu M, Speed R, Taggart M, et al. The mouse *Dazla* gene encodes a cytoplasmic protein essential for gametogenesis. *Nature* 389:73, 1997.

54 McNeilly JR, Saunders PTK, Taggart M, et al. Loss of oocytes in *Dazl* knockout mice results in maintained ovarian steroidogenic function but altered gonadotropin secretion in adult animals. *Endocrinology* 141:4284, 2000.

55 Dorfman DM, Genest DR, Reijo Pera RA. Human *DAZL1* encodes a candidate fertility factor in women that localizes to the prenatal and postnatal germ cells. *Hum Reprod* 14:2531, 1999.

56 Tsai MY, Chang SY, Lo HY, et al. The expression of DAZL1 in the ovary of the human female fetus. *Fertil Steril* 73:627, 2000.

57 Xu EY, Moore FL, Reijo Pera RA. A gene family required for human germ cell development evolved from an ancient meiotic gene conserved in all metazoans. *Proc Natl Acad Sci U S A* 98:7414, 2001.

58 Schork NJ, Fallin D, Thiel B, et al. The future of genetic case-control studies. *Adv Genet* 14:191, 2001.

59 Risch N, Merikangas K. The future of genetic studies of complex human diseases. *Science* 273:1516, 1996.

60 Ranade K, Wu KD, Hwu CM, et al. Genetic variation in the human urea transporter-2 is associated with variation in blood pressure. *Hum Mol Genet* 10:2157, 2001.

61 Ranade K, Wu KD, Risch N, et al. Genetic variation in aldosterone synthase predicts plasma glucose levels. *Proc Natl Acad Sci U S A* 98:13219, 2001.

62 Tiepolo L, Zuffardi O. Localization of factors controlling spermatogenesis in the nonfluorescent portion of the human Y chromosome long arm. *Hum Genet* 34:119, 1976.

63 Elliot DJ, Cooke HJ. The molecular genetics of male infertility. *Bioessays* 19:801, 1997.

64 Cooke HJ. Y chromosome and male infertility. *Rev Reprod* 4:5, 1999.

65 Vogt PH, Edelmann A, Kirsch S, et al. Human Y chromosome azoospermia factors (AZF) mapped to different subregions in Yq11. *Hum Mol Genet* 5:933, 1996.

66 Sun C, Skaletsky H, Rozen S, et al. Deletion of *azoospermia factor a (AZFa)* region of human Y chromosome caused by recombination between HERV15 proviruses. *Hum Mol Genet* 9:2291, 2000.

67 Sun C, Skaletsky H, Birren B, et al. An azoospermic man with a de novo point mutation in the Y-chromosomal gene *USP9Y*. *Nat Genet* 23:429, 1999.

68 Blagosklonova O, Fellmann F, Roux M-CC, et al. AZFa deletions in Sertoli cell-only syndrome: a retrospective study. *Mol Hum Reprod* 6:795, 2000.

69 Ma K, Inglis JD, Sharkey A, et al. A Y chromosome gene family with RNA-binding protein homology: Candidates for the azoospermia factor AZF controlling human spermatogenesis. *Cell* 75:1287, 1993.

70 Elliot DJ, Millar MR, Oghene K, et al. Expression of *RBM* in the nuclei of human germ cells is dependent on a critical region of the Y chromosome long arm. *Proc Natl Acad Sci U S A* 94:3848, 1997.

71 Reijo R, Lee TY, Salo P, et al. Diverse spermatogenic defects in humans caused by Y chromosome deletions encompassing a novel RNA-binding protein gene. *Nat Genet* 10:383, 1995.

72 Reijo R, Alagappan RK, Patrizio P, et al. Severe oligospermia resulting from deletions of the *Azoospermia Factor* gene on the Y chromosome. *Lancet* 347:1290, 1996.

73 Girardi SK, Mielnik A, Schlegel PN. Submicroscopic deletions in the Y chromosome of infertile men. *Hum Reprod* 12:1635, 1997.

74 Saxena R, Brown LG, Hawkins T, et al. The *DAZ* gene cluster on the human Y chromosome arose from an autosomal gene that was transposed, repeatedly amplified and pruned. *Nat Genet* 14:292, 1996.

75 Saxena R, Vries JWAD, Repping S, et al. Four *DAZ* genes in two clusters found in the *AZFc* region of the human Y chromosome. *Genomics* 67:256, 2000.

76 Reijo RA, Dorfman DM, Slee R, et al. DAZ family proteins exist throughout male germ cell development and transit from nucleus to cytoplasm at meiosis in humans and mice. *Biol Reprod* 63:1490, 2000.

77 Skaletsky H, Kuroda-Kawaguchi T, Minx PJ, et al. The male-specific region of the human Y chromosome is a mosaic of discrete sequence classes. *Nature* 423:825, 2003.

78 Simoni M. Molecular diagnosis of Y chromosome microdeletions in Europe: state-of-the-art and quality control. *Hum Reprod* 16:402, 2001.

79 Kostiner DR, Turek PJ, Reijo RA. Male infertility: analysis of the markers and genes on the human Y chromosome. *Hum Reprod* 13:3032, 1998.

80 Pryor JL, Kent-First M, Muallem A, et al. Microdeletions in the Y chromosome of infertile men. *N Engl J Med* 336:534, 1997.

81 Kretser DMD. Male infertility. *Lancet* 349:787, 1997.

82 Roeder GS. Meiotic chromosomes: it takes two to tango. *Genes Dev* 11:2600, 1997.

83 Baker SM, Bronner CE, Zhang L, et al. Male mice defective in the DNA mismatch repair gene PMS2 exhibit abnormal chromosome synapsis in meiosis. *Cell* 82:309, 1995.

84 Baker SM, Plug AW, Prolla TA, et al. Involvement of mouse Mlh1 in DNA mismatch repair and meiotic crossing over. *Nat Genet* 13:336, 1996.

85 Pittman D, Cobb J, Schimenti KJ, et al. Meiotic prophase arrest with failure of chromosome synapsis in mice deficient for *Dmc1*, a germline-specific RecA homolog. *Mol Cell* 1:697, 1998.

86 Yoshida K, Kondoh G, Matsuda Y, et al. The mouse *RecA-like* gene *Dmc1* is required for homologous chromosome synapsis during meiosis. *Mol Cell* 1:707, 1998.

87 Chaganti RSK, German J. Human male infertility, probably genetically determined, due to defective meiosis and spermatogenic arrest. *Am J Hum Genet* 31:634, 1979.

88 Chaganti RSK, Jhanwar SC, Ehrenbard LT, et al. Genetically determined asynapsis, spermatogenic degeneration, and infertility in men. *Am J Hum Genet* 32:833, 1980.

89 Pearson P, Ellis J, Evans H. A gross reduction in chiasma formation during meiotic prophase and a defective DNA repair mechanism associated with a case of human male infertility. *Cytogenetics* 9:460, 1970.

90 Nudell D, Castillo M, Turek PJ, et al. Increased frequency of mutations in DNA from infertile men with meiotic arrest. *Hum Reprod* 15:1289, 2000.

91 Schmid TE, Kamischke A, Bollwein H, et al. Genetic damage in oligozoospermic patients detected by fluorescence in-situ hybridization, inverse restriction site mutation assay, sperm chromatin structure assay and the comet assay. *Hum Reprod* 18:1474, 2003.

92 Findlay I. Pre-implantation genetic diagnosis. *Br Med Bull* 56:672, 2000.

93 Hardenbol P, Baner J, Jain M, et al. Multiplexed genotyping with sequence-tagged molecular inversion probes. *Nat Biotechnol* 21:673, 2003.

94 Jain KK. Applications of biochip and microarray systems in pharmacogenomics. *Pharmacogenomics* 1:289, 2000.

95 Wells D, Levy B. Cytogenetics in reproductive medicine: the contribution of comparative genomic hybridization (CGH). *Bioessays* 25:289, 2003.

96 Maher ER, Brueton LA, Bowdin SC, et al. Beckwith-Wiedemann syndrome and assisted reproduction technology (ART). *J Med Genet* 40:62, 2003.

97 Cox GF, Burger J, Lip V, et al. Intracytoplasmic sperm injection may increase the risk of imprinting defects. *Am J Hum Genet* 71:162, 2002.

98 Reik W, Walter J. Genomic imprinting: Parental influence on the genome. *Nat Rev Genet* 2:21, 2001.

99 Humpherys D, Eggan K, Akutsu H, et al. Abnormal gene expression in cloned mice derived from embryonic stem cell and cumulus cell nuclei. *Proc Natl Acad Sci U S A* 99:12889, 2002.

100 Workshop ESHRE. Infertility revisited: the state of the art today and tomorrow. *Hum Reprod* 11:1779, 1996.

101 Workshop ESHRE. Female infertility: treatment options for complicated cases. *Hum Reprod* 12:1191, 1997.

102 Workshop ESHRE. Consensus workshop on advanced diagnostic andrology techniques. *Hum Reprod* 12:873, 1997.

103 Crosignani PG, Collins J, Cooke ID, et al. Recommendations of the ESHRE workshop on 'Unexplained Infertility.' *Hum Reprod* 8:977, 1993.

104 Lander ES, Schork NJ. Genetic dissection of complex traits. *Science* 265:2037, 1994.

105 Kruglyak L, Lander ES. High-resolution genetic mapping of complex traits. *Am J Hum Genet* 56:1212, 1995.

106 Kruglyak L, Lander ES. Complete multipoint sib-pair analysis of qualitative and quantitative traits. *Am J Hum Genet* 57:439, 1995.

107 Khoury MJ, Flanders WD, Lipton RB, et al. Commentary: the affected sib-pair method in the context of an epidemiologic study design. *Genet Epidemiol* 8:277, 1991.

108 Risch NJ. Searching for genetic determinants in the new millennium. *Nature* 405:847, 2000.

109 Lohmueller KE, Pearce CL, Pike M, et al. Meta-analysis of genetic association studies supports a contribution of common variants to susceptibility to common disease. *Nat Genet* 33:177, 2003.

110 Reich DE, Cargill M, Bolk S, et al. Linkage disequilibrium in the human genome. *Nature* 411:199, 2001.

111 Glazier AM, Nadeau JH, Aitman TJ. Finding genes that underlie complex traits. *Science* 298:2345, 2002.

112 Cardon LR, Abecasis GR. Using haplotype blocks to map human complex trait loci. *Trends Genet* 19:135, 2003.

113 Phillips MS, Lawrence R, Sachidanandam R, et al. Chromosome-wide distribution of haplotype blocks and the role of recombination hot spots. *Nat Genet* 33:382, 2003.

114 Daly MJ, Rioux JD, Schaffner SF, et al. High-resolution haplotype structure in the human genome. *Nat Genet* 29:229, 2001.

115 Garbriel SB, et al. The structure of haplotype blocks in the human genome. *Science* 296:2225, 2002.

116 Vogt PH. Human Y chromosome deletions in Yq11 and male fertility. *Adv Exp Med Biol* 424:17, 1997.

117 Davison RM, Davis CJ, Conway GS. The X chromosome and ovarian failure. *Clin Endocrinol* 51:673, 1999.

Recurrent Pregnancy Loss

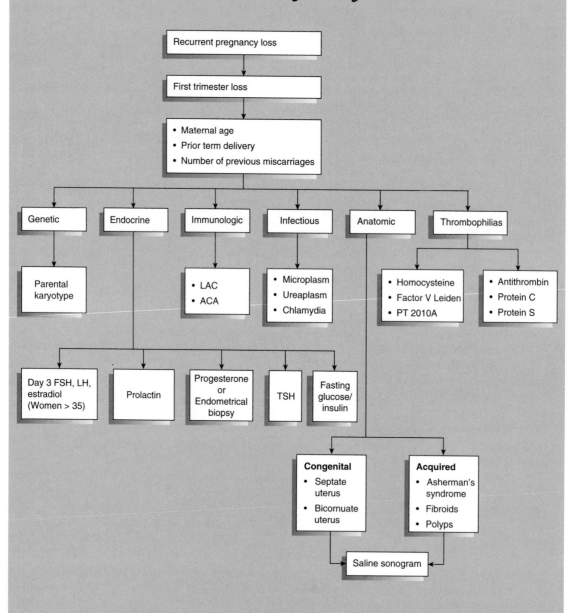

19 Recurrent Pregnancy Loss

William H. Kutteh

Introduction

Recurrent pregnancy loss is a profound personal tragedy to the couples seeking parenthood and a formidable clinical challenge to their physician. While spontaneous abortion occurs in approximately 15% of clinically diagnosed pregnancies of reproductive aged women, recurrent pregnancy loss occurs in about 1–2% of this same population.[1] Great strides have been made in characterizing the incidence and diversity of this heterogeneous disorder and a definite cause of pregnancy loss can be established in approximately 65% of couples after a thorough evaluation.[2] A complete evaluation will include investigations into genetic, endocrinologic, anatomic, immunologic, microbiologic, thrombophilic and iatrogenic causes. In cases of idiopathic recurrent miscarriage, intense supportive care is indicated and successful outcomes will occur in over two-thirds of all couples.[3]

Definition of Pregnancy Loss

The traditional definition of recurrent pregnancy loss included those couples with three or more spontaneous, consecutive pregnancy losses. However, several studies have recently indicated that the risk of recurrent miscarriage after two successive losses is similar to the risk of miscarriage in women after three successive losses; thus, couples with two or more consecutive spontaneous miscarriages warrant an evaluation to determine the etiology of their pregnancy loss.[4,5] Any loss before 20 gestational weeks is considered a miscarriage. Miscarriages can be further divided into embryonic losses, which occur before the ninth gestational week, and fetal losses, which occur at or after the ninth gestational week to 20 weeks. Those couples with primary recurrent loss have never had a previous viable infant, while those with secondary recurrent loss have previously delivered a pregnancy beyond 20 weeks and then suffered subsequent losses.

Recurrence Risk

The risk of recurrence depends on several factors, including maternal age, the number of previous miscarriages, and the history of previous term deliveries. Recent studies evaluating the frequency of pregnancy loss, based on highly sensitive tests for quantitative hCG, indicate that the total clinical and preclinical losses in women aged 20–30 are approximately 25%, while the loss rate in women aged 40 or more is at least double that figure.[6,7] Similarly, a greater number of prior losses is associated with an increased risk of recurrence in most studies. A patient with two prior losses has a recurrence risk of at least 25% and after four losses that figure is at least doubled. Most studies have indicated a more favorable prognosis in women with secondary recurrent pregnancy loss.

Etiologies of Recurrent Pregnancy Loss

GENETIC ABNORMALITIES

Structural abnormalities in parental chromosomes occur in 3–5% of couples with recurrent pregnancy loss. The most common chromosomal abnormality is a balanced translocation, an event that occurs at meiosis with an abnormal genetic complement in the germ cells. In recurrent pregnancy loss, this abnormality is found more frequently in the female partner at a ratio of 2:1 up to 3:1 (female:male). Other parental chromosome abnormalities occur less frequently, such as Robertsonian translocations, inversions, sex chromosome aneuploidies, and supernumerary chromosomes. Treatment includes genetic counseling, prenatal diagnoses by amniocentesis or chorionic villus sampling, donor gametes, or preimplantation genetic diagnosis.

ENDOCRINOLOGIC FACTORS

LUTEAL PHASE DEFICIENCY Progesterone produced from the corpus luteum is necessary for successful implantation and maintenance of early pregnancy until progesterone production by the placenta takes over. Luteal phase deficiency has been described as a cause of pregnancy loss. Classically, diagnosis was obtained after an endometrial biopsy on day 26 or day 27 of the cycle that was more than 2 days out of phase and, more recently, the use of a mid-luteal progesterone of <10 ng/mL has been suggested to be diagnostic. Women with out of phase endometrial biopsies are unable to maintain endometrial progesterone receptors and have abnormal expression of the αVβ3 integrin, a biomarker of uterine receptivity.[8] The αVβ3 integrin normally appears in the endometrial glands on cycle days 20–21 during the "window of implantation." The majority of these patients, when treated with supplemental progesterone or low-dose clomiphene citrate, will have restoration of normal histologic endometrium and normal αVβ3 expression. Late implantation of the embryo has also been associated with an increased miscarriage rate.[9]

UNTREATED HYPOTHYROIDISM Untreated hypothyroidism may increase the risk of miscarriage. A recent study of over 700 patients with recurrent pregnancy loss identified 7.6% with hypothyroidism.[10] Hypothyroidism is easily diagnosed with a sensitive thyroid-stimulating hormone (TSH) test and patients should be treated to become euthyroid before attempting a next pregnancy.

INSULIN RESISTANCE Patients with poorly controlled diabetes are known to have an increased risk of spontaneous miscarriage, which is reduced to normal spontaneous loss rates when women are euglycemic preconceptually.[6] It is known that women with polycystic ovarian syndrome have an increased risk of miscarriage. The high prevalence of insulin resistance in women with polycystic ovarian syndrome may account for the increased risk of miscarriage in this group.[11,11a] Testing for fasting insulin and glucose is simple and treatment with insulin-sensitizing agents can reduce the risk of recurrent miscarriage.

ELEVATED DAY 3 FSH Elevated day 3 FSH levels have been associated with decreased pregnancy rates in women undergoing *in vitro* fertilization. Although the frequency of elevated day 3 FSH levels in women with recurrent miscarriage is similar to the frequency in the infertile population, the prognosis for recurrent miscarriage is increased with increased day 3 FSH levels.[12] Although no treatment is available, testing should be performed in women over the age of 35 with recurrent pregnancy loss and appropriate counseling should follow.

ANATOMIC ABNORMALITIES

CONGENITAL UTERINE ANOMALIES Congenital uterine anomalies associated with Müllerian fusion defects have been associated with an increased risk of pregnancy loss. The most common abnormality associated with pregnancy loss is the septate uterus. Uncontrolled studies suggest that resection of the uterine septum results in higher delivery rates than in women without treatment. Other congenital abnormalities, such as bicornuate and unicornuate uterus are more frequently associated with later trimester losses or preterm delivery.

ACQUIRED ABNORMALITIES Intrauterine synechiae (Asherman's syndrome) have been associated with recurrent miscarriage. The most common causes of intrauterine adhesions are curettages occurring postabortion or postpartum. The adhesions are thought to interfere with the normal placentation and are treated with hysteroscopic resection. Intrauterine cavity abnormalities, such as leiomyomas and polyps, can contribute to pregnancy loss by interfering with implantation. Until recently, it was felt that only submucous leiomyomas should be surgically removed prior to subsequent attempts at pregnancy. However, several recent studies investigating the implantation rate in women undergoing *in vitro* fertilization have clearly demonstrated decreased implantation with intramural myomas in the range of 30 mm.[13] When smaller myomas are identified, it is unclear if myomectomy is beneficial.[14]

IMMUNOLOGIC FACTORS

AUTOIMMUNE CAUSES

Antiphospholipid Antibodies Autoantibodies to phospholipids, thyroid antigens, nuclear antigens, and others have been investigated as possible causes for pregnancy loss.[10] Antiphospholipid antibodies include both the lupus anticoagulant and anticardiolipin antibodies. The occurrence of recurrent pregnancy loss, fetal death, and/or thrombosis in conjunction with antiphospholipid antibodies is termed the antiphospholipid antibody syndrome[15] (Table 19-1). There is still controversy concerning testing

Table 19-1. CLINICAL AND LABORATORY CHARACTERISTICS OF ANTIPHOSPHOLIPID ANTIBODY SYNDROME

CLINICAL CHARACTERISTIC	LABORATORY CHARACTERISTIC

Pregnancy morbidity
  ≥1 unexplained death at ≥10 weeks or
  delivery at ≤34 weeks with severe
  pregnancy induced hypertension or
  three or more losses before 10 weeks
Thrombosis
  Venous
  Arterial, including stroke
	IgG aCL (≥20 GPL)
	IgM aCL (≥20 MPL)
	Positive lupus anticoagulant test

*a*Patients should have at least one clinical and one laboratory feature at some time in the course of their disease. Laboratory tests should be positive on at least two occasions more than 6 weeks apart.

Abbreviations: GPL, IgG phospholipid units; MPL, IgM phospholipid units.

for other phospholipids, but an increasing number of studies suggest that antibodies to phosphatidyl serine are also associated with pregnancy loss. In the past, treatment with low-dose steroids was advocated; however, recent studies indicate that this treatment significantly increases maternal and fetal complications without enhancing live birth rate.[16,17] Independent, prospective investigations have indicated the efficacy of subcutaneous heparin and aspirin for the treatment of antiphospholipid antibody syndrome.[18–20]

Antithyroid Antibodies Antithyroid antibodies (antithyroid peroxidase, antithyroglobulin) have been reported in an increased frequency in women with recurrent pregnancy loss. However, if the patient is euthyroid, the presence of antithyroid antibodies does not affect pregnancy outcome.[21] Women who have positive antithyroid antibodies and are euthyroid are at an increased risk for hypothyroidism during and after pregnancy. These women should have their TSH tested during each trimester and postpartum for thyroiditis.[22]

Antinuclear Antibodies Approximately 10–15% of all women will have detectable antinuclear antibodies regardless of their history of pregnancy loss. Their chance of successful pregnancy outcome is not dependent on the presence or absence of antinuclear antibodies. Treatments such as steroids have been shown to increase the maternal and fetal complications without benefiting live births[17]; thus, testing and treatment for antinuclear antibodies is not indicated.

ALLOIMMUNE CAUSES Alloimmune factors have been suggested to be associated with recurrent pregnancy loss. Human leukocyte antigen (HLA) sharing was thought to be associated with recurrent pregnancy loss based on a decreased maternal immune response and, thus, decreased production of blocking antibodies. Recent large studies, however, reveal no association among HLA (and HLA-DQα), homozygosity, and recurrent pregnancy loss.[23] Other investigators have implicated certain embryotoxic factors, such as TNF-α and interferon-δ, identified in the supernatants of peripheral blood lymphocytes from women with pregnancy loss; however, this has not been confirmed by independent studies. Immunophenotypes of endometrial cells from women with recurrent pregnancy loss demonstrate altered natural killer cell (CD56+) populations. Some have suggested that increased natural killer cells are associated with pregnancy loss, while others have indicated that decreased natural killer cells are associated with pregnancy loss. None of these tests have been clearly associated with pregnancy loss; thus, there are no recommended tests or treatments at this time.[24] Therapies such as leukocyte immunotherapy and intravenous immunoglobulin have not been shown to be efficacious.[25,23]

MICROBIOLOGIC CAUSES

Certain infectious agents have been identified more frequently in cultures from women who have had spontaneous pregnancy losses.[25a] These include *Ureaplasma urealyticum*, *Mycoplasma hominus*, *Chlamydia*, and other less frequent pathogens. Although no studies have associated any infectious agent with recurrent pregnancy loss, it is unthinkable that a clinician would leave a patient untreated to determine this association. Because of the clear association with sporadic pregnancy losses and the ease of diagnosis, women with recurrent pregnancy loss should be cultured for these organisms and both partners should be treated if positive.

THROMBOPHILIC PROBLEMS

Recent attention has focused on certain inherited disorders that may predispose to arterial and/or venous thrombosis and their possible association with pregnancy complications.[26,27] These include the group of mutations leading to a hypercoagulable state, such as factor V Leiden (G1691A), factor II prothrombin mutation (G20210A), and hyperhomocysteinemia (thermolabile MTHFR C677T). Another group of deficiencies leading to hypercoagulable states include the antithrombin III deficiency, protein C deficiency, and protein S deficiency. Studies are not in agreement at this time, although it appears that some of these hypercoagulable states are more commonly found in late trimester pregnancy losses rather than early pregnancy losses.[28] However, two recent meta-analyses have established a significant association between certain thrombophilias and early recurrent pregnancy loss.[28a,28b] Hyperhomocysteinemia has been reported in early pregnancy losses and is treated with folic acid supplementation.[29]

Lifestyle Issues

Tobacco use of more than 15 cigarettes a day has been associated with an increased risk of pregnancy loss by 1.5- to 2-fold, as well as alcohol consumption of greater than four drinks per week. When both personal habits are prevalent in the same individual, the risk of pregnancy loss may increase fourfold. Couples should be counseled concerning these habits and strongly encouraged to discontinue these prior to attempting subsequent conception.[30]

Evaluation for Pregnancy Loss

When the clinician makes the decision to initiate an evaluation for recurrent pregnancy loss, it is recommended that the complete diagnostic testing be performed. This obviously includes a complete history, including documentation of prior pregnancies, any pathologic tests that were performed on prior miscarriages, any evidence of chronic or acute infections or diseases, any recent physical or emotional trauma, a history of cramping or bleeding with a previous miscarriage, any family history of pregnancy loss, and any previous gynecologic surgery or complicating factor. A summary of the diagnosis and management of recurrent pregnancy loss includes an investigation of genetic, endocrinologic, anatomic, immunologic, microbiologic, iatrogenic, and possible thrombophilic causes (Table 19-2).

Table 19-2. **DIAGNOSIS AND MANAGEMENT OF RECURRENT PREGNANCY LOSS**

ETIOLOGY	DIAGNOSTIC EVALUATION	ABNORMAL RESULT	THERAPY
Genetic	Karyotype partners	3–5%	Genetic counseling
			Donor gametes
Anatomic	Hysterosalpingogram	15–20%	Septum transection
	Hysteroscopy		Myomectomy
	Sonohysterography		Lysis of adhesions
Endocrinologic	Midluteal progesterone	8–12%	Progesterone
	TSH		Levothyroxine
	Prolactin		Bromocriptine, Dostinex
	Fasting insulin:glucose		Metformin
	Day 3 FSH, estradiol		Counseling
Immunologic	Lupus anticoagulant	15–25%	Aspirin
	Antiphospholipid antibodies		Heparin + aspirin
	? Embryotoxicity assay		? IV gamma globulin
	? Immunophenotypes		
Microbiologic	Cervical cultures	5–10%	Antibiotics
Thrombophilic	Antithrombin Activity	? 5%	Aspirin
	Protein C, protein S Activity		Heparin + aspirin
	Factor V Leiden mutation		LMW heparin
	Factor II Prothrombin mutation		
	Fasting Hyperhomocysteine		Folic acid
Psychologic	Interview	Varies	Support groups
	Questionnaire		Counseling
Iatrogenic	Tobacco, alcohol use	5%	Eliminate consumption
	Exposure to toxins, chemicals		Eliminate exposure

? = uncertain value of testing and treatment

Outcome

In approximately 65% of all cases of recurrent pregnancy loss, a complete evaluation will reveal a possible etiology.[2] If no cause can be found, the majority of couples will eventually have a successful pregnancy outcome with supportive therapy alone.[3] Couples who have experienced recurrent pregnancy loss want to know what caused the miscarriage. Unexplained reproductive failure can lead to anger, guilt, and depression. Anger may be directed toward their physician for not being able to solve their reproductive problems. Feelings of grief and guilt following an early loss are often as intense as those following a stillbirth and parents experience a grief reaction similar to that associated with the death of an adult. The couple should be assured that exercise, intercourse, and dietary indiscretions do not cause miscarriage. Any questions or concerns that the couple may have about personal habits should be discussed.

Women who suffer recurrent pregnancy loss have already begun to prepare for their baby, both emotionally and physically, as compared to couples with infertility who have never conceived. When a miscarriage occurs, a couple may have great difficulty informing friends or family about the loss. Feelings of hopelessness may continue long after the loss. Patients may continue to grieve and have episodes of depression on the expected due date or the date of the pregnancy loss. Participation in support groups or referral for grief counseling may be beneficial in many cases.[31]

REFERENCES

1 Kutteh WH. Recurrent pregnancy loss. In: Carr BR, Blackwell RE, Azziz R. (eds.), *Essential Reproductive Medicine*, McGraw-Hill, NY, NY-2005. 34:585–592.

2 Stephenson M. Frequency of factors associated with habitual abortion in 197 couples. *Fertil Steril* 66:24–29, 1996.

3 Brigham SA, Conlon C, Farguharson RG. A longitudinal study of pregnancy outcome following idiopathic recurrent miscarriage. *Hum Reprod* 14:2868–2871, 1999.

4 Branch DW, Silver RM. Antiphospholipid syndrome. *ACOG Educ Bull* 244:302–211, 1998.

5 Carson SA, Branch DW. Management of recurrent early pregnancy loss. *ACOG Pract Bull* 24:1–12, 2001.

6 Mills JL, Simpson JL, Driscoll SG, et al. Incidence of spontaneous abortion among normal women and insulin-dependent diabetic women whose pregnancies were identified within 21 days of conception. *N Engl J Med* 319:1617–1623, 1988.

7 Clifford K, Rai R, Regan L. Future pregnancy outcome in unexplained recurrent first trimester miscarriage. *Hum Reprod* 12:387–389, 1997.

8 Castelbaum AJ, Lessy BA. Infertility and implantation defects. *Infertil Reprod Med Clin North Am* 12:427–446, 2001.

9 Wilcox AJ, Baird DD, Weinberg CR. Time of implantation of the conception and loss of a pregnancy. *N Engl J Med* 340:1796–1799, 1999.

10   Ghazeeri GS, Clark DA, Kutteh WH. Immunologic factors in implantation. *Infertil Reprod Med Clin North Am* 12:315–337, 2001.

11   Sills ES, Perloe M, Palermo GD. Correction of hyperinsulinemia in oligoovulatory women with clomiphene-resistant polycystic ovary syndrome: a review of therapeutic rationale and reproductive outcomes. *Eur J Obstet Gynecol Reprod Biol* 91:135–141, 2000.

11a   Craig LB, Ke RW, Kutteh WH. Increased prevalence of insulin resistance in women with a history of recurrent pregnancy loss. *Fertil Steril* 78:487–490, 2002.

12   Hoffman GE, Khoury J, Thie J. Recurrent pregnancy loss and diminished ovarian reserve. *Fertil Steril* 74:1192–1195, 2000.

13   Stovall DW, Parrish SB, Van Voorhis BJ, et al. Uterine leiomyomas reduce the efficacy of assisted reproduction cycles: results of a matched follow-up study. *Hum Reprod* 13:192–197, 1998.

14   Surrey ES, Lietz AK, Schoolcraft WB. Impact of intramural leiomyomate in patients with a normal endometrial cavity on in vitro fertilization-embryo transfer cycle outcome. *Fertil Steril* 75:405–410, 2001.

15   Wilson WA, Ghavari AK, Piette JC. International classification criteria for antiphospholipid syndrome: synopsis of a post-conference workshop held at the Ninth International (Tours) APL Symposium. *Lupus* 10:457–460, 2001.

16   Cowchock FS, Reece EA, Balaban D. Repeated fetal losses associated with antiphospholipid antibodies: a collaborative randomized trial comparing prednisone with low-dose aspirin treatment. *Am J Obstet Gynecol* 166:1318–1323, 1992.

17   Laskin CA, Bombardier C, Hanna ME, et al. Prednisone and aspirin in women with autoantibodies and unexplained recurrent fetal loss. *N Engl J Med* 337:148–153, 1997.

18   Kutteh WH. Antiphospholipid antibody-associated recurrent pregnancy loss: treatment with heparin and low dose aspirin is superior to low dose aspirin alone. *Am J Obstet Gynecol* 174:1584–1589, 1996.

19   Rai R, Cohen H, Dave M, et al. Randomized controlled trial of aspirin and aspirin plus heparin in pregnant women with recurrent miscarriage associated with phospholipid antibodies. *Br Med J* 314:253–257, 1997.

20   Empson M, Lassere M, Craig JC, et al. Recurrent pregnancy loss with antiphospholipid antibody: a systematic review of therapeutic trials. *Obstet Gynecol* 99:135–144, 2002.

21   Rushworth FH, Bakos M, Rai R, et al. Prospective pregnancy outcome in untreated recurrent miscarriers with thyroid antibodies. *Hum Reprod* 15:1637–1639, 2000.

22 Esplin MS, Branch DW, Silver R, et al. Thyroid antibodies are not associated with recurrent pregnancy loss. *Am J Obstet Gynecol* 179:1583–1586, 1998.

23 Ober C, Karrison T, Odem RR, et al. Mononuclear-cell immunisation in prevention of recurrent miscarriages: a randomised trial. *Lancet* 354:365–369, 1999.

24 Kutteh WH, Stovall DW, Scott JR. The immunologic diagnosis and treatment of recurrent pregnancy loss. *Infertil Reprod Med Clin North Am* 8:267–287, 1997.

25 Daya S, Gunby J, Porter F, et al. Critical analysis of intravenous immunoglobulin therapy for recurrent miscarriage. *Hum Reprod Update* 5:475–482, 1999.

25a Penta M, Lukic A. Infectious agents in tissues from spontaneous abortions in the first trimester of pregnancy. *New Microbiology* 26:329–337, 2003.

26 Blumenfeld Z, Brenner B. Thrombophilia-associated pregnancy wastage. *Fertil Steril* 72:765–774, 1999.

27 Regan L, Rai R. Thrombophilia and pregnancy loss. *J Reprod Immunol* 55:163–180, 2002.

28 Lockwood CJ. Inherited thrombophilias in pregnant patients: detection and treatment paradigm. *Obstet Gynecol* 99:333–341, 2002.

28a Rey E, Kahn S, David M, Shrier I. Thrombophilic disorders and fetal loss. A meta-analysis. *Lancet* 361:901–908, 2003.

28b Kovalevsky G, Garcia CR, Berlin JA, Sammel MD, Barnhant KT. Evaluation of the association between hereditary thrombophilias and recurrent pregnancy loss. A meta-analysis. *Arab Intern Med* 164:558–563, 2004.

29 Quéré I, Mercier E, Bellet H, et al. Vitamin supplementation and pregnancy outcome in women with recurrent early pregnancy loss and hyperhomocysteinemia. *Fertil Steril* 75:823–825, 2001.

30 Ness RB, Grisso JA, Hirschinger N, et al. Cocaine and tobacco use and the risk of spontaneous abortion. *N Engl J Med* 340:333–339, 1999.

31 SHARE, Pregnancy and Infant Loss Support, Inc., St. Joseph Health Center, 300 First Capitol Drive, St. Charles, MO, www.nationalshareoffice.com.

20

Legal Issues

Susan L. Crockin
Karen E. Dumser

Introduction

Twenty-five years after the birth of the world's first *in vitro* fertilization (IVF) baby, advancing medical technologies continue to both broaden options for infertility patients and create unprecedented challenges for the legal system. The expanding array of assisted reproductive technology (ART) procedures, embryo and gamete cryopreservation, the involvement of multiple parties in collaborative reproductive arrangements, and nontraditional families all create novel complexities for the legal structures that define family relationships and guide practitioners.

Medical and mental health professionals involved with patients and third-parties attempting to create children through these technologies will want to have a general understanding of the legal issues, competing interests, and varying degrees of vulnerabilities for themselves and all involved. This chapter will primarily examine how the legal system characterizes various ART arrangements and participants, with an emphasis on collaborative reproduction, including traditional surrogacy; gestational carrier arrangements; and gamete and embryo use, donation, and dispositions. The developing law of provider liability and access to infertility treatments will also be examined. Regulatory issues, currently more the subject of ongoing and interdisciplinary debates than clearly developed federal and state law, are largely beyond the scope of this chapter.

Applicable Law

In the United States, the majority of laws affecting children and families predate IVF and most of the other developments in assisted reproduction. More recently enacted state laws intended to address the ARTs and the families they create vary considerably from state to state and are largely untested. In many instances, both the forced application or extension of antiquated laws and the judicial interpretations of new laws have created inconsistent and unpredictable results. While trends appear to be emerging in some areas, in others the legal framework for the ARTs is a virtual patchwork quilt from state to state and even court to court.

The U.S. Constitution grants certain fundamental rights that apply in every state, including the right to privacy. The right to procreate or not procreate has been recognized as an aspect of the right to privacy in a long line of Supreme Court cases involving sterilization, contraception, and abortion.[1] The debate over the regulation of procreation has centered on the degree of acceptable limitations on individual autonomy to make procreative decisions without governmental restriction. Regulations that limit fundamental rights must both advance a compelling governmental interest and be drafted in a manner that least imposes on an individual's rights. No consensus exists on the extent to which an individual's right to procreate includes using medical technology or collaborative arrangements.

KEY POINT

Regulations that limit fundamental rights (like the right to procreate) must both advance a compelling governmental interest and be drafted in a manner that least imposes on an individual's rights.

In general, the law refrains from interfering in family relationships absent overriding public policy concerns. Thus, parents are presumed fit to parent their children without public interference, except in narrow areas where oversight has been deemed necessary. For instance, every state has enacted comprehensive statutory schemes defining and governing the parent-child relationship, including specific laws regulating paternity, custody, child support, and adoption.

Statutes addressing the assisted reproductive technologies are both less common and usually less comprehensive, including defining the parentage of the resulting children. In the absence of comprehensive statutory schemes, case law has developed applying, interpreting, and extending existing laws to more and more novel fact patterns.

Some practical guidance for ART professionals may be found in medical and mental health Practice Guidelines and Ethics Reports issued by the American Society for Reproductive Medicine (ASRM).[2] These various guidelines and reports address multiple aspects of the reproductive technologies, including IVF, gamete donation, embryo donation, and informed consent. While not legally binding, they suggest at least minimum professional standards on a number of issues, such as donor compensation and mental health screening practices.

Collaborative Reproductive Arrangements

DONOR INSEMINATION AND SPERM STORAGE   Donor insemination is by far the oldest and consequently most widely regulated form of assisted conception. Although not considered by most medical professionals to be an ART procedure, statutes addressing "artificial insemination," as most are termed, are often cited by courts and extended by analogy to, or distinguished from, other ART contexts. Forty-two states regulate the practice in varying degrees.[3] Seven of those state statutes are limited in scope to the regulation of human immunodeficiency virus (HIV) screening or HIV transmission through donated semen.[4] The remaining 35 statutes focus on the parentage of the resulting child. The statutes that address parentage generally provide that the recipient and her consenting husband are the child's legal parents. Beyond that basic premise, the statutes vary in their detailed requirements, such as written consent or the involvement of a licensed physician.

Two-thirds of these state statutes refer only to a married woman or wife.[5] The exclusion of single women and nontraditional couples from statutory parentage protections creates legal vulnerabilities and necessitates additional steps to establish parentage, such as adoption where available.

Litigation involving donor insemination has included suits brought over the parent-child relationship of the resulting child, access to sperm during or after the donor's lifetime, or liability claims against medical providers or storage banks.

There have been numerous estate-related lawsuits involving attempts by a family member to preclude a child born through donor insemination from sharing in an inheritance based on arguments of illegitimacy. Although courts have almost uniformly rejected such suits,[6] trust and estate lawyers routinely recommend specifically identifying or naming all heirs to avoid any such vulnerability.[7]

To date, there have been no known cases of an anonymous sperm donor asserting parental rights, and relatively few cases where a known sperm donor has asserted a claim for paternity, primarily involving donations to single women or lesbian couples, with varied results. Courts have looked to both state law and any written expressions of intention.

In a 1994 case from New York, a known sperm donor successfully obtained a paternity order.[8] The child, who was 12 at the time of the court decision, had been living with her mother and partner since birth, but visited periodically with the sperm donor. The court found that the child's mother had "initiated and encouraged, over a substantial period of time, the relationship between the [donor] and his daughter," noted that preserving the donor's paternity rights would have "the advantage of supplying a further source of support, should the necessity arise, together with the potential for substantial inheritance," and found the sperm donor was entitled to an order of "filiation" (or paternity) as a matter of constitutional due process, in order to give him standing to seek visitation.

More recently, a Florida court rejected a similar claim involving a lesbian couple, their twins, and their friend who contributed sperm. The women were vulnerable to such a claim because Florida's extensive ART statute fails to define "donor" and Florida law prohibits adoptions by same sex couples. After several protracted rounds of court hearings, the final court to hear the case ruled definitively, ". . . this is a simple case that can be resolved in a one-sentence opinion, to wit: Danny A. Lucas is a sperm donor, not a parent, and has no parental rights. . . ."[9] The parties had entered into an unambiguous written contract in which the donor agreed to provide sperm to enable a pregnancy and have no parental rights. The court relied on both the contract between the parties and the Florida statute in finding the sperm donor had no parental rights.

To minimize potential vulnerabilities such as these, donor insemination participants will want to take all available precautions, including physician-facilitated insemination and written spousal/partner consents. Due to their added risks, unmarried

KEY POINT

> *While most states have statutes pertaining to sperm donation, legal counsel, especially for nontraditional couples and single women, is advisable.*

prospective recipients, nontraditional families, and prospective recipients using known donors would be particularly well-advised to consult independent legal counsel before proceeding with sperm donation, both to understand whether a written agreement may be advisable and enforceable, and whether there are other legal steps available to protect the intended family. In a growing number of states, a coparent adoption may be an option to establish legal parentage after the child is born. If available, and although possibly dependent on a sperm donor's continued cooperation, such a step is highly recommended and may protect both the couple from future claims by a sperm donor and the nonbiological parent/partner from future changes of circumstances. ART professionals will want to proceed cautiously by recommending or requiring patients to seek outside legal counsel, rather than by rendering legal assurances or advice themselves.

Posthumous reproduction presents another unusual situation with significant legal uncertainties for patients and providers. Physicians or courts may be presented with either an emergency request to extract sperm from a man who died suddenly, or, more likely, a request by a woman for insemination with a deceased partner's previously banked sperm. Documentation may or may not exist indicating whether the decedent consented to posthumous use of his sperm or intended to essentially become a parent after death.

A small but growing number of cases have arisen where a woman, who becomes pregnant using the banked sperm of her deceased partner, subsequently seeks to establish legal paternity and therefore federal benefits for the child or children. Since federal benefits are given to those considered "heirs" under the relevant state law,[10] inconsistent decisions have resulted.

In 2002, the highest state court in Massachusetts decided the novel question of whether a posthumously conceived child would "enjoy the inheritance rights of natural children under Massachusetts' law of intestate succession,"[11] and thus be eligible for Social Security survivor benefits. The court established a three-prong test: proof of the decedent's genetic paternity and "both that the decedent affirmatively consented to posthumous conception and to the support of any resulting child." The court added that time limitations, and presumably competing claims by other prospective heirs, might still preclude a claim on behalf of a posthumously conceived child.

With varying inheritance laws from state to state, and differing judicial biases and perspectives, inconsistent rulings are to be expected. For example, a New Jersey court, interpreting its inheritance laws, came to the same conclusion as the Massachusetts court,[12] while a federal court in Arizona denied Social Security survivor's benefits to twins conceived more than 10 months after their genetic father's death.[13] The latter court based its ruling on an interpretation of Arizona's intestacy laws which expressly provided that only a child surviving the deceased parent or in gestation at the time of death may inherit.

Posthumous parenthood raises significant issues of law and ethics, including concerns about how to ascertain the deceased's intentions with respect to any use of his sperm after his death. Patients and providers will want to be aware of, and act as consistently as possible with applicable law in their jurisdiction. Since the law is likely to remain unsettled for some time, it is also advisable for the adult male to put his intentions in writing, as clearly and unambiguously as possible, when preserving his sperm, both in any clinical consent form and in a separate agreement with any intended recipient. Patients should be encouraged to consult with independent legal counsel for these purposes. Such anticipatory steps and documentation may avoid the need to seek court orders by surviving widows, fiancées, and parents, all of which have occurred. Even with such clearly stated intentions, legal recognition of posthumous paternity will depend on both applicable state laws and judicially ascertained public policy.

KEY POINT

Posthumous conception faces significant legal uncertainties. Specific intentions should be documented, in advance, whenever possible.

EGG DONATION

Only eight states have enacted egg donation statutes to date: Colorado, Delaware, Florida, North Dakota, Oklahoma, Texas, Virginia, and Washington.[14] All explicitly state that an egg donor has no parental rights (or in the case of Florida, that the donor "shall relinquish all maternal rights and obligations with respect to the donation or the resulting children"). Beyond this central tenet, the complexity and requirements of each state vary considerably.[15] The statutes differ as to the circumstances under which the recipient(s) are presumed to be parents, whether written consent is required, whether the absence of consent always precludes a paternity finding, and whether the legally presumed father has a limited time frame to commence an action disputing his paternity.

Of the eight state laws, Delaware, Florida, Texas, and North Dakota address and expressly or impliedly allow compensation to egg donors.[16] Florida's statute provides, "[o]nly reasonable compensation directly related to the donation of eggs . . . shall be permitted."[17] Louisiana, by contrast, explicitly forbids payment to egg donors.[18]

ASRM guidelines suggest that monetary compensation to a donor should reflect "the time, inconvenience, and physical and emotional demands and risks associated with oocyte donation and should be at a level that minimizes the possibility of undue inducement of donors and the suggestion that payment is for the oocytes themselves."[19] Though it is common for actual dollar amounts to vary widely, compensation that is abnormally high within a geographic area raises not only the concern of undue inducement, but also ethical issues regarding payment for certain genetic attributes, such as intelligence or desirable physical characteristics. An ASRM Ethics Committee Report stated that while there is no consensus on the precise payment egg donors should receive, "at this time [August 2000] sums of $5,000 or more require justification and sums above $10,000 go beyond what is appropriate."[20]

In determining parentage in states without explicit egg donation statutes, a court may look to other parentage-related statutes or case law for guidance. Prior to the advent of medical technology allowing otherwise, courts and legislatures could safely assume that a woman giving birth to a child was the child's mother. Further, the law has traditionally presumed that the husband of a woman who gives birth to a child is the child's father.[21] In states with a sperm donation statute and equal protections laws in place, a strong argument should be available that a recipient of donated eggs should be treated the same as a recipient of donated sperm. Arguably, where a woman receives donated eggs and also gestates the child, given her gestational connection, she should be in an even stronger position than a man, with no gestational or genetic connection, whose wife bears a child using donated sperm.

There are no known cases involving egg donors attempting to assert parentage of children born through egg donation. The only known custody disputes involving children born via egg donation were two separate divorce cases where the husbands unsuccessfully sought custody claiming to be the better parent due to being the sole genetic parent. The courts ruled the egg donation was irrelevant to custody.[22] In 2002, media attention focused on interrelated lawsuits filed involving an egg donor's claims that two couples shared her donated eggs without her knowledge or consent, and despite a written legal agreement with the first couple that precluded any further use of her eggs.[23] The second couple sued the egg donor, the doctor who had reportedly used the eggs based on his understanding of Texas law, and the clinic after being told they could not use the frozen embryos absent the egg donor's consent. While the final outcome of this litigation is not yet known, the disputes highlight the importance of legal agreements and a clear written record of consent and intent in all egg donation arrangements.

Given the very limited laws and consequential legal uncertainties surrounding egg donation, legal contracts between egg donors and intended recipients are highly recommended and serve multiple purposes. Although enforceability cannot be guaranteed, in the event of any future maternity claim by an egg donor, an agreement should be evidence of her consent and intent to donate rather than parent, and of her waiver of any present or future parental rights. As discussed earlier, in sperm donor litigation courts have looked to just such evidence.[24]

A contract also creates a clear record of the parties' agreement on numerous other issues, such as the financial aspects of the arrangement (including any circumstances under which a donor may not be entitled to full compensation), future contact by either party either for medical reasons or subsequent donations, confidentiality provisions, allocation of risk amongst the parties, and responsibility for medical expenses, including complications. Occasionally, the process of negotiating an agreement, with separate independent counsel for each party, uncovers irreconcilable underlying differences that suggest the parties not go forward.

KEY POINT

While in most states, an analogy with the sperm donation statutes and the acceptance of the birth mother as the legal mother are supportive of oocyte donation arrangements, legal contracts are strongly recommended.

EMBRYO DONATION

A recent study revealed that, as of April, 2002, there were nearly 400,000 frozen human embryos stored in the United States.[25] The vast majority, about 88%, is designated for family-building use by the patients who created them. Only approximately 2%, or around

8000, of these embryos are in storage reportedly for the purpose of donation to another patient. The study indicates that 338 of the 340 responding practices require patients to sign a consent form before their embryos are frozen. It does not, however, state whether the clinics' reported classifications of embryos were based on such precryopreservation consent forms or whether separate embryo donation consent forms were subsequently signed after the patients own family-building efforts were completed, and the patients had then decided or redecided to donate their embryos. ASRM guidelines state that, "embryo donors must sign an informed consent document indicating their permission to use their embryos for embryo donation," but do not specify a timeframe for doing so.[26]

Beyond mere semantics, the terminology applied to embryo donation is laden with significant political and legal implications. With the sole exception of Louisiana's reference to "adoptive implantation," no state laws recognize "adoption" of an embryo, whether *in utero* or in cryopreserved storage,[27] and those who embrace the term do not apply existing adoption laws and structures. Notwithstanding this fact, following hearings on the available frozen embryos for stem cell research in the summer of 2002, the federal government authorized $1million in educational grants to promote "embryo adoption."[28] Whether artless diction or a deliberate political statement, these terms imply very different legal frameworks. An arrangement construed as a "donation" may be treated legally akin to gamete donation, whereas an arrangement construed as a true "adoption" would be subject to more extensive state requirements for the adoption of children, and would raise significant and unanswered concerns as to the legal status of embryos, the timing of relinquishments (which under traditional adoption law cannot be prior to birth and a subsequent *cooling off* period for birth parents), and other legal protections and restrictions. For the most part, those who use the term "embryo adoption," including those who believe that life begins at conception, are neither literally referring to, nor intending to invoke or use the legal framework and protections of, the adoption laws.

Eight state statutes address embryo donation, including the egg donation statutes (except Colorado) and Louisiana, which addresses only embryos.[29] Embryo donors are uniformly relieved of parental rights. Beyond this, the state laws vary as to the specific requirements for legal parentage of the recipient(s), the need for consent, and the applicability to unmarried patients.

While the number of cases involving the use of frozen embryos by fighting ex-spouses has been growing (discussed below), there is little precedent for establishing parentage of a child born through embryo donation. No reported judicial decisions exist where consenting embryo donors have sought parental rights. There have been, however, a small number of contested parentage cases involving children born after inadvertent embryo transfers to the wrong patients, as discussed in the Section "Gamete and Embryo Mishandling" below.

Additional complexity and potential vulnerability arise in cases where the patients who originally created the embryos used donor gametes to do so. Limited research studies suggest that a majority of embryos offered for donation were created with either donor egg or sperm.[30] Speculation as to the reasons for this have included suggestions that the donating couple may have less attachment to such embryos or that they are more sensitized to donation issues from their own treatments. Whatever the reason, donating embryos originally created with donor egg or donor sperm should be approached cautiously. While there is virtually no case law yet developed in this area, learning from informed consent issues in other ART areas, it would seem that absent either an express consent or agreement from the original donor to redonate the embryos or an original consent broad enough to cover the contemplated redonation, proceeding is a risk to all involved.

Thus, any agreement between the initial patients and their gamete donor(s) and that donor's prior consent should be carefully scrutinized to ensure that the embryos are, in fact, legally available for redonation to another patient(s). Unless such consent is indicated in a donor's clinical consent form or in their private contract with the recipient patients, or the initial consent is drafted sufficiently broadly to cover redonation to another patient, it is these authors' practice to recontact the gamete donor(s) for contemporaneous consent to the anticipated embryo donation or decline to use the embryos. On a prospective basis, it is recommended that this issue be raised with any donor prior to a donation and recorded in any contract with a recipient patient(s).

On first consideration, many patients may consider embryo donation a relatively simple, easy, and loving solution to the question of what to do with their excess embryos. Significant, long-term issues can be frequently overlooked, suggesting the need and significant role for an experienced mental health professional. ASRM's 2002 guidelines for embryo donation provide detailed, albeit minimum, psychologic recommendations for addressing the complex issues that confront participants.[31] Somewhat surprisingly, the guidelines recommend but do not require a minimal mental health consultation, as is required to be done in egg donation.

In these authors' limited experience, mental health intervention has been critical and often the determinative factor in prospective embryo donors' ultimate decision as to whether they are truly prepared to proceed with their donation. In our practice, in approximately a dozen prospective cases in a 1-year period, one half of prospective embryo donors ultimately elected not to donate after comprehensive mental health consultations. Frequently, spouses had differing views that could not always be reconciled, suggesting the importance of not only a single consult, but of an opportunity for prospective donors to explore their individual concerns.

Due to the lack of clear legal precedent in embryo donation, prudent practice dictates that participants enter a legal contract with each other to outline their intentions and the terms of their arrangement. Donor/recipient contracts should address the same types of issues as in egg donation, including parentage, confidentiality, future contact, and financial arrangements. Since it is quite likely that two or more genetically related children may ultimately be involved, many of these issues will involve more sensitivity and planning.

The financial arrangements in embryo donation also require close scrutiny. Unlike sperm and egg donation, payments to embryo donors are strictly limited to expense reimbursement. At least 20 states prohibit compensation for embryo or tissue donation, generally in the context of public health and safety laws and regulations.[32] ASRM practice guidelines recommend that donors should receive no compensation for the donation other than reimbursement for specific expenses (e.g., obligatory blood tests or extended storage costs attributed to the potential donation).[33]

KEY POINT

Embryo donation, while appearing as a loving alternative use for stored embryos, is rife with unresolved legal issues and requires careful counseling of the couples involved.

Establishing or challenging parentage of children born via embryo donation is another legal unknown. Longstanding assumptions that a woman who delivers a child is that child's mother have already been successfully challenged in the context of both gestational carrier arrangements and mistransferred embryos, as discussed in Sections Embryo Donation and Gamete and Embryo Mishandling below. This suggests that couples may want to take additional steps to protect their legal parentage, such as seeking a court order of parentage, even in the absence of an explicitly applicable state law. Because of the significant novel issues raised by embryo donation, both prospective donors and recipients should be strongly advised, if not required, to consult with both a mental health professional and experienced independent legal counsel before proceeding.

TRADITIONAL SURROGACY AND GESTATIONAL CARRIER ARRANGEMENTS

Although sometimes referred to loosely as "surrogacy," the distinct practices of "traditional surrogacy" and "gestational carrier arrangements" (sometimes referred to as *gestational surrogacy*) should be defined and distinguished for purposes of clarity and discussion. Only the former refers to women with a genetic link to the child, a frequently critical distinction for courts and lawmakers alike. "Traditional surrogates" are women who are artificially inseminated with sperm, usually that of the intended father, to bear a child to be raised by the intended parent(s). "Gestational carriers," the term many legal practitioners (including these authors) prefer, are women who have an embryo transferred to their uterus, usually created by the intended parents, to bear a child to be raised by the intended parent(s).

At least 24 states have enacted laws governing surrogacy which vary widely in breadth and substance.[34] For example, one very restrictive statute enacted in the District of Columbia prohibits any oral or written agreement for traditional or gestational surrogacy and imposes a civil penalty and/or imprisonment for violating the law.[35] Several other states ban paid traditional and/or gestational surrogacy, including Michigan, New York, Utah, New Hampshire, Nevada, and Kentucky.[36] In addition, some states declare surrogacy contracts void as contrary to public policy, although they vary on whether they refer to paid or unpaid and traditional or gestational surrogacy.[37] An Arizona statute that attempted to prohibit all forms of surrogacy arrangements was successfully challenged as unconstitutional on equal protection grounds, because only men could challenge the parentage presumptions.[38]

In states that allow some types of surrogacy, the level of statutory regulation varies widely. For instance, statutes in Florida, Nevada, New Hampshire, and Virginia provide mandatory terms for valid surrogacy contracts.[39] Several state statutes address the legal parentage of intended parents, either by stating a presumption or by providing a mechanism for establishing legal parentage: Connecticut (by court petition), Florida (by court petition), Illinois (by state public health department procedure), Nebraska (paternity presumption), Nevada (presumption), New Hampshire (by court involvement), Tennessee (presumption), and Virginia (by court involvement).[40]

Some state statutes are more minimal, addressing neither contracts nor parentage. For example, in Wisconsin and Wyoming, surrogacy is only addressed in the states' birth registration statutes, which provide that a traditional surrogate or gestational carrier is named on the child's birth certificate unless a court orders otherwise.[41] In Alabama, Iowa, and West Virginia, surrogacy is merely mentioned as an exception in those states' statutes prohibiting baby-selling or payments to birth mothers in adoptions.[42]

Several courts have also ruled on various aspects of traditional surrogacy and gestational carrier arrangements. Both genetics and intent have been key factors in the determination of legal parenthood in the courts that have decided these cases. Traditional surrogates, dating back to the 1988 landmark decision, *In re Baby M*, are often treated in the eyes of the law as birth mothers and entitled to the protections of a state's adoption laws.

In *Baby M*, after the traditional surrogate changed her mind during the pregnancy, the New Jersey Supreme Court held that a traditional surrogacy contract between a married couple and a traditional surrogate was void, and that the genetic, intended father and the surrogate were the child's legal parents.[43] The court ultimately awarded custody to the father and granted the surrogate visitation rights as the legal mother. Since *Baby M*, absent a contrary state surrogacy statute, courts have generally treated traditional surrogates as birth mothers and found traditional surrogacy contracts unenforceable as against public policy which prohibits birth mothers from contracting to relinquish their unborn children or accepting money to do so.[44]

Gestational carrier arrangements have become more common in recent years, in part due to the availability of IVF, and in part due to their reduced legal risk. The few reported decisions reflect a general consensus that the couple providing the gametes and intending to parent the child are the child's legal parents, overcoming any common law presumption of maternity based on giving birth.

In the 1993 seminal case of *Johnson v. Calvert*, the California Supreme Court adopted a parentage determination analysis that essentially used intent as a maternity tiebreaker between genetics and gestation.[45] A gestational carrier, with no genetic connection to the child, refused to relinquish the child to his genetic, intended parents. The court held that, under existing California law, parentage could be determined by either genetic determination or giving birth, and that, "when the two means do not coincide in one woman, she who intended to procreate the child—that is, she who intended to bring about the birth of a child that she intended to raise as her own—is the natural mother under California law."

Following *Johnson v. Calvert*, intent to procreate played a decisive role in one well-publicized child support case involving both a gestational carrier and donor gametes, *In re Buzzanca*.[46] In the context of a divorce, a California appellate court ordered the husband to pay child support although he was not the genetic father and his wife did not carry the child. The court found that he was one of the intended parents of a child carried by a married gestational carrier created using donated sperm and eggs. Parentage and child support flowed from the fact that, 'but for' the intended parents' intention to create the child, as reflected in a written agreement with the carrier (who was not asserting a maternity claim), the child would not have been born.

As a practical matter, for noncontested cases seeking to clarify parentage in gestational carrier cases (including with donated gametes in some cases and states), an increasing number of states allow cases to be filed during the pregnancy or immediately after the birth to establish the legal parentage of the intended parents.[47] Some state courts, even without explicit precedent in their jurisdiction, have also acknowledged the legal maternity of an intended, but nongenetic, mother in gestational carrier cases where donated eggs were used.[48] Where allowed, these actions eliminate or reduce the need for traditional step-parent adoptions after the child's birth. The availability, nature, timing, and requirements for such actions vary widely from state to state. Thus, patients considering entering into these complex family-building arrangements will want to consult experienced legal counsel in the relevant state or states on the issue of establishing parentage prior to deciding whether to enter into a legal agreement.

A legal agreement between a gestational carrier, her husband if married, and the intended parents, negotiated by independent, separate legal counsel, is highly recommended, except in states banning or voiding such contracts by statute.[49] Some state laws include detailed guidance for the terms of such contracts. Florida law provides that a contract for gestational surrogacy shall not be binding and enforceable unless the parties are 18 years of age or older and the intended parents are married.[50] The statute lists specific provisions that must be in every contract, including the carrier's agreement to adhere to medical instructions and relinquish any parental rights, the intended parents' agreement to accept custody of the child regardless of the child's health, and that the intended parents may pay only reasonable living, legal, medical, psychologic, and psychiatric expenses of the carrier that are directly related to the pregnancy.[51]

Even in states without specific requirements, a gestational carrier contract should be as comprehensive as possible, setting forth, for example, the parties' intentions with respect to the parentage of the child, their financial arrangements, prenatal care, delivery plans, selective reduction, abortion, future contact among the parties, and cooperation on legal steps to establish parentage. Because of constitutional procreative rights and protections, specific performance of certain critical aspects of an agreement, such as selective reduction and abortion, is highly unlikely. Should a carrier breach that aspect of an agreement, provisions for damages may be appropriate and enforceable.

Even though the enforceability of such contracts cannot be guaranteed in states lacking legal precedent, at a minimum the process forces parties to discuss, negotiate, and reach a thoughtful agreement on many significant details of their arrangement. The document itself provides both a guide for the parties and evidence of intent for a court in any future dispute.

KEY POINT

Traditional and gestational surrogacy are distinct, with respect to genetic parentage, as well as legal implications.

Frozen Embryos

Frozen embryos have been the subject of a growing number of cases dating back over a decade. Most, but not all, involve divorcing spouses who disagree over the disposition of their excess embryos. Many of such former patients have previously recorded consent forms in which they indicated some choice of disposition in the event of future, divorce, or death. Possible dispositions for excess embryos typically include discard, donation for research, or donation to another patient for family-building purposes. Most of the reported cases involve divorcing couples who no longer agree on their previously recorded, jointly reached, decision as to disposition.

Starting in the early 1990s with the Tennessee case of *Davis v. Davis*,[52] a growing number of state courts have been forced to both interpret and determine the enforceability of such prior consents or agreements in disputes between divorcing spouses with leftover cryopreserved embryos. Cases have arisen in Louisiana, Massachusetts, Texas, New Jersey, and New York, and certain trends appear to be emerging.[53] First, those courts that have characterized human embryos or preembryos have trended toward referring to them as entities "deserving of special respect" due to their potential for life (rather than as property), and to those who create them as having "dispositional authority" over them (rather than owners).[54]

With respect to their creators' differing views on disposition, a trend also seems to be emerging to honor prior agreements that do not relate to procreation (i.e., destruction or research), but to refuse to honor those that would now violate one of the creator's expressed desire not to procreate. Thus, for example, where no prior agreement was in place and Junior Davis objected to his ex-wife's subsequent desire to use the embryos, the Louisiana court ultimately ruled that his constitutional right not to procreate trumped his ex-wife's right to procreate, especially given her remarriage and ability to conceive again.

One subsequent case refused to allow an ex-wife to retract her prior agreement to donate excess embryos to the IVF program for research,[55] while two other subsequent cases have allowed one ex-spouse to prevent the other's use or donation of the embryos for procreation, notwithstanding a prior agreement for just that purpose.[56]

The significant and decisive factor for the courts appears to be not allowing the creation of a child over a contemporaneous objection by one potential biological parent. In allowing an ex-husband to prevent his ex-wife from using embryos despite his seven previous written consents to her use, the Massachusetts court ruled very clearly that "forced procreation is not amenable to judicial enforcement."[57] Relying on the Massachusetts precedent, the New Jersey court allowed a wife to prevent the donation of embryos to her sister-in-law, despite an earlier agreement to do so.[58]

ART programs will thus want to ensure that their consent forms and cryopreservation agreements are clearly written, with choices thoughtfully considered, clearly articulated, and unambiguously recorded in writing. At the same time, developing case law suggests programs will also want to recognize and acknowledge to their patients that they cannot guarantee that all choices, and at least those involving procreation, will be able to be honored under all future circumstances. If this trend away from enforcing procreative choices in the face of subsequent disagreement continues, as the New Jersey decision suggests in refusing to enforce an agreement to donate, even embryos created with donor sperm or egg may be vulnerable to a change of mind by either a donor or ex-spouse.

KEY POINT

Disposition, of frozen embryos, in case of death or divorce, should be discussed and documented prior to embryo freezing. However, couples should be aware that decisions involving procreation may not be enforceable.

Provider Liability

STANDARD OF CARE AND CIVIL LIABILITY

Infertility patients are owed the same standard of care as all other patients, and traditional medical malpractice standards, not reviewed here, apply. Standard practice and professional guidelines promulgated by ASRM may provide some guidance or minimum practice standards to follow.[59] In addition, at least as to third-parties, such as donors, surrogates, or carriers, a few courts have suggested that ART professionals may be held to an even higher duty and standard of care.[60] In separate cases dating back several years, two courts found that traditional surrogacy brokers, as well as the medical and legal professionals involved, owed a higher, "affirmative duty of care" to two healthy traditional surrogates the brokers had recruited. Those decisions may suggest a higher standard of care in other ART arrangements, and professionals will want to be aware of the courts' expressed concerns.

In a 1992 federal case, *Stiver v. Parker*, a traditional surrogate was inseminated with the sperm of an intended father. He had not been screened for cytomegalovirus, and the surrogate, Judith Stiver, gave birth to a severely affected child. The court ruled that the broker, doctor, and lawyers involved all owed her an affirmative duty of protection to keep her from harm. The court explained, "[t]his . . . affirmative duty of protection, marked by heightened diligence, arises out of a special relationship because the defendants engaged in the surrogacy business and expected to profit thereby." The court articulated that duty to include designing and administering a program to protect the parties, including a requirement for appropriate testing, in order to protect the surrogate mother as well as the child and contracting parents from foreseeable harm caused by the surrogacy undertaking.

In 1997, a Pennsylvania court relied on the *Stiver* court's reasoning to also apply a higher affirmative duty of protection due to the "special relationship" created between a surrogacy business and its recruited traditional surrogates in a wrongful death suit. That surrogate argued that the surrogacy broker, by failing to investigate or counsel the intended parent to ensure his fitness as a parent, breached its duty to her. The father, a single 26 year old, killed the child at 6 weeks by shaking him to death; the autopsy confirmed preexisting injuries to the child as well. After the fact, the surrogate learned that the father had recently lost his mother and had no child care experience. Although her lawsuit was initially dismissed, it was reinstated on appeal with the court citing *Stiver*. The appellate court applied a higher, affirmative standard and ruled that brokers should be liable for the foreseeable consequences of a surrogacy arrangement, which it held included child abuse.

It remains to be seen whether a similar affirmative duty may be extended by other courts and to other areas of collaborative reproduction, such as gamete donation, embryo donation, or gestational carrier arrangements.

PREGNANCY AND BIRTH-RELATED CLAIMS

Claims against physicians outside of the arena of ART cases alleging the tort of wrongful birth have been brought for decades, resulting in well-developed legal precedent. A cause of action for wrongful birth is a lawsuit brought by parents against a defendant whose negligence allegedly led to the birth of a child with birth defects.[61] Most states allow such actions for wrongful birth, which claims typically involve errors or omissions in parental or prenatal testing.

An action for wrongful life, on the other hand, is brought by or on behalf of a child born with birth defects or other medical problems against a defendant whose negligence allegedly caused the child's birth. Most jurisdictions that have considered such claims have not permitted them on the theory that any life has more value than none.[62] A minority of states, however, has recognized wrongful life actions, including California, New Jersey, and Washington.[63]

At least two states, New Mexico and Ohio, have allowed claims for wrongful pregnancy brought by a child or a child's parents. Wrongful pregnancy claims allege that a healthy child's birth resulted from negligence, such as incorrectly performing a sterilization procedure.[64]

More recently, and of particular significance for ART providers, successful claims have been brought for multifetal pregnancies and births resulting from infertility treatment. In one such case, a U.K. woman claimed that her doctor prescribed an incorrect dose of the infertility drug metrodin, resulting in a quadruplet pregnancy.[65] The children were born at 26 weeks gestation, with one child dying 34 hours after birth. Of the three surviving children, the parents alleged one is healthy, one has cerebral palsy, and one has behavioral problems that the parents attribute to his premature birth. The U.K. court awarded £2 million to the surviving three children.

In 2001, a Yorkshire woman settled another multifetal pregnancy case for a reported £20,000.[66] After giving birth to triplets, she alleged that a fertility clinic transferred three embryos to her instead of two as she requested. The settlement was meant to compensate her for the trauma of giving birth to a third baby.

Such cases may open the door to more claims in the United States against infertility specialists who transfer a high number of embryos to a patient. ASRM guidelines provide guidance as to the appropriate number of embryos to transfer for patients in different age and prognosis categories, yet also state that, "strict limitations, such as a maximum replacement of three embryos as required by law in some countries, do not allow individual variation according to each patient's circumstances. These guidelines may be varied according to individual clinical conditions . . . and as clinical data is accumulated with newer techniques."[67] Procedures far outside this norm may create potential wrongful birth or life liability if the tort is so extended.

GAMETE AND EMBRYO MISHANDLING

Another potential liability source for infertility providers, and often the subject of widespread media attention, involves gamete and embryo mishandling. The late 1990s brought at least two high-publicity gamete and embryo mix-up cases, and a number of other clinic liability cases as well.

Physicians at the University of California-Irvine were accused of having mishandled hundreds of gametes and embryos in their care, creating embryos without the knowledge or consent of the gamete providers and, in some cases, transferring such embryos to other patients.[68] Criminal charges were brought against the physicians and more than 100 civil lawsuits were filed by former patients against the University. By 1999, the University had agreed to pay claimants nearly $17 million to settle their claims. At least six children were reportedly born to couples from erroneously created or mistransferred embryos, using gametes from patients who allegedly never consented to their "donation" to another couple. In all known reported parental rights cases that arose, however, the genetic parents eventually settled or withdrew their claims to protect the children from the trauma that would have resulted from custody litigation.[69]

Another embryo mix-up came to light during the twin pregnancy of Donna Fasano, when the Fasanos and the Rogers, another family using the same clinic for IVF treatment, were notified by the clinic that a vial of the Rogers' embryos were mistakenly transferred to Ms. Fasano along with her own embryos. Amniocentesis tests revealed that one of the fetuses was genetically related to the Rogers.

After the birth, the Rogers filed suit against the Fasanos to obtain physical and legal custody of the second child. After ultimately overturning the common law presumption of maternity for Ms. Fasano, and a series of lengthy court battles and out-of-court negotiations, the Rogers were ultimately awarded exclusive custody of their child and the Fasanos denied any parental or visitation rights.[70]

In addition to the custody litigation, each family sued their doctors and the laboratory for mixing the embryos.[71] The Fasanos brought a negligence action alleging physical and emotional injury, based on their need to decide whether to carry a fetus to term that was not theirs, to undergo a cesarean section birth because of the multifetal pregnancy, and to decide whether to relinquish custody to the genetic parents. The Rogers brought a medical malpractice action against the obstetricians and laboratory. The court found the Rogers had suffered emotional harm by having been deprived of the opportunity to experience pregnancy and childbirth and deprived of custody of their son for approximately 4 months after his birth. In both cases, the court found that the families had viable claims.

Another embryo mix-up case was decided by the Court of Appeal of California, where a single woman, Susan B, gave birth to a child after the clinic allegedly implanted the wrong embryos.[72] Susan B's intent was to use embryos created with donor egg and donor sperm; instead, the clinic implanted the embryos of a married couple using the same clinic, which the couple had created for their own use with the husband's sperm and donated eggs. The couple also had a child from the same group of embryos. In the parentage action filed by the married couple, the trial court ruled that the husband could not be characterized as a "donor" within the meaning of California's statute because he did not intend to inseminate anyone other than his wife, that Susan B's claim for sole parentage was better suited to the legislation, and that any constitutional claims by the child to a stable, permanent placement were arguments better suited for a potential future custody claim by the father and his wife. The wife was held to have no parental rights, a decision affirmed an appeal.

Another pending child custody case involves two women who created twins using eggs from one and carried by the other.[73] The trial court has characterized the egg provider as a donor, not a mother, in large part based on her having signed the IVF program's general egg donor consent form. It is disputed whether they presented to the IVF program as a couple, but the standard consent forms were apparently neither amended nor supplemented with more specific and accurate language argued to be applicable to their factual circumstances. That case is also currently on appeal.

While cases like these may arise as actions among the parties to adjudicate parentage, custody, or visitation, it would seem inevitable that the programs whose practices may have arguably contributed to the vulnerability of their patients' parentage will be involved in these ongoing disputes.

In other cases where parentage has not been an issue, patients have alleged claims against programs directly. In one such case, a sperm bank allegedly failed to pass on information purportedly disclosed by a donor about a kidney disorder in his family history.[74] The California appellate court found that the sperm bank and physicians did not cause the child's inherited abnormalities by improperly approving the sperm donor to donate. Rather, the child's kidney condition "was caused by the gene contained within the sperm provided by Donor No. 276." The parents of the child had also brought fraud claims against the sperm bank based on alleged alterations of the donor's profile. The court concluded that the trial court had fairly characterized the cause of action as one for wrongful life, and that under prior California judicial precedent, the child was thus not entitled to recover general damages or damages for lost earnings.

In another lawsuit brought against a sperm bank, parents of healthy triplets brought a claim against the sperm bank for negligent infliction of emotional distress resulting from the clinic using the wrong donor's sperm to inseminate the wife. The couple selected a particular donor based on his matching blood type and hair color; after the birth, it was determined that the children did not have the same blood type and physical appearance. The Utah Supreme Court rejected the case based on the couple's failure to demonstrate any injury, and thus left undecided the issue of whether there was any negligence by the sperm bank in the sperm donation process.

KEY POINT

Medical and legal professionals involved in ART procedures may require a higher "affirmative duty of care" in the course of participating in the creation of families with alternative ART.

Access to Infertility Treatment

Patient access to infertility treatment, and the various legal bases available to argue in favor of such access, is a legally complex and still evolving area of the law involving constitutional, federal, and state insurance, health, and discrimination laws. A full treatment of this topic is beyond the scope of this chapter and the reader is referred to multiple scholarly articles and chapters on various aspects of these laws.[75] An overview identifying the relevant sources of law in this area is set out here.

In the late 1970s and 1980s, as the prevalence of medical intervention to treat infertility began to rise in response to medical advancements, insurance companies commonly excluded many such treatments from their coverage plans. In response, consumer advocacy movements arose in the mid-1980s to advocate for infertility coverage. At least 13 states have since enacted laws that require health insurers to either cover or offer to cover some degree of infertility treatment.[76] The statutory mandates differ widely from state to state in the range of treatments insurers are required to cover or offer and those they may permissibly exclude.

As one example, Massachusetts' infertility mandate requires most insurers to provide, "to the same extent that benefits are provided for other pregnancy-related procedures, coverage for medically necessary expenses of diagnosis and treatment of infertility."[77] Massachusetts regulations promulgated in connection with the statute allow insurers to create both appropriate eligibility requirements and certain exclusions.[78]

A threshold question is whether a state's statutory mandate applies to the particular health insurance plan. Under the federal Employee Retirement Income Security Act of 1974 (ERISA), self-insured health plans are exempt from state regulation.[79] State law may also allow certain exemptions, based on employer size or otherwise. Legal counsel experienced in infertility and insurance law may be of assistance in obtaining insurance coverage and any appeals of denials, in order to ensure that all legal remedies and claims are properly pursued.

Regardless of whether a state has enacted an insurance mandate, a patient's access to infertility treatment may be protected under the relevant policy or through federal laws prohibiting discrimination based on disability. Such federal statutory protection may be found under the Americans With Disabilities Act (ADA),[80] the Civil Rights Act of 1964,[81] or the Pregnancy Discrimination Act (PDA) of 1978.[82]

The ADA prohibits discrimination in regard to employee compensation and "other terms, conditions, and privileges of employment."[83] The ADA prohibits such discrimination in any place of "public accommodation," which by statutory definition includes insurance and health care providers' offices.[84] A person is considered to have a disability—and thus afforded protections against disability discrimination—if the person: (1) has a physical or mental impairment that substantially limits one or more of his or her "major life activities"; (2) has a record of such an impairment; or (3) is regarded as having such an impairment.[85]

In 1998, in *Bragdon v. Abbott*, the U.S. Supreme Court held that reproduction constitutes a major life activity under the ADA.[86] An HIV-positive woman alleging discrimination in the denial of dental care filed suit and the Court found HIV is a "disability" that substantially limited a major life activity, namely reproduction. While this decision did not directly involve infertility or insurance coverage, it may be argued to apply in the context of employer-sponsored health insurance discrimination against those with infertility.

In addition to seeking protection under the ADA, a person denied access to infertility treatment as a result of discrimination may also seek protection under Title VII of the Civil Rights Act of 1964, which prohibits employment practices that "discriminate against any individual with respect to his compensation, terms, conditions, or privileges of employment, because of such individual's race, color, religion, sex, or national origin."[87] This prohibition extends to discrimination in providing health insurance and other fringe benefits.[88] In 1978, the Civil Rights Act was amended by the PDA which added discrimination based on "pregnancy, childbirth, or related medical conditions" within its definition of sex discrimination.[89]

Judicial opinions vary as to whether infertility is a medical condition related to pregnancy or childbirth under the PDA. Some courts have found that the PDA applies to discrimination based on potential or intended pregnancy, in additional to actual pregnancy.[90] On the other hand, at least one court has found that infertility is not a pregnancy-related medical condition, ruling that infertility prevents conception, while pregnancy and childbirth occur after conception.[91] Another court has denied the protections of the PDA on the grounds that infertility affects equal numbers of each sex.[92] Thus, the amount of protection offered by the PDA to those denied access to infertility treatment remains uncertain.

Regulation: A Brief Overview

Little current regulation exists within the United States and a discussion of the current efforts to increase or streamline any such regulation is beyond the scope of this chapter. The Fertility Clinic Success Rate and Certification Act of 1992 requires statistical reporting by ART programs.[93] The federal government, in the form of not only Clinical Laboratory Improvement Amendments, but also the Food and Drug Administration, the Center for Disease Control, and multidisciplinary professional groups such as the American Bar Association, the National Conference of Commissioners on Uniform State Laws, the National Coalition for Oversight of Assisted Reproductive Technologies among others, are studying ways in which to regulate, impact, or shape the ARTs. Parallel efforts and models also exist in other states, such as the Human Fertilization and Embryology Authority in the United Kingdom and the National Health & Medical Research Council in Australia. With ever-increasing medical options and challenges, these debates and efforts will certainly continue and intensify.

The Future of Assisted Reproduction: A Legal Perspective

Family building has long left the privacy of the bedroom, and entered not only the doctor's office but also courtrooms and legislatures around the country. As treatment options for infertility patients continue to expand, they bring new challenges for patients, third-parties, providers, lawmakers, and policymakers alike. As techniques such as preimplantation genetic diagnosis (PGD) and egg freezing become more prevalent, new legal responses and frameworks will need to be crafted. Already, the growing number of children born via sperm and egg donation has brought calls for national registries or other means to ensure the ability of those children to share information about and with one another. Embryo donation possibilities have piqued both the interest and concerns of multiple law and policy makers.

Courts, legislatures, federal and state regulators from multiple disciplines, and professional organizations, are all weighing in on the perceived needs to shape, regulate, guide, and limit the availability and scope of treatments for infertile patients. Professionals who provide infertility services to patients and third-parties will want to have an appreciation of the legal issues and vulnerabilities surrounding their practices in order to better serve their patients, third-parties, and ultimately the resulting children. It is hoped that this overview has provided insights into the laws affecting ART professionals, patients, third-parties, and children they all seek to create.

ENDNOTES

1 Skinner v. Oklahoma, 316 U.S. 535 (1942); *Griswold v. Connecticut*, 381 U.S. 479 (1965); *Eisenstadt v. Baird*, 405 U.S. 438 (1972); *Roe v. Wade*, 410 U.S. 113 (1973); *Stanley v. Illinois*, 405 U.S. 645 (1972); *Planned Parenthood of Southeastern Pennsylvania v. Carey*, 112 S.Ct. 2791 (1992).

2 See www.asrm.org

3 Alabama, Alaska, Arizona, Arkansas, California, Colorado, Connecticut, Delaware, Florida, Georgia, Idaho, Illinois, Indiana, Iowa, Kansas, Kentucky, Louisiana, Maryland, Massachusetts, Michigan, Minnesota, Missouri, Montana, Nevada, New Hampshire, New Jersey, New Mexico, New York, North Carolina, North Dakota, Ohio, Oklahoma, Oregon, Rhode Island, South Carolina, Tennessee, Texas, Virginia, Washington, West Virginia, Wisconsin, Wyoming.

4 Del.Code Ann. Tit.16, §§1202, 1203, 2801 (1999); Ind. Code Ann. §16-41-14-1 to 20 (1999); Iowa Code Ann. §141.23 (1999); Ky.Rev.Stat.Ann. §§214.181, 214.625 (1998); R.I.Gen.Laws §23-1-38 (1999); S.C. Code Ann. §44-29-145 (1998).

5 For example, Massachusetts law provides: "Any child born to a married woman as a result of artificial insemination with the consent of her husband, shall be considered the legitimate child of the mother and such husband." G.L. c.46, §4B. Exceptions include the District of Columbia, Louisiana, New Hampshire, New Jersey, North Carolina, North Dakota, Ohio, Oklahoma, and Oregon, which do not specifically refer to a married woman or wife.

6 See, e.g., *Anonymous v. Anonymous*, 246 N.Y.S.2d 835 (Sup.Ct. 1964); *K.S. v. G.S.*, 440 A.2d 64 (N.J. Super.Ct.Ch.Div. 1981); *People v. Sorenson*, 437 P.2d 495 (Cal. 1968); *Gursky v. Gursky*, 242 N.Y.S.2d 406 (Sup.Ct. 1963).

7 Levitan S. Inheritance and estate planning issues for adoptive and reproductive technology assisted families. *Adoption & Reproductive Technology in Massachusetts*, MCLE, 2000.

8 *Thomas S. v. Robin Y.*, 618 N.Y.S.2d 356 (1994).

9 *Lamaritata v. Lucas*, 823 So.2d 316 (Fla.2d DCA 2002).

10 *Woodward v. Comm'r of Social Security*, 435 Mass. 536, n.4 (2002).

11 *Woodward v. Comm'r of Social Security*, 435 Mass. 536 (2002).

12 *In re Estate of Kolacy*, 2000 N.J. Super. LEXIS 275 (4/19/00).

13 *Gillett-Netting v. Comm'r of Social Security*, No. CV 02-014 TUC JMR (10/24/02).

14 Colo.Stat. §19-4-106; 13 Del.C. §§8-101 *et seq.*; Fla.Stat.Ann. §§742.11 and 742.14; N.D.Cent.Code Chapter 14-18; Okla.Stat.Ann.Tit.10, §§554-555; Tex.Fam.Code Ann. §§160.701-160.707; Va.Code Ann. §20-158; and Wash.Rev.Code §§26.26.705 *et seq.*

15 Colorado's statute states that if, under the supervision of a licensed physician with the consent of her husband, a wife consents to assisted reproduction with an egg donated by another woman to conceive a child for herself, not as a surrogate, the wife is treated in law as if she were the natural mother of the child.

Delaware's statute states that a man who provides sperm for, or consents to, assisted reproduction by a woman with intent to be the parent of the child, is a parent of the child.

Florida's statute applies only to children "born within wedlock," and provides that such children are irrebuttably presumed to be the children of the recipient married couple, provided both have consented in writing to the use of donated eggs.

Oklahoma provides that the child is presumed to be the child of married recipients where both consent to the egg donation.

North Dakota provides that the husband is presumed to be the father unless within 2 years of learning of the child's birth the husband commences an action in which it is determined that he did not consent to the assisted conception.

Texas provides that if a husband provides sperm for or consents to egg donation by his wife, he is the father of the resulting child. The husband's failure to sign a consent does not preclude a finding that the husband is the father if the wife and husband openly treated the child as their own.

Virginia provides that the gestational mother using egg donation is the child's mother, and her husband, if she is married, is the father unless he commences an action within 2 years after his discovery of the child's birth in which it is determined that he did not consent to the assisted conception.

Washington provides that if a husband provides sperm or consents to assisted reproduction by his wife, he is the father of the child. The consent must be in writing. The failure of the husband to sign a consent does not preclude a finding that the husband is the father of the child if the husband and wife openly treated the child as their own.

16 Fla.Stat. §742.14; Delaware, Texas, and North Dakota define "donor" to include either compensated or uncompensated donors, thus indirectly sanctioning payment. 13 Del.C. §8-102(8); Tex.Fam.Code Ann. §160.102; and N.D.Cent.Code Chapter 14-18-01.

17 Fla.Stat. §742.14 (2002).

18 La.Rev.Stat.Ann. §9:122 (1999).

19 2002 Guidelines for gamete and embryo donation. *Fertil Steril* 77(6 Suppl. 5), 2002.

20 Ethics Committee Report. Financial incentives in recruitment of oocyte donors. *Fertil Steril* 74(2), 2000.

21 See, e.g., Massachusetts General Laws, c.209C, §6 (". . . a man is presumed to be the father of a child . . . if: (1) he is or has been married to the mother and the child was born during the marriage, or within 300 days after the marriage was terminated by death, annulment, or divorce. . . .").

22 *MacDonald v. MacDonald*, 608 N.Y.S.2d 477 (App.Div.1994); *Ezzone v. Ezzone*, No. 96-DR-000359 (Ohio Lake County Ct. C.P. 1996).

23 J.A. Zuniga, Houston Chronicle, 5/31/02.

24 See *Thomas*; *Lucas, supra n.8, 9.*

25 Hoffman, et al. Cryopreserved embryos in the United States and their availability for research. *Fertil Steril* 79(5), 2003.

26 See Guidelines for cryopreserved embryo donation. *Fertil Steril* 77(6 Suppl. 5), 2002.

27 With the possible exception of Louisiana, with a statute stating in pertinent part, "[I]f the *in vitro* fertilization patients renounce by notarial act, their parental rights for *in utero* implantation, then the *in vitro* fertilized human ovum shall be available for adoptive implantation in accordance with written procedures of the facility where it is housed or stored." LA RS 9:130 (Acts 1986, No. 964 Sec. 1).

28 Department of Health and Human Services Program Announcement No. OPHS 2002/01; Federal Register, Vol. 67, No. 143 (7/25/02).

29 Four of the seven states (Delaware, Florida, Oklahoma, and Washington) refer explicitly to embryo donation, whereas the other three (North Dakota, Texas, and Virginia) apply by the inference that "assisted conception" includes embryo donation and a gamete "donor" includes an embryo donor(s). Louisiana refers to an "*in vitro* fertilized human ovum," and declare it to be a "juridical person," the parental rights to which may be renounced, without compensation. Several states also regulate payment for embryos, generally in the context of their public health and safety statutes. See Section III(B), note 14, *infra.*

30 Klock SC, Sheinin S, Kaser RR. The disposition of unused frozen embryos. *N Engl J Med* 345(1):69–70, 2001.

31 2002 Guidelines for gamete and embryo donation. *Fertil Steril* 77(6 Suppl. 5):S10, 2002. "The decision to proceed with embryo donation is complex and patients may benefit from psychologic counseling to aid in this decision. Psychologic counseling should be offered to all couples. The physician should require psychologic consultation for couples in whom there appear to be factors that warrant further evaluation."

32 California, Connecticut, Delaware, Washington, DC, Georgia, Illinois, Louisiana, Maine, Michigan, Minnesota, Nevada, New Mexico, North Dakota, Pennsylvania, Rhode Island, Texas, Virginia, West Virginia, Wisconsin, and Wyoming. Assisted reproductive technologies, collaborative reproduction, and adoption. In: Hollinger JH (ed.), *Adoption Law and Practice*, 2002.

33 2002 Guidelines for gamete and embryo donation. *Fertil Steril* 77(6 Suppl. 5), 2002.

34 Alabama, Arizona, Arkansas, Connecticut, Washington, DC, Florida, Illinois, Indiana, Iowa, Kentucky, Louisiana, Michigan, Nebraska, Nevada, New Hampshire, New York, North Dakota, Tennessee, Utah, Virginia, Washington, West Virginia, and Wisconsin.

35 D.C. Code Ann. §16-401 and §16-402 (1999).

36 Mich.Comp.Laws Ann. §722.859 (1999); N.Y. Dom. Rel. Law §123 (1999); Utah Code Ann. §76-7-204(1)(a) (1999); N.H. Rev. Stat. Ann. §168-B:16 (2000); Nev.Rev.Stat.Ann. §126.045 (2000); Ky. Rev. Stat. Ann. §199.590(4) (1998).

37 Indiana, Kentucky, Louisiana, Michigan, Nebraska, New York, North Dakota, Utah, and Washington.

38 Ariz.Rev.Stat.Ann. §25-218 (2000); *Soos v. Sup.Ct.*, 182 Ariz. 470, 897 P.2d 1356 (1994).

39 Fla.Stat.Ann. §742.15 (1999); Nev.Rev.Stat.Ann. §126.045 (2000); N.H. Rev.Stat.Ann. §168-B *et seq.* (2000); Va. Code Ann. §20-160 (1999).

40 2001 Conn.Acts 01-163 (Reg.Sess.); Fla.Stat.Ann. §742.16 (1999); 1999 Ill.P.A. 91-308; Neb.Rev.Stat. §25-21,200 (1999); Nev.Rev.Stat.Ann. §126.045(2) (2000); N.H. Rev.Stat.Ann. §168-B *et seq.*(2000); Tenn.Code Ann. §36-1-102(48)(A) (1999); Va.Code Ann. §120-160(D) (1999).

41 Wis.Stat.Ann. §69.14(1)(h) (1999); Wyo.Stat. §35-1-410(d) (2000).

42 Ala.Code §26-10A-34 (1999); Iowa Code Ann. §710.11 (1999); W.Va.Code §48-22-803(e) (2000).

43 *In re Baby M.*, 537 A.2d 1227 (N.J. 1988).

44 *R.R. v. M.H.*, 426 Mass. 501, 689 N.E.2d 790 (1998).

45 *Johnson v. Calvert*, 851 P.2d 776 (1993).

46 *In re Buzzanca*, 61 Cal.App. 4th 1410, 72 Cal.Rptr.2d 280 (1998).

47 See, e.g., *Culliton v. Beth Israel Deaconess Medical Center*, 435 Mass. 285 (2001).

48 Multiple, unreported trial court cases within Massachusetts and California.

49 See notes 36-38, *supra*.

50 Fla. Stat. §742.15(1) (2002).

51 Fla. Stat. §742.15(3) (2002).

52 *Davis v. Davis*, 842 S.W.2d 588 (Tenn. 1992).

53 Detailed discussions and reviews of those cases may be found in multiple texts, including those of these authors and others. Elster N. ARTistic license: should assisted reproductive technologies be regulated? In: Dejonge C, Barratt C (eds.), *ART: Today and Beyond*. Cambridge: Cambridge University Press, 2002, pp. 366–375); Crockin SL et al. Embryo law. In: *Adoption and Reproductive Technology Law in Massachusetts*. MCLE, 2000.

54 *Davis v. Davis*, 842 S.W.2d 588 (Tenn. 1992).

55 *Kass v. Kass*, 696 N.E.2d 174 (N.Y. 1998).

56 *A.Z. v. B.Z.*, 431 Mass. 150 (2000); *J.B. v. M.B.*, 751 A.2d 613 (N.J.Super.App.Div. 2000).

57 *A.Z. v. B.Z.*, 431 Mass. 150 (2000).

58 *J.B. v. M.B.*, 751 A.2d 613 (N.J.Super.App.Div. 2000).

59 See www.asrm.org.

60 *Stiver v. Parker*, 975 F.2d 261 (6th Cir. 1992); *Huddleston v. Infertility Ctr. of America Inc.*, 700 A.2d 453 (Pa.Super.Ct. 1997).

61 *Siemieniec v. Lutheran General Hospital*, 117 Ill.2d 230, 512 N.E.2d 691 (Ill. 1987); *Berman v. Allan*, 80 N.J. 421, 404 A.2d 8 (1979); *James v. Caserta*, 332 S.E.2d 872 (W.Va. 1985); *Becker V. Schwartz*, 46 N.Y.2d 401, 413 N.Y.S.2d 895, 386 N.E.2d 807 (1987); *Reed v. Campagnolo*, 810 F.Supp. 167 (D.Md. 1993).

62 *Lininger v. Eisenbaum*, 764 P.2d 1202 (Colo. 1988); *Gildiner v. Thomas Jefferson Univ. Hospital*, 451 F.Supp 692 (E.D.Pa. 1978); *Flanagan v. Williams*, 623 N.E.2d 185 (Ohio App. 1993).

63 *Turpin v. Sortini*, 31 Cal.3d 220, 182 Cal.Rptr. 337, 643 P.2d 954 (1982); *Procanik v. Cillo*, 97 N.J. 339, 478 A.2d 755 (1984); *Harbeson v. Parke-Davis, Inc.*, 98 Wash.2d 460, 656 P.2d 483 (1983).

64 *Lovelace Medical Center v. Mendez*, 11 N.M. 336, 805 P.2d 603 (N.M. 1991); *Johnson v. University Hospitals of Cleveland*, 540 N.E.2d 1370 (Ohio 1989).

65 BBC News, 6/19/03.

66 BBC News, 6/19/03.

67 *Guidelines on Number of Embryos Transferred*, ASRM Practice Committee Report, November 1999.

68 *Stone v. Regents of the Univ. of Cal*, 77 Cal.App.4th 736, 92 Cal.Rptr.2d 94 (1999); Moore v. UCI, Clay v. UCI, No. 752293-94 (Cal.Orange County Super.Ct. settlements allowed Aug. 1996).

69 Crockin SL (ed.). *Adoption and Reproductive Technology Law in Massachusetts*. MCLE, §11.7.1.

70 *Perry-Rogers v. Fasano*, 276 A.D.2d 67 (N.Y. 2000).

71 *Fasano v. Nash*, 723 N.Y.S.2d 181 (App.Div. 2001); *Perry-Rogers v. Obasaju*, 723 N.Y.S. 2d 28 (App.Div. 2001).

72 *Robert B. v. Susan B.*, 109 Cal.App.4th 1109 (2003); *rev. den'd*, 2003, Cal. LEXIS 6671 (September 10, 2003).

73 *K.M. v. E.G.*, 118 Cal.App.4th 477 (2004); *rev. granted*, 2004, Cal. LEXIS 8199 (September 1, 2004).

74 *Johnson v. Sup.Ct.of LA*, 101 Cal.App.4th 869 (2002).

75 Shorge Sato, *Note: A Little Bit Disabled: Infertility and the Americans With Disabilities Act*, 5 N.Y.U.J.Legis. & Pub.Pol'y 189 (2001/2002); Julie Manning Magid, *Pregnant with Possibility: Reexamining the Pregnancy Discrimination Act*, 38 Am.Bus.L.J. 819 (Summer, 2001).

76 Arkansas, California, Connecticut, Hawaii, Illinois, Maryland, Massachusetts, Montana, New Jersey, New York, Ohio, Rhode Island, and Texas.

77 M.G.L. Chapter 175, §47H.

78 211 C.M.R. 37:00 *et seq.*

79 Employee Retirement Income Security Act of 1974, 29 U.S.C. §§1001, *et seq.*

80 Americans With Disabilities Act of 1990, 42 U.S.C. §§12101-12213.

81 Title VII of the Civil Rights Act of 1964, 42 U.S.C. §2000e *et seq.*

82 Pregnancy Discrimination Act of 1978, 42 U.S.C. §2000e(k).

83 42 U.S.C. §12112(a).

84 42 U.S.C. §12181(7)(F).

85 42 U.S.C. §12102(2).

86 *Bragdon v. Abbott*, 524 U.S. 624, 118 S.Ct. 2196 (1998).

87 42 U.S.C. §2000e-2(a)(1).

88 *Saks v. Franklin Covey Co.*, 315 F.3d 337 (2nd Cir. 2003); *Newport News Shipbuilding & Dry Dock Co. v. EEOC*, 462 U.S. 669 (1983).

89 42 U.S.C. 2000e(k).

90 *Erickson v. Bd. of Governors*, 911 F.Supp. 316 (N.D.Ill. 1995), rev'd on other grounds, 207 F.3d 945 (7th Cir. 2000); *Pacourek v. Inland Steel Co.*, 858 F.Supp. 1393 (N.D. Ill. 1994).

91 *Krauel v. Iowa Methhodist Med. Ctr.*, 95 F.3d 674 (8th Cir. 1996).

92 *Saks v. Franklin Covey Co.*, 315 F.3d 337 (2nd Cir. 2003).

93 Pub.L. 102-493, 42 U.S.C. 263a-1 *et seq.*

21

Ethical Issues in Using ART: What Your Patients Need to Consider

Elena Gates

Introduction

The ethical issues arising with the use of assisted reproductive technologies (ART) have received attention for decades, starting with the initial use of donor semen, moving through the beginnings of IVF with the birth of Louise Brown, and more recently with innovations including intracytoplasmic sperm injection (ICSI) and preimplantation genetic diagnosis (PGD). As of 2002, most nations and organizations that have examined the issue of ART, and most ethical commentary, find that basic IVF is morally acceptable.

The evolution of new technologies and interventions in ART has, for the most part, outpaced the examination of the ethical questions that they raise. In the 1970s and 1980s, in response to reports of births after IVF, ethical guidelines for the use of ART were developed in many countries, including the United Kingdom, Australia, and The Netherlands.[1] Despite a fair degree of ethical analysis emerging from academic and professional sources, the United States remains one of the few western countries that still has not reached agreement on a national policy regarding assisted reproduction. Although federally sponsored bioethics committees have met and generated guidelines, the political process has kept their policy recommendations from being adopted. In large part this is the result of the diversity of moral views held by U.S. citizens on the subject of early human embryos and from the connection that is repeatedly drawn in political circles between embryo manipulation and abortion.

An important result of the absence of federal policy on assisted reproduction is the lack of support for embryo and ART research by federal funding agencies. In most areas of research, the process of federal funding brings with it a substantial degree of ethical analysis and procedural regulation aimed at protecting human subjects. This has been absent in ART except to the degree that professional organizations have attempted to address ethical issues and establish voluntary reporting systems and standards of practice. The American Society for Reproductive Medicine (ASRM) has, through its committee structure, developed and published a number of guidelines that can be useful in considering both the practical and the ethical issues that arise when ART is used.[2-9] This organization also collaborates with the Centers for Disease Control and Prevention (CDC) in supporting the ART outcomes reporting system of the Society for Assisted Reproductive Technology (SART).

This chapter will take a practical rather than a policy focus. It will address the ethical issues and questions that most commonly arise in the use of ART and that are of importance both to those who are using the technology for family building and to the generalist obstetrician-gynecologist referring them for care.

KEY POINT

The lack of acceptance of formal ethical guidelines, with respect to ART, in the United States has prohibited federal support for embryo and ART research, and its attendant oversight for human subject protection.

BASIC ETHICS CONCEPTS

There are a number of ways of thinking about ethical decision-making. The one with which many physicians are familiar relies on basic ethical principles and their corollary obligations, including respect for autonomy, beneficence, and justice.[10]

Central to the practice of medicine is the obligation of beneficence, to promote the best interests and well-being of the patient, and the corollary obligation of nonmaleficence, to prevent harm to the patient. In the context of treatment for infertility, well-being is not limited to the achievement of a successful pregnancy, but also includes consideration of the physical health of a particular patient, her psychologic well-being, as well as the physical and psychologic well-being of her future children. Historically, these two obligations embodied the ethical foundation of the physician-patient relationship, with a patient's best interests being defined by the physician, from a medical perspective. In the last half-century, however, physicians have come to understand beneficence as involving good, or benefit, as defined primarily from the perspective of the patient.

This shift reflects the increasing importance of another ethical obligation, respect for patient autonomy. This refers to a physician's obligation to recognize the patient as the ultimate authority when it comes to her own health needs, goals, and the means chosen to achieve them. In the context of reproduction, individual autonomy is closely tied to the concept of procreative liberty, or freedom to make choices about whether, when, and how to bear children. In the United States this includes a right to use contraception to prevent pregnancy and a right to choose abortion in the event of an undesired pregnancy. To what degree this right extends to one's right to *assistance* in conception is a matter of debate. The distinction that has been drawn between a liberty right (the right to freedom from interference in pursuing a goal) and a welfare right (the right to assistance in attaining a goal) is useful here. While most would claim that individuals should be free to use new technologies in pursuit of a successful conception and pregnancy, fewer would argue that those individuals should be provided with whatever financial or medical support they require in pursuit of those goals.

Providers of health care to women should bear in mind some historical points about women and the health care system. Physicians have historically viewed female patients as objects of treatment rather than as respected consumers of health care services and have not always regarded their opinions as worthy of serious consideration. This history underscores the important role of obstetrician-gynecologists today not only as health care providers for women, but also as their advocates in the health care arena.

Issues of justice also figure prominently in discussions about infertility treatment and the use of assisted reproductive technologies. This principle requires that individuals be treated "according to what is fair, due or owed."[11] In the health care setting it means that the treatment patients receive should be determined by their medical need, not by other factors such as financial considerations, personal influence, race, or gender. Issues of access to and reimbursement for fertility service can be examined using the principle of justice, as can inequities between countries in which millions are spent on fertility services and countries (as well as communities within the United States) where basic medical and humanitarian needs are not met.

This approach to ethical analysis, focusing as it does on abstract rules and principles, has been criticized for the fact that it does not account for individual differences and for the personal context in which decisions are made. This includes attention to the experiences of those involved and to the impact of decisions that are made on the relationships fundamental to the participants' lives and on their community. For example, a focus on "autonomy" puts self-interest and self-determination first, often losing sight of the fact that one's values and choices are largely determined by current and past experiences and relationships.

The contributions of feminist scholars are particularly relevant to thinking about ethical decision-making in the contexts of infertility treatment and family building. As Susan Sherwin describes this,

> Feminism teaches that moral theories are partial and defective when they speak of the interests, values and rational choices of individuals as abstract entities, as if the personal histories and social contexts of persons are irrelevant. Feminists are very aware that persons are not all situated so as to be independent and equal; many are disadvantaged, dependent, exploited, responsible for the care of others, or otherwise limited in their ability to assert their rights in competition with the claims of other persons.[12]

KEY POINT

Any discussion of the ethical implications of ART, should begin by considering the basic ethical principles of respect for autonomy, beneficence, and justice, but should not lose sight of the individual's experiences and relationships.

Informed Consent

Informed consent is the way that the principle of respect for autonomy is operationalized in the context of medical care, as it supports a patient's autonomy by enabling her to understand and make decisions about interventions that affect her health. It has been defined as "the willing and uncoerced acceptance of a medical intervention by a patient after adequate disclosure by the physician of the nature of the intervention, its risks and benefits, as well as of alternatives with their risks and benefits."[13] Ideally, the process of informed consent will be collaborative, with the relationship of trust between physician and woman/couple enabling all parties to speak honestly and address issues and concerns openly, in making decisions about treatment.

The number of issues that must be considered in the process of deciding about the use of ART can be daunting. They include decisions about how aggressive to be in pursuing a pregnancy, what to do in the case of a high-order multiple gestation, whether to use donor gametes, and what to do with excess embryos. Decision-making will be informed by beliefs about the moral status of the embryo, attitudes about the importance of the genetic contribution to family building, and how much physical, psychologic, and financial risk is warranted in pursuit of a child. The general gynecologist can play an important role in setting the stage for the complex decisions that a woman or couple will face when they embark on ART. As patient advocate, the gynecologist should assure him or herself that the practice to which patients are referred provides adequate counseling about the choices that must be made. This counseling should include a discussion of pretreatment screening tests, the methods a practice uses to maintain confidential information, pregnancy and childbirth rates for the practice, an individual woman's likelihood of success, the costs of various aspects of care, and the disposition of any embryos in excess of those required for family building.

The fact that a woman or couple's choices about treatment are determined primarily by the desire to have a child can pose significant challenges when it comes to promoting voluntary choice about treatment and optimizing the process of informed consent. Reame has pointed out that "some consumer advocates would argue that middle-class, college-educated, White infertile couples may be some of the most vulnerable patients in the medical system today."[14] The more treatment options there are available for an infertile woman or couple, the harder it can be to make a decision to stop trying to conceive. The generalist gynecologist's role as consultant and advocate becomes particularly valuable when treatments have failed.

Innovations in ART are attractive to patients because they increase hope that treatment will lead to the desired-for successful pregnancy. As they can't be introduced through federally funded research programs, new techniques are introduced and

The general gynecologist can play a central role of advocacy for an infertile couple.

developed in a clinical setting, with financial support coming largely from fees paid by those who are hoping to conceive. As a result, the boundaries between research and clinical infertility care can become blurred, with patients not always understanding to what degree the procedures they choose are evidence-based, or whether they have been proven effective and safe. ART clinicians, in a quest for high success rates and satisfied clientele, face pressure to try new approaches when standard ones have not succeeded. As Shanner has noted, "New techniques are rapidly introduced into clinical use without patients (and many clinicians) appreciating that they are still experimental. Explicit clarification must be made among procedures that are experimental, innovative, common but not yet validated, and truly validated."[15] As women or couples are referred for fertility treatment, general gynecologists can prepare them for the challenge of distinguishing promising but untested interventions from the "tried and true."

THE MORAL STATUS OF THE EMBRYO

The moral status of the embryo is a matter of debate in our society. At one end of the spectrum of opinion is the conviction, typically grounded in religious belief, that from the moment of conception the human embryo has the same moral status as a child or an adult. At the other extreme lies the view that the human embryo is a cluster of cells with a moral standing no different than that of any other cluster of human cells. The 1999 National Bioethics Advisory Commission report, "Ethical Issues in Stem Cell Research," took a moderate stance in concluding that "the embryo merits respect as a form of human life, but not the same level of respect accorded to persons."[16]

Disagreement about the moral status of the human embryo leads to conflict regarding applicability of treatment alternatives.

Why should the moral status of the embryo matter to women or couples considering IVF as a means of having a child? As members of our society, those using IVF to pursue family building may hold views of the embryo that lie at any point along the spectrum just described. Their decisions at many points in the treatment process will depend on these views. Because they will be asked to make decisions regarding the disposition of their embryos, including choices about cryopreservation, discard and donation to research, patients should be encouraged to consider their own views on the moral status of the embryo as they embark on IVF.

BALANCING HEALTH RISKS WITH DESIRE FOR A SUCCESSFUL PREGNANCY

It is important that a woman balance risks to her health and to that of her future child or children with her desire for a successful pregnancy. Given that a woman or couple's primary, and sometimes overwhelming, interest is in having a child, it can be difficult for them to realistically assess risks to the woman or her offspring. Nevertheless, a woman embarking on the use of ART will assume a number of physical and psychologic risks. These include the risks of ovarian hyperstimulation, the complications of oocyte retrieval, and the potential long-term sequelae of ovulation induction. Multiple gestation, which occurs in more than a third of IVF pregnancies, is physically riskier than singleton gestation. Further, the whole process of ART can be psychologically stressful for a woman and her partner and can strain their relationship (see Chap. 7).

When newer interventions are used in ART, one can be less confident about their long-term safety for women and children. From the onset of their clinical use, these new interventions can lead to pregnancy and the birth of a child; there is no "preclinical" phase in which one can examine safety without risking harm to a newborn. Data from Australia indicate that infants conceived using IVF with or without ICSI have twice the rate of major birth defects as do infants conceived naturally.[17] In addition, there has been concern over the well-being of children conceived through IVF using ICSI because of an increased rate of sex chromosome abnormalities and the unforeseeable consequences of overcoming nature's attempt to prevent, through male infertility, the perpetuation of certain genetic conditions like cystic fibrosis.[18]

KEY POINT

Due to the lack of funded research, new innovations in ART are brought quickly into the clinical arena. Safety for the mother, and the resultant child, may not always be assured and potential risks should be discussed with couples undergoing ART.

Multiple gestation is the most common preventable risk to the children of women using ART, bringing with it the risk of premature birth and subsequent neonatal and childhood morbidity. In contrast to the guidelines issued by the ASRM in 1998 in an effort to reduce the rate of multiples, CDC/SART data for 1998 indicated a 29% rate of twinning and an 8% rate of triplets or greater.[19] Both ART providers and individual women or couples may vary in terms of how high a risk of multiple pregnancy they are willing to accept, and, consequently, how many embryos they are willing to transfer or when to consider abandoning a cycle of ovarian stimulation. Embryo reduction is an option which some women or couples may wish to use in the event of a multiple gestation. This procedure involves the destruction of one or more intrauterine embryos, yielding, in general, a pregnancy with one or two surviving fetuses.

The Use of Donor Gametes

Some women or couples using ART will decide to incorporate donor gametes into their treatment. This may be due to male factor infertility, as a consequence of ovarian aging or oophorectomy, or because there is no male partner. Our society's emphasis on genetic relationships with children complicates the decision to use a donor gamete.

Selecting a donor can be challenging. One of the areas in which commercialism has made the greatest inroads into assisted reproductive technology is in the use of donor gametes. While most gamete donations are anonymous, some agencies provide donors with specific profiles: athlete, scholar, Nobel laureate, highly attractive physical appearance. Siblings or other family members can also be considered as gamete donors. Some families prefer this as a means of maintaining a genetic connection with their offspring. Use of family members does raise questions that are avoided when unrelated or anonymous donors are used. There is the potential for confused family relationships, for example, if a child's aunt is also its biological "mother." Disagreements may arise as to whether and when to disclose the fact of gamete donation to the child. It is important that both donor and recipient explore the unique challenges and opportunities that come with the use of a known or related gamete donor with a counselor or other professional.

Early ethics commentary on gamete donation focused on concerns raised by the presence of three, four, or even five parties in the conception, gestation, and parenting of a child.[20] Before cryopreservation became available, excess oocytes were available for donation, to other infertile couples, after fresh IVF cycles. Now, most women choose to fertilize as many retrieved oocytes as possible and to freeze any excess embryos. As a result, most oocytes now come from donors who undergo ovulation stimulation and ooctye retrieval solely for the purposes of donation.

Some gynecologists will have patients who consider donating oocytes. This situation raises particular ethical concerns. Though altruistic motives are certainly common among oocyte donors, many women are attracted by the financial compensation offered by the agencies that coordinate donation. While gamete donors are not to be paid for the gametes themselves, they are generally compensated for their time and physical inconvenience. Oocyte donors typically are reimbursed at a much higher level than are sperm donors, in recognition of the greater physical risk and time commitment required. Women considering becoming oocyte donors should be encouraged to think about the psychologic ramifications of making a genetic contribution to a child who will not be theirs, particularly if they do not have children of their own. Counselors are often available through the donor agencies or through the IVF practices where the donations are actually made. Some practices require counseling prior to donation. Physical risks should also be considered, including the side effects of ovulation induction, the possibility of ovarian hyperstimulation, and the potential complications of oocyte retrieval. Potential donors should ascertain whether they will be cared for and compensated in the event of a complication or injury. Finally, donors must decide whether their donation will be anonymous or through a more open mechanism that might allow future contact with children created from their oocytes.

Issues related to disclosure are challenging to recipient families as well. The anonymous nature of most donations, and the measures taken to protect the privacy of both donor and recipient may be barriers to the communication of information important to the health of one or both parties. For example, the knowledge of an inborn error of metabolism in a child created using a donor ooctye might be important to the ooctye donor in making her own reproductive plans.

Families differ as to whether, when, and how much to tell a child about the circumstances of his or her conception. Some parents prefer that their children remain ignorant of the use of donor gametes although current thinking argues against withholding this information from resultant children. In 1998, Nachtigall et al. reported that only 54% of respondent couples in their San Francisco practice planned to disclose the fact of donor insemination to their children.[21] It may not be feasible to maintain secrecy over the lifetime of the child, particularly if several family members are aware that donor gametes were used, or if a couple disagrees about the appropriateness of disclosure. Significant

KEY POINT

The use of donor gametes raises issues of informed consent, especially for the donors, and issues regarding the definition of "family" and protection of children's rights to information regarding their birth.

harm might result from an inadvertent or poorly planned disclosure. Debate continues about whether adult offspring have a right to information about their beginnings in life. Donor anonymity, while it may protect the donor, limits the interests of the offspring in understanding their genetic heritage.[15]

DISPOSITION OF EXCESS EMBRYOS

As the IVF process is initiated, women or couples will be asked to decide which possible uses of their excess embryos are acceptable to them. Options include cryopreservation, donation to another couple, and donation to research. While cryopreservation allows excess embryos from one IVF cycle to be saved for use later, the disposition of stored embryos must be determined eventually.[22] Couples who had intended to bear and raise children using the embryos in question may divorce, or one potential parent may die, making it important to have a clear sense of intent in advance. Prefreeze agreements, required by most IVF practices that offer cryopreservation, enable those with an interest in a particular embryo to agree to acceptable options for its eventual disposition, maximizing the chances that their wishes will be respected when future decisions are made.

Discussions regarding disposition of embryos will occur twice—once at the onset of treatment, and again when woman or couple has decided not to use remaining cryopreserved embryos for her/their own reproductive needs. Women or couples should be reassured that their fertility treatment will not be affected by their decision whether or not to donate excess embryos. A decision that remaining embryos are no longer needed for family building should precede any decision about donation.

One option available to women or couples who have completed their families but who are in possession of excess embryos is to have those embryos destroyed, generally by allowing them to thaw. A second option is to donate the embryos to another individual or couple to use in their fertility treatment. SART data from 2000 indicate that 72% of the 108 programs responding to a survey offered embryo donation and 35% had actually performed donations.[23] These arrangements are similar in many ways to adoption. In general, donation is anonymous and there is no payment involved. More rarely, a woman or couple may decide to donate embryos to a known recipient. In these cases, counseling is important so that donors are aware of the potential complications that may ensue if an embryo which they created for their own childbearing needs develops instead into a child to be raised by someone with whom they maintain an ongoing relationship.

A third option is donation of embryos for research. Most would agree that the status of embryos as potential human beings means that they should not be used for trivial purposes. Research in which human embryos are used should address scientifically important questions in ways that are likely to yield meaningful results. In addition, studies involving human embryos should undergo ethical review by an institutional review board.

The nature of the research to be performed may be relevant to an individual's decision about donation. It would be most efficient for participants to give general consent to the use of their embryos for research, with the particular research for which their embryos are used be determined by current research needs and by the characteristics of their embryos. However, individuals may be willing to donate embryos for one type of research but not for others. They may feel differently about research that will enhance the treatment of infertility, such as research on early embryo development and implantation, than they do about research on less directly relevant areas, such as the development of stem cell lines for the treatment of juvenile diabetes or Parkinson's disease. Couples will need to agree on the kinds of research for which they are willing to donate. Embryos should not be used in research to which one member of a couple has an objection.

The disposition of excess embryos becomes more complicated when donor gametes are used. If a woman donated oocytes in order to assist a family in having a child, it should not be assumed that she would agree that embryos made using those oocytes be donated for developmental or stem cell research. Anonymous donation, a step taken to protect the privacy of both gamete donors and recipients, limits the donors' ability to participate in decisions about the disposition of the embryos created from their gametes.

Efforts are underway to include a discussion of embryo donation for research in the process of sperm and oocyte donation, so that the moral views of gamete donors can be respected when decisions are made about the disposition of embryos created from their gametes.[24] Gamete donors should be given the opportunity at the time of donation to consider and consent to the use of their gametes, or the resulting embryos, for research purposes.

Given the current value placed on maintaining the privacy of gamete donors, it is typically not feasible to contact donors years after their donation to inquire about their desires.

Currently, anonymous sperm donors usually are not asked their views regarding such research. As oocyte donors must be treated in ART practices, the opportunity to obtain their consent for research is greater. It is appropriate that individual institutional review boards require consent from gamete donors in order for research using donated embryos to proceed.

CONCERN FOR CHILDREN RESULTING FROM ART

When weighing the interests of the various parties involved when ART is used, it is the interests of the offspring that should concern us most. Adult users of ART are more able to safeguard their own interests, and have access to counselors and other professionals during the process of donation or of treatment. They have knowingly given consent for involvement in ART. The children who result from the process cannot consent to it. Their interests have to be protected by the adults involved in the process, both parent(s) and ART providers. Future parents generally are assumed to have the best interests of their, yet to be born, children at heart. It also is appropriate for professionals involved in using assisted reproductive technologies to take steps to safeguard the interests of the children they help to create. Acknowledging responsibility for the well-being of the children being created is consistent with the ART physician's obligation of beneficence. Physicians are morally responsible for the outcomes of the treatments they provide.

ART extends the possibility of reproduction to individuals who might otherwise not be able to bear or raise genetically related children. Women who have passed menopause can now become pregnant. Lesbian couples can build families through insemination with donor semen. Single women can use the same technique to become pregnant with the intention of parenting a child without a partner. Gay men can build families with the involvement of a gestational surrogate. HIV discordant couples can more safely have children using insemination of an infected female or ICSI with the sperm of an infected male.[25] Providers of ART differ in their willingness to provide treatment to individuals along this wide spectrum of potential clients. Some may claim that concern for the welfare of the future child precludes using ART to assist certain kinds of individuals in their family building. Examination of available data on, for example, same sex couples, supports the argument that their parenting is of at least equivalent quality to that of heterosexual couples.[26] It is important that providers of ART distinguish legitimate concern for the well-being of the children being created from social biases that are not based in fact and that may limit the ability of some individuals to achieve their reproductive goals.[15] Pennings has pointed out the inconsistency in denying access to ART because of concerns about the parenting ability of individuals with certain characteristics, while risking multiple birth with its serious sequelae in the quest to achieve high pregnancy rates."[27]

THE FUTURE

Each new development in ART brings with it ethical questions that both general obstetrician-gynecologists and ART providers will need to consider. Ooplasmic transfer is being explored as a mechanism for enhancing fertility for women whose oocytes fail to implant but who desire a genetically related child. The potential harm to a child that might result from inheriting mitochondrial DNA from two sources remains unclear.[28] While preimplantation genetic diagnosis may enable individuals to reproduce without risking the birth of children with an inherited disease, it provides the opportunity to select for gender and, potentially, other physical attributes.[29] Other approaches to preconception gender selection are also being developed. Professional organizations such as the ASRM continue to debate this particular issue.[6] It is important that obstetrician-gynecologists remain well-informed about the ethical issues that arise in using ART so that they can serve as effective health care providers and advocates for patients who elect to use these technologies in building their families or in helping others to do so.

REFERENCES

1 Walters L. Ethics and new reproductive technologies: an international review of committee statements. *Hastings Cent Rep* 17(3):S3–S9, 1987.

2 Informed consent and the use of gametes and embryos for research. The Ethics Committee of the American Society for Reproductive Medicine. *Fertil Steril* 68(5):780–781, 1997.

3 Disposition of abandoned embryos. Ethics Committee of the American Society for Reproductive Medicine. *Fertil Steril* 67S:1S, 1997.

4 Oocyte donation to postmenopausal women. Ethics Committee of the American Society for Reproductive Medicine. *Fertil Steril* 67S:2S–3S, 1997.

5 Financial incentives in recruitment of oocyte donors. The Ethics Committee of the American Society for Reproductive Medicine. *Fertil Steril* 74(2):216–220, 2000.

6 *ASRM Position on Gender Selection.* http://www.asrm.org/Media/Press/genderselection.html: American Society for Reproductive Medicine, 2001.

7 Preconception gender selection for non-medical reasons. Ethics Committee of the American Society for Reproductive Medicine. *Fertil Steril* 75:861–864, 2001.

8 Donating spare embryos for embryonic stem-cell research. Ethics Committee of the American Society for Reproductive Medicine. *Fertil Steril* 78:957–960, 2002.

9 Ethical considerations of assisted reproductive technologies. By the Ethics Committee of the American Fertility Society. *Fertil Steril* 62(5 Suppl 1):1S–125S, 1994.

10 American College of Obstetricians and Gynecologists. Ethical decision making on obstetrics and gynecology. In: *Ethics in Obstetrics and Gynecology.* Washington, DC: ACOG, 2004, pp. 3–9.

11 Faden RR, Beauchamp TL. *A History and Theory of Informed Consent.* New York, NY: Oxford University Press, 1986.

12 Sherwin S. Feminism and bioethics. In: Wolf S (ed.), *Feminism and Bioethics: Beyond Reproduction.* New York, NY: Oxford University Press, 1996, p. 52.

13 Jonsen AR, Siegler M, Winslade WJ. *Clinical Ethics,* 2nd ed. New York, NY: Macmillan, 1986, p. 62.

14 Reame NK. Making babies in the 21st century: new strategies, old dilemmas. *Womens Health Issues* 10(3):152–159, 2000.

15 Shanner L, Nisker J. Bioethics for clinicians: 26. Assisted reproductive technologies. *CMAJ* 164(11):1589–1594, 2001.

16 *Ethical Issues in Human Stem Cell Research.* Rockville, MD: National Bioethics Advisory Commission, 1999.

17 Hansen M, Kurinczuk JJ, Bower C, Webb S. The risk of major birth defects after intracytoplasmic sperm injection and in vitro fertilization. *N Engl J Med* 346(10):725–730, 2002.

18 te Velde ER, van Baar AL, van Kooij RJ. Concerns about assisted reproduction. *Lancet North Am Ed* 351(9115):1524–1525, 1998.

19 *Society for Assisted Reproductive Technologies/Centers for Disease Control National Summary and Fertility Clinics Report 2000:* US Department of Health and Human Services, Centers for Disease Control and Prevention, 2000.

20 Capron AM. Too many parents. *Hastings Cent Rep* 28(5):22–24, 1998.

21 Nachtigall RD, Becker G, Quiroga SS, Tschann JM. The disclosure decision: concerns and issues of parents of children conceived through donor insemination. *Am J Obstet Gynecol* 178(6):1165–1170, 1998.

22 Annas GJ. Ulysses and the fate of frozen embryos—reproduction, research, or destruction? *N Engl J Med* 343(5):373–376, 2000.

23 Kingsberg SA, Applegarth LD, Janata JW. Embryo donation programs and policies in North America: survey results and implications for health and mental health professionals. *Fertil Steril* 73(2):215–220, 2000.

24 Lo B, Chou V, Cedars MI, et al. Consent from donors for embryo and stem cell research. *Science* 301:921–921, 2003.

25 Human immunodeficiency virus and infertility treatment. *Fertil Steril* 77:218–222, 2002.

26 Anderssen N, Amlie C, Ytteroy EA. Outcomes for children with lesbian or gay parents. A review of studies from 1978 to 2000. *Scand J Psychol* 43(4):335–351, 2002.

27 Pennings G. Avoiding multiple pregnancies in ART: multiple pregnancies: a test case for the moral quality of medically assisted reproduction. *Hum Reprod.* 15(12):2466–2469, 2000.

28 Templeton A. Ooplasmic transfer—proceed with care. *N Engl J Med* 346(10):773–775, 2002.

29 Sex selection and preimplantation genetic diagnosis. The Ethics Committee of the American Society of Reproductive Medicine. *Fertil Steril.* 72(4):595–598, 1999.

Index

Page numbers followed by italic *f* or *t* denote figures or tables, respectively.